Manual of ENDOSCOPY

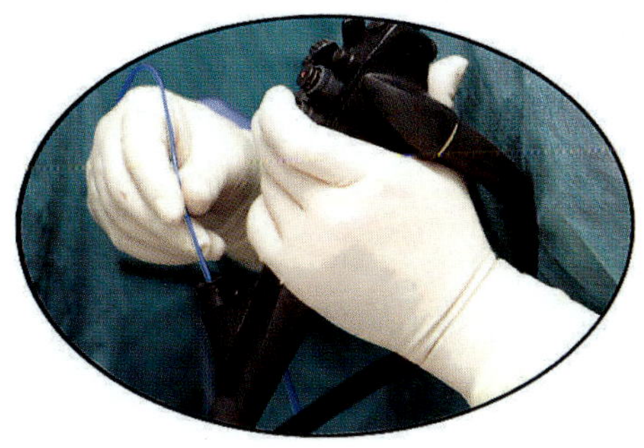

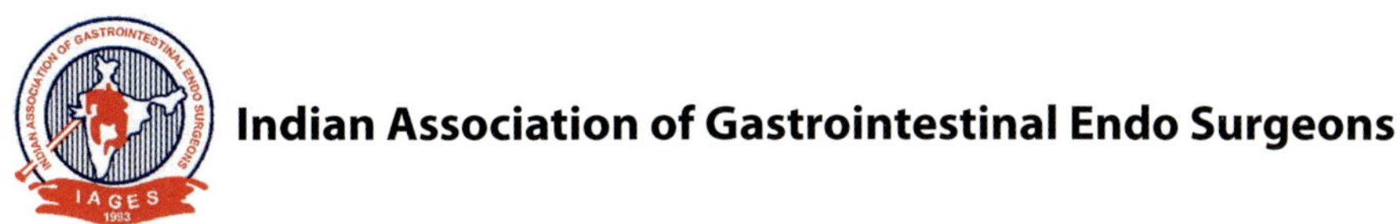

Manual of ENDOSCOPY

Editor

S Easwaramoorthy

MS FRCS (England) FRCS (Glasgow) Hon FRCS (Edinburgh)

Intercollegiate FRCS CSST (UK) FIAGES FMAS FAGIE

Professor of Surgery

Department of Minimal Access Surgery

Lotus Hospital and Research Centre

Erode, Tamil Nadu, India

Advisor, IAGES Endoscopy Board

In Association with

Endoscopy Board
IAGES

Foreword

Prof (Dr) B Krishna Rau

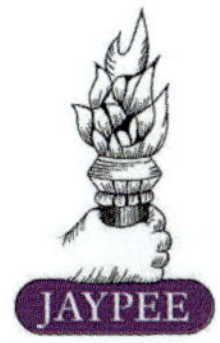

JAYPEE BROTHERS MEDICAL PUBLISHERS

The Health Sciences Publisher

New Delhi | London

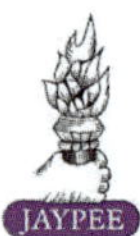

Jaypee Brothers Medical Publishers (P) Ltd

Headquarters
EMCA House, 23/23-B
Ansari Road, Daryaganj
New Delhi 110 002, India
Landline: +91-11-23272143, +91-11-23272703
+91-11-23282021, +91-11-23245672
e-mail: jaypee@jaypeebrothers.com

Corporate Office
4838/24, Ansari Road, Daryaganj
New Delhi 110 002, India
Phone: +91-11-43574357
Fax: +91-11-43574314
e-mail: jaypee@jaypeebrothers.com

Overseas Office
JP Medical Ltd.
83, Victoria Street, London
SW1H 0HW (UK)
Phone: +44-20 3170 8910
e-mail: info@jpmedpub.com

EU GPSR Authorised Representative
Logos Europe, 9 rue Nicolas Poussin
17000, La Rochelle, France
Phone: +33 (0) 6 67 93 73 78
e-mail: contact@logoseurope.eu

Website: www.jaypeebrothers.com
Website: www.jaypeedigital.com

Inquiries for bulk sales may be solicited at: jaypee@jaypeebrothers.com

Manual of Endoscopy

First Edition: **2026**

ISBN: 978-93-6616-565-3

Printed at: Samrat Offset Pvt. Ltd.

Contributors

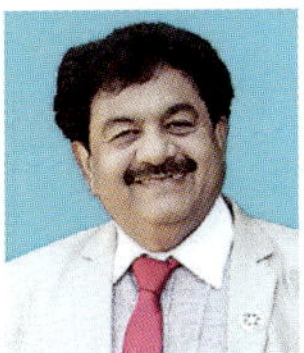

A Zameer Pasha MS FRCS (England)
General and Laparoscopic Surgeon
Shanawaz Nursing Home
Tiruchirappalli, Tamil Nadu, India
Past President, IAGES
Trustee, IAGES

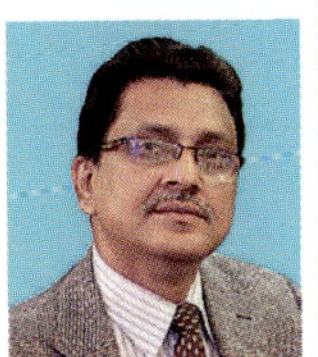

AHM Towhidul Alam MBBS FCPS FRCS FACS
Chief Surgeon
Green Life Endo-Laparoscopic Centre
Dhaka, Bangladesh
Governor ELSA, Member SAGES, APHS and ACS
Past President, SOSB and SELSB

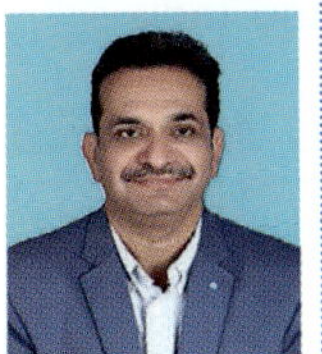

Amol Bapaye MBBS MS (Pune) FISG MSGEI FASGE (USA) FJGES (Japan)
Head (Digestive Diseases and Endoscopy)
Deenanath Mangeshkar Hospital and Research Center
Pune, Maharashtra, India
Fellowship of the American Society of Gastrointestinal Endoscopy (FASGE)

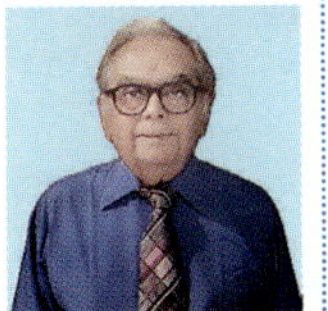

B Krishna Rau MS FRCS (Eng and Edin) FIAMS FACG FICS FIGSC
Hon Fellow American Surgical Association
Past President: ASI, IAGES, ISLAM, World Federation of Society for Laser Surgery and Medicine (WFSLMS)
BC Roy Awardee

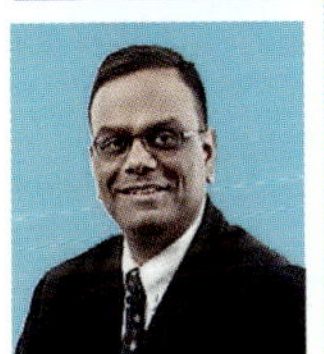

Chelliah Selvasekar
MD FRCS (Edinburgh) (Gen) MFSTEd PG Cert (Med Ed) MBA
Consultant General, Colorectal, Laparoscopic and Robotic Surgeon
Director of Surgery
The Christie NHS Foundation Trust, Manchester
Accredited Colonoscopist, National Bowel Cancer Screening Programme, UK
Hon Sr Lecturer, University of Manchester
MCh Pathway Lead, Minimal Access Surgery and Surgical Oncology
Edge Hill University, Chair, NW BAPIO

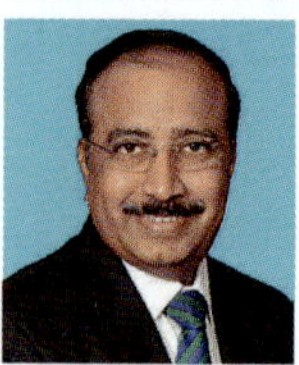

G Siddesh MS FAIS
Consultant Laparoscopic Surgeon and Endoscopist
Sharada Clinic
Formerly Professor and Head
Department of Surgery and Endoscopy
JSS Medical College Hospital
Mysuru, Karnataka, India

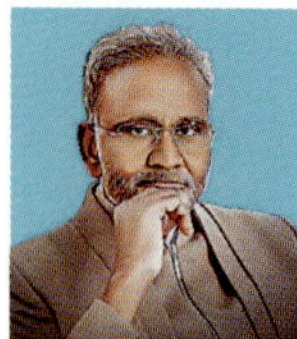

Ganni Bhaskara Rao MS FICS FIAGES EFIAGES
Professor and Head
Department of Surgery
Founder and Chairman
GSL Educational Institute
Rajahmundry, Andhra Pradesh, India
Vice President, Central Zone IAGES
Course Director, GSL Smart Lab

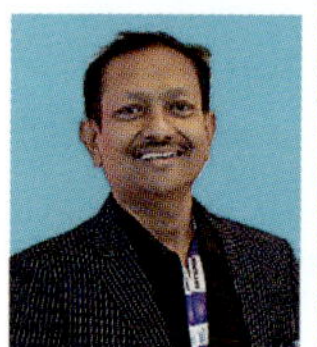

K Govindaraj MS FRCS (Glasg) FIAGES FICS Dip MIS Dip Lap FAGIE
Endoscopy Country Lead for ASI
Course Director, Post Doctoral Endoscopy Training
Dr MGR University
Dr G Viswanathan Specialty Hospital, Trichy, Tamil Nadu, India
President Elect, IAGES (2026)
Past Chairman, Association of Surgeons of India (2022–2024)

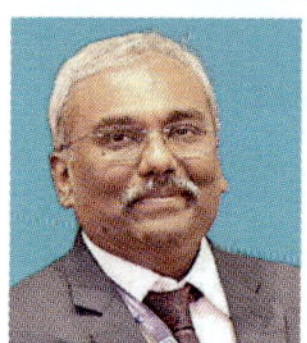

M Kanagavel DNB (Surgery) MRCS (Edinburgh) MNAMS FAIS FIAGES FALS (Bariatric and Hernia) EFIAGES FAGIE
Senior Consultant and PG Faculty
Department of General, GI and Minimal Access Surgery
St Isabel Hospital
Chennai, Tamil Nadu, India
EC Member and Academic Council Member, IAGES

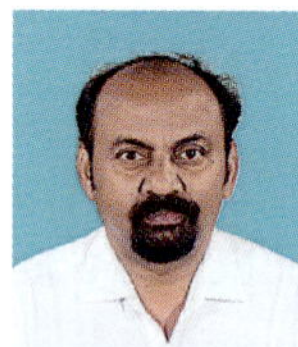

M Senthil MS (General Surgery) FIAGES FALS EFIAGES FAGIE
Director
Gunam Super Speciality Hospital
Krishnagiri, Tamil Nadu, India
EC Member, IAGES

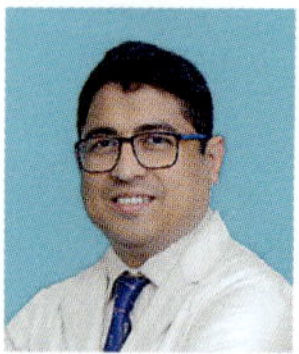

Masfique Ahmed Bhuiyan MBBS (DMC) FCPS (Surgery) FACS FMAS
Laparoscopy and Endoscopy Surgeon
Dhaka Medical College
Dhaka, Bangladesh
Life Member, Endoscopic and Laparoscopic Surgeons of Asia (ELSA)
International Member, SAGES

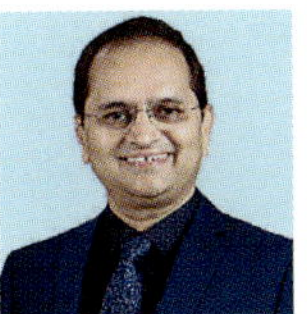

Pravin Suryawanshi MBBS DNB (General Surgery) FRCS (Glasgow) FMAS FAIS FIAGES FICS (GI Surgery)
President
Association of Surgeons of India
Deputy Dean, Professor and Head
Department of HPB Surgery MGM Medical College and Hospital
Chief Endoscopist, Advanced Laparoscopic, Hepato Pancreatico Biliary and Liver Transplant Surgeon
Center of Excellence for Gastroenterology and Advanced Minimally Access Surgery
Chief Executive Officer
MGM Medical Centre and Research Institute

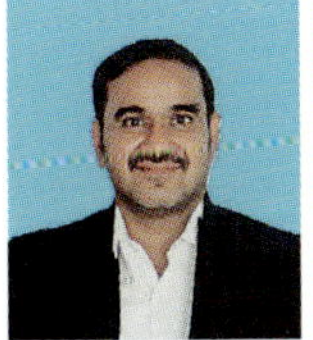

Sakthivel Chandrasekar
DNB (General Surgery) EFIAGES FIAGES FAGIE FALS-Hernia
Consultant, Laparoscopic Surgeon and Endoscopist
Lotus Hospital and Research Centre
Erode, Tamil Nadu, India

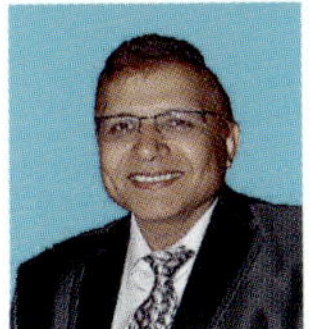

Satish Midha MBBS MS (General Surgery)
CEO and Founder
Vivekanand Hospital
Ranchi, Jharkhand, India
Hon President, IAGES (2025)

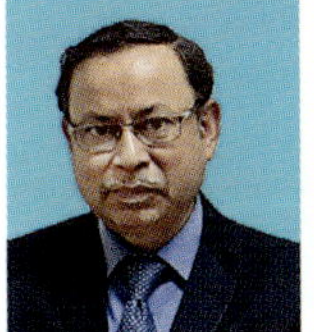

Satyapriya De Sarkar MS FIAGES EFIAGES FAGIE
Head
Department of Gastroenterology
GD Hospital and Diabetes Institute
Kolkata, West Bengal, India
International Member, American College Gastroenterology
Chairman, Endoscopy Board, EFIAGES

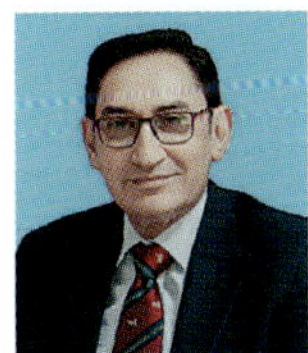

Subhash Khanna MS FRCS (Ed) FIAGES FICS FALS FICLS FAGIE
Dean
Swagat Academy of Medical Science
Guwahati, Assam, India
Hon Professor of SGE
GSL Medical College
Rajahmundry, Andhra Pradesh, India
Past President, IAGES
Congress President, World Congress of Endoscopic Surgery (WCES, 2024)

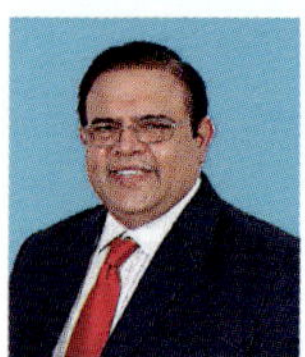

Sunil D Popat MS FRCS (Ed) FIAGES FICS FALS FMAS FAIS EFIAGES FAGIE
Gastrointestinal and Laparoscopic Surgeon
Nidhi Hospital
Ahmedabad, Gujarat, India
Hon Professor of SGE
GSL Medical College
Rajahmundry, Andhra Pradesh, India
Past President, IAGES
Past President, Ahmedabad Surgeons Association

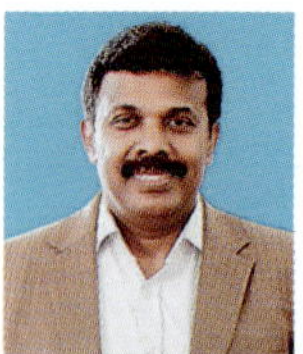

T Sivakumar MS Dip (Lap) FIAGES FMAS FALS
Founder Chairman and CEO
Siva Hospital, Nagercoil, Tamil Nadu, India
Head
Department of Minimal Access Surgery
Course Director, FMAS

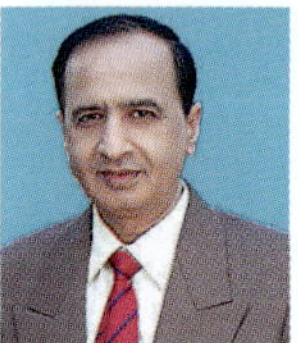

Vijay Borgaonkar MS MNAMS FIAGES
Founder and Director
Krupamayi Hospitals
Aurangabad, Maharashtra, India

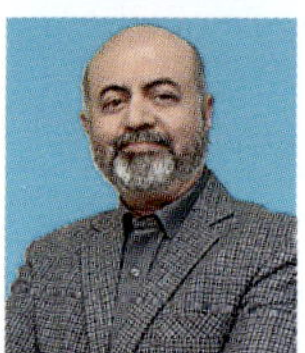

Vipulroy Rathod MS FASGE FSGEI
Director of Gastroenterology
Fortis Hospital
Mumbai, Maharashtra, India

Foreword

Dear Dr S Easwaramoorthy,

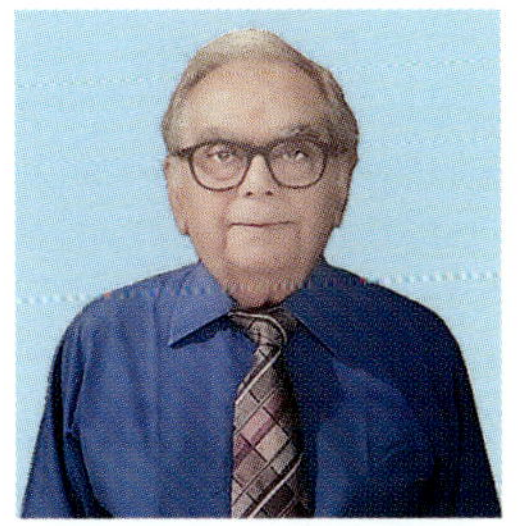

It was a great pleasure to review the *Manual of Endoscopy*.

It demonstrates your intense dedication to teaching and writing it down in the form of a book for posterity. I appreciate your desire to pass on your knowledge to the next generation.

The chapters are well thought out, written in simple text with many illustrations and photographs. Each chapter has a brief history of prominent endoscopists who contributed to that knowledge. The chapters emphasize the important technical aspects, complications, and how to avoid them. Further, the references are apt and informative. The observations of the specialists are well-directed and emphatic. Overall, the manuscript has far exceeded my expectations.

I have not, to this date, come across any manual of this expertise. I have no hesitation in advising all budding endoscopists and those doing advanced procedures to have this manual in their endoscopic suites.

I wish you continued excellence in teaching and also greatly appreciate the members of the IAGES Endoscopy Board for their continued support in teaching and training the young surgeons in the art and science of endoscopy.

Prof (Dr) B Krishna Rau
MS FRCS (Eng and Edin) FIAMS FACG FICS FIGSC
Hon Fellow American Surgical Association
Past President: ASI, IAGES, ISLAM, World Federation of Society for Laser Surgery and Medicine (WFSLMS)
BC Roy Awardee
Chairman, 21st Congress of the International Society for Laser Surgery and Medicine 2015

Preface

Dear Friends,

It gives us immense pleasure to bring out this *Manual of Endoscopy* under the auspices of IAGES to benefit the surgical fraternity.

A structured endoscopy training course is the need of the hour. Flexible endoscopy has a vast array of diagnostic and therapeutic potentials. All general and gastrointestinal (GI) surgeons should strive to acquire the skillset of safe endoscopy.

We take this opportunity to thank the Indian Association of Gastrointestinal Endosurgeons (IAGES) for providing the perfect platform to teach and train budding surgeons in the art and science of endoscopy since 2016. This has helped hundreds of surgeons to gain knowledge and experience in basic and advanced endoscopy.

We have carefully chosen 20 important topics in flexible endoscopy and given all the important practical points with ample illustrations. This manual would be invaluable for surgeons taking endoscopy training courses like EFIAGES and FAGIE Colonoscopy. We thank our endoscopy board members and faculty for their help and expertise.

We sincerely hope this manual will benefit every enthusiastic endoscopic surgeon to learn the art and science of flexible endoscopy.

There is more scope if we have the skillset of a flexible endoscope!

Thank you

Endoscopy Board
IAGES

Acknowledgments

We thank Drs Sakthivel Chandrasekar, Gurusamy Govindan, and Pranesh Sridhar from Lotus Hospital and Research Centre, Erode, Tamil Nadu, for their invaluable efforts toward manuscript writing and image archiving.

We profoundly thank Professor B Krishna Rau for his constant encouragement and help toward this mammoth task. We thank all our past and present members of the Endoscopy Board of IAGES for their valuable input to bring this endoscopy training manual.

Please refer to the following YouTube link for demonstration https://www.youtube.com/@SEMMasterclass.

We dedicate this book to all our patients who helped us to impart the endoscopy skills to all budding surgeons.

We thank M/s Jaypee Brothers Medical Publishers (P) Ltd, New Delhi, India, for bringing out this beautifully crafted manual in record time.

Endoscopy Board
IAGES

Contents

CHAPTER 1

Evolution of Endoscopy

Chapter Outline

Keywords: Evolution of endoscopy, history of gastroscopy, era of video endoscopy, birth of endoscopy

INTRODUCTION

Decades of hard work, innovation, and dedication by scores of scientists and doctors have led to the developments we are witnessing today in the field of flexible endoscopy.

EVOLUTION OF ENDOSCOPY

The evolution of endoscopy is a fascinating story and can be studied under the following 10 headings.

1. Concept of Endoscopy

- *Philipp Bozzini (1806)* ***(Figs. 1A and B)****:* He designed a light conductor known as "Lichtleiter" with a light source, reflecting mirrors, and a speculum. It allowed direct visual examination of various internal body cavities including the bladder and rectum which was not otherwise possible then. Hence, he has been considered the father of the concept of endoscopy.

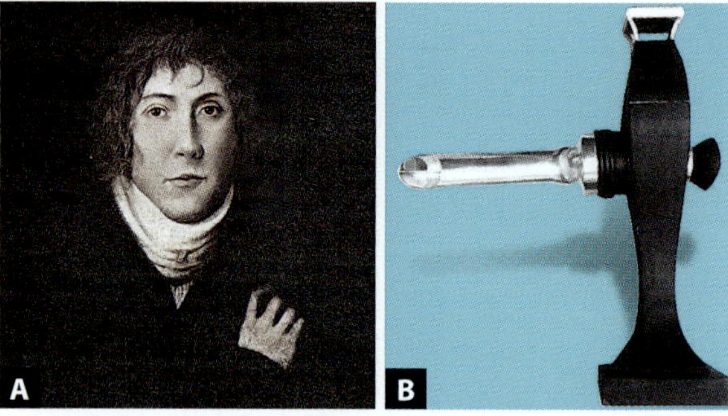

Figs. 1A and B: Philipp Bozzini and Lichtleiter.

- *Antonin Desormeaux (1853)* ***(Figs. 2 and 3)****:* With the help of the Charriere company in France, he designed a scope lit by turpentine oil. He is believed to be the person who coined the term "endoscope".

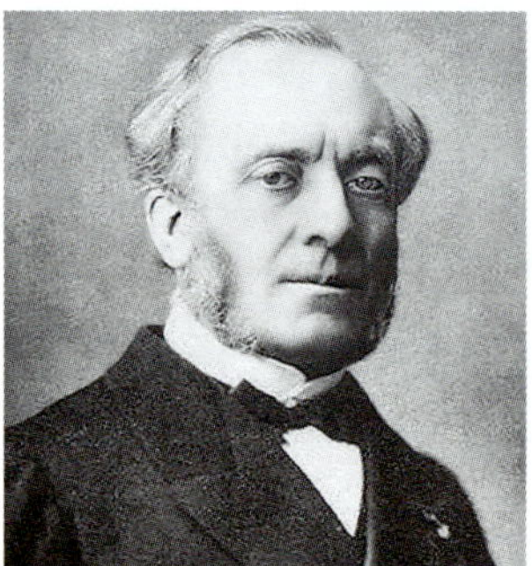

Fig. 2: Antonin Desormeaux.

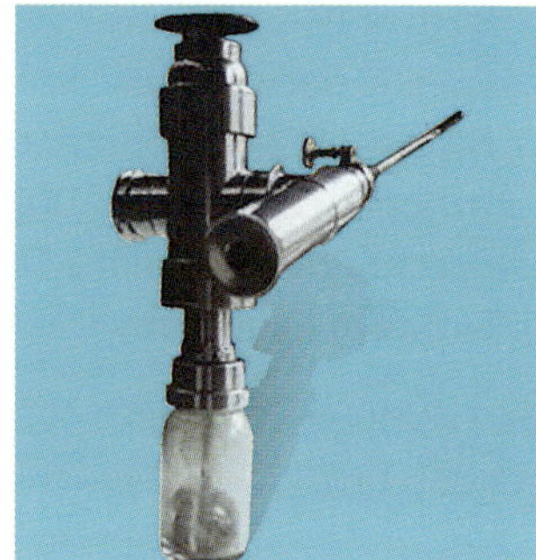

Fig. 3: Rigid endoscope.

2. History of Gastroscopy

- *Adolf Kussmaul (1868)* ***(Figs. 4 and 5)****:* Impressed by the ease and finesse with which the sword swallowers performed in their show, he designed and initially performed the rigid endoscopy in them to look inside the gullet. However, he had several problems with many of his subsequent patients due to a lack of insufflation and good view.

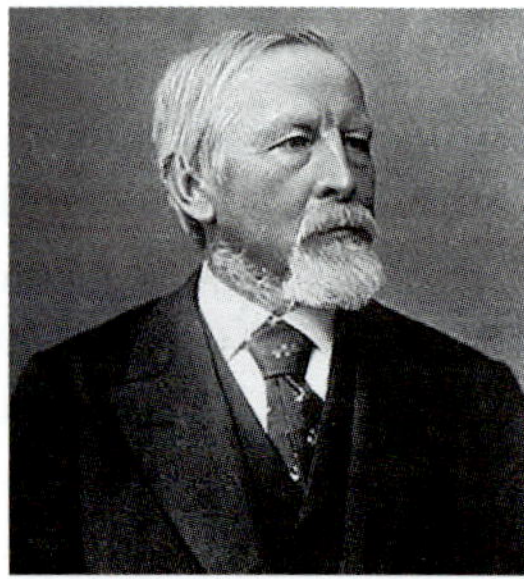

Fig. 4: Adolf Kussmaul.

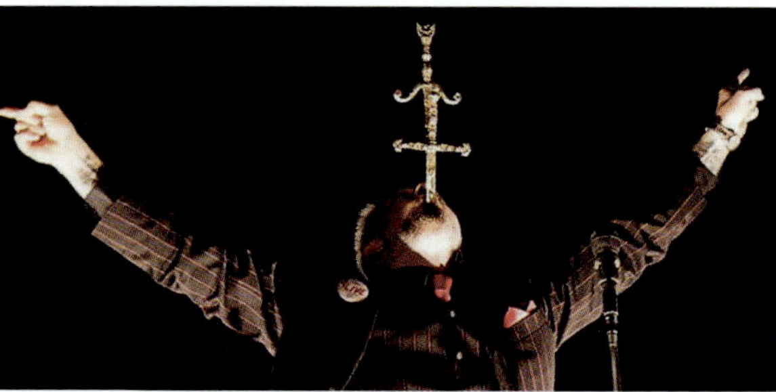

Fig. 5: Sword swallower.

- *Jan Mikulicz-Radecki (1850–1905):* This Polish physician can be considered as the "father of rigid gastroscopy" because of his monumental work in the endoscope design involving provisions for insufflation and removal of secretion **(Fig. 6)**.

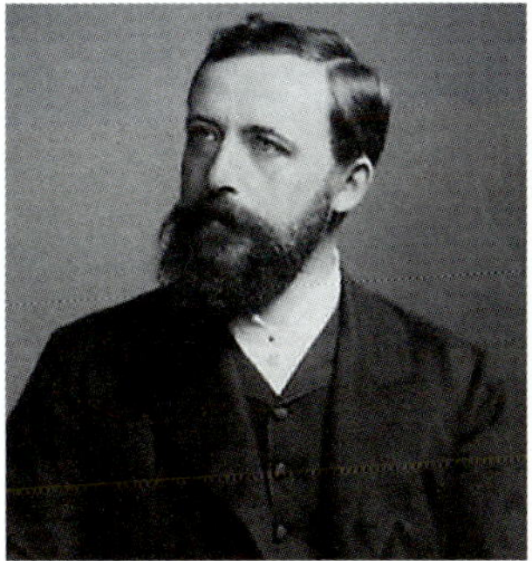

Fig. 6: Jan Mikulicz-Radecki.

- *Rudolf Schindler, Germany (1888–1968)* ***(Figs. 7 and 8)****:* He popularized semiflexible endoscopy across the globe. He designed his novel semiflexible endoscopy with the help of the company "Wolf". It was a tube of 75 cm length and 11 mm diameter. About one-third of the entire length of the tube toward the tip could bend to a certain degree. Rudolph Schindler examined the inside of a stomach through numerous lenses positioned throughout the tube with a miniature light. Ms Gabriella, his staff nurse, helped him during all endoscopic procedures, elegantly holding their head and observing and reassuring them while Schindler did the endoscopy. He subsequently married his nurse to retain her as a permanent invaluable assistant. Schindler meticulously recorded all the endoscopic findings by vivid pictures for the benefit of teaching future generations. He traveled worldwide to teach the art of endoscopy.

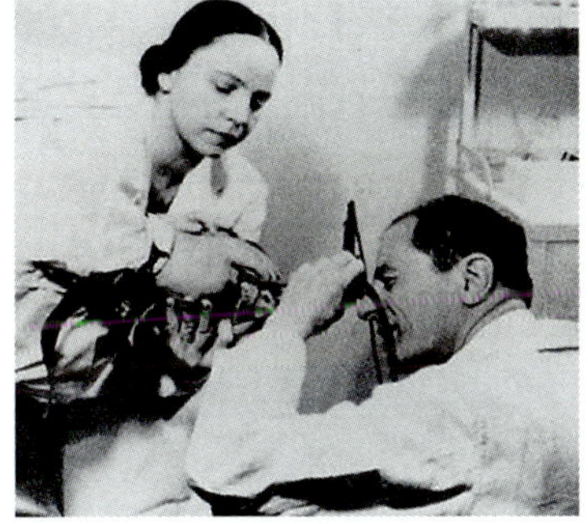

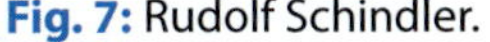

Fig. 7: Rudolf Schindler.

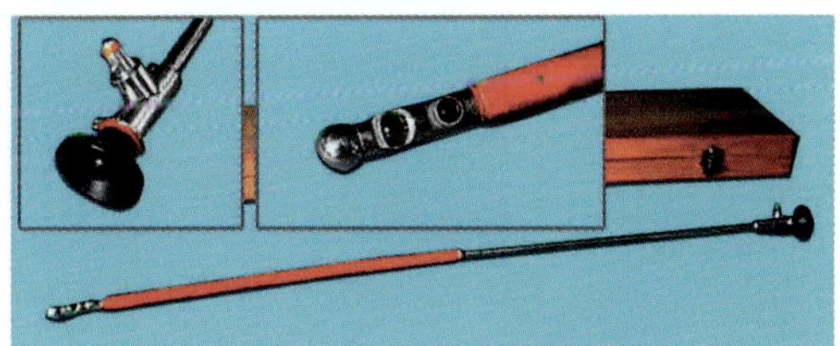

Fig. 8: Semiflexible endoscope.

- *Eyeless gastrocamera (1950)* ***(Fig. 9)****:* Doctors working at the University of Tokyo Medical Center requested Olympus Optical Company to develop a camera that could photograph and examine the interior of stomach to detect rampant gastric cancers found in Japan. Olympus came out with this novel device in 1950.

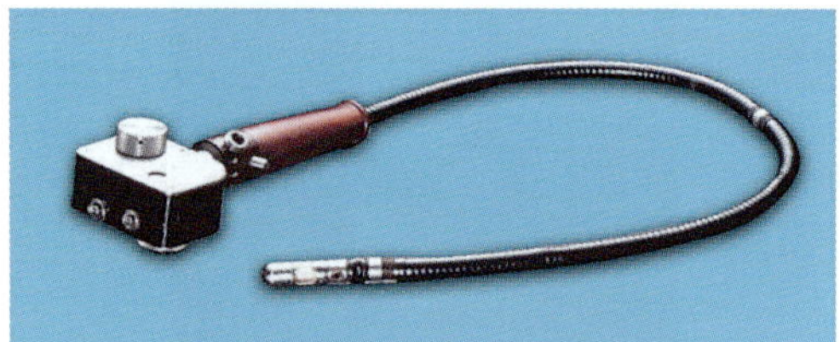

Fig. 9: Eyeless gastrocamera.

- *Harold Hopkins and Narinder Singh Kapany from UK* ***(Fig. 10)****:* Both were credited for design and development of the fiberoptic cable which was composed of thousands of tiny glass fibers. It helps to transmit light and image from one end of the fiber to the other end even when it is bent, due to total internal reflection.

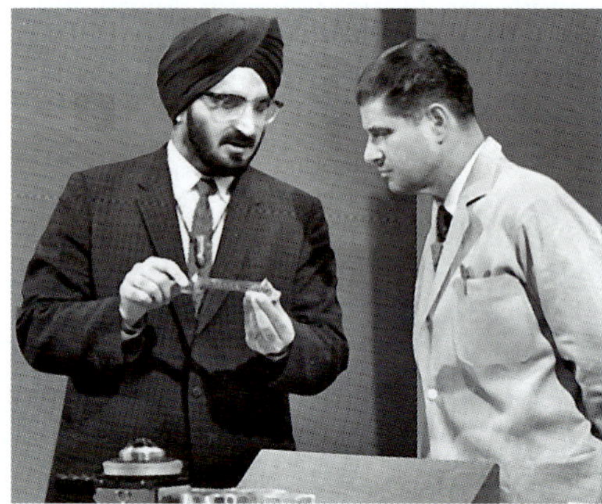

Fig. 10: Harold Hopkins and Narinder Singh Kapany.

- *Basil Hirschowitz (1960)* ***(Figs. 11 and 12)****:* He was considered the father of "fiberoptic endoscopy" and credited both for designing and for the clinical application of fiberoptic endoscopy. He got the concept of fiberoptics from Kapany and flew to the United States to seek the help of Larry Curtiss, a physicist, and Corning Glass company to design a flexible fiberoptic endoscope. He did endoscopy in scores of patients and flashed the pictures worldwide. He presented his impressive work in an original article "Gastroscopy in Gastroenterology" in 1958 and became world-famous overnight.

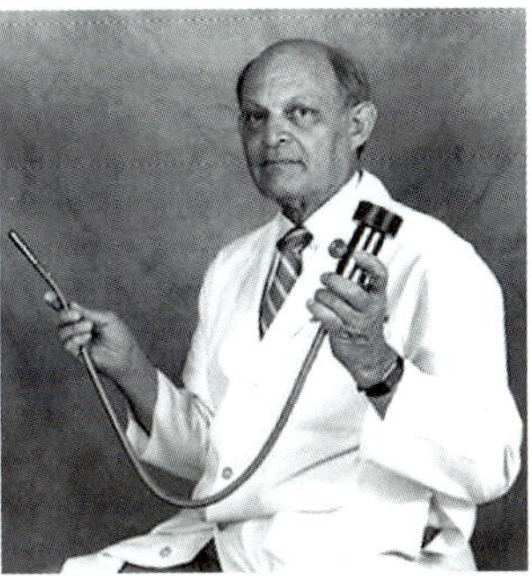

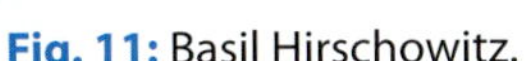

Fig. 11: Basil Hirschowitz.

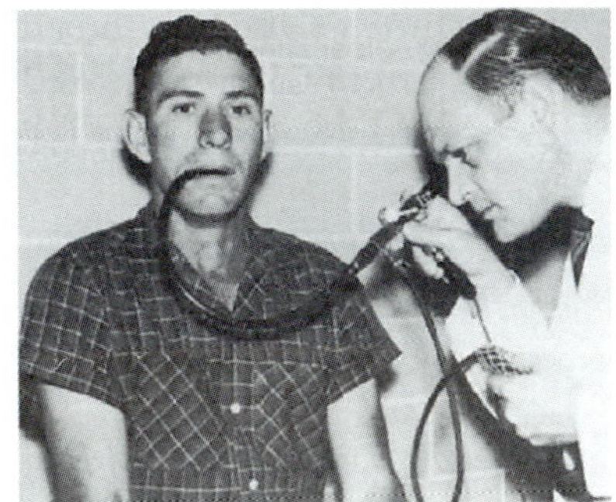

Fig. 12: Fiberoptic endoscope.

- The *gastrocamera* with a fiberscope designed in 1964 eliminated the weaknesses associated with earlier "eyeless" gastrocameras.
- With the advent of the charge-coupled device (CCD) chip and video processing unit and good halogen and subsequent xenon light source, video endoscopy became a reality. Thanks to the work of companies such as Olympus, Pentax, and Fujinon. We are fortunate to live in the era of video endoscopy. The benefits of video endoscopy are obvious. The image quality is better. Teamwork is facilitated, and hence, therapeutic endoscopy has become a simplified task. Transmission of image to the monitor, then to the storage device, to the next room, or even to the neighboring continent is possible.

3. History of Rigid Sigmoidoscopy

- *Strauss rigid sigmoidoscope (1903)* **(Fig. 13)** consisted 2 cm diameter metal tube with an obturator and a miniature light bulb at the tip and a rubber hand pump to distend the bowel.
- While lithotomy and left lateral positions were commonly followed, Kelly was the first to describe the knee-elbow position to perform a sigmoidoscopy.

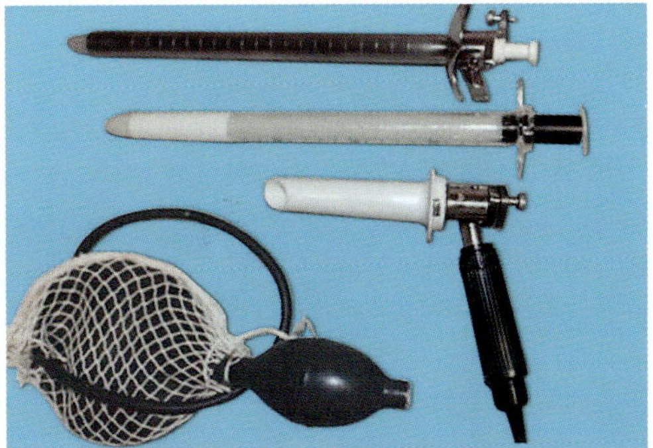

Fig. 13: Rigid sigmoidoscope.

- *Sakita and Niwa (1960)* developed a picture-taking sigmoidoscope.
- *Regenbogen from Germany (1966)* designed a novel sigmoidoscope that could observe even the proximal sigmoid colon.

4. History of Fiberoptic Colonoscopy

- *Niwa (1960)* developed the colon camera, a modification of the type V gastrocamera but with a longer shaft.
- *American fiberscope development:*
  - 10 years after Hirschowitz's successful gastroscopy, in 1967 Overholt at Illinois reported a series of 40 successful flexible sigmoidoscopies.
  - American Cystoscope Makers Inc. (ACMI) designed a scope with an innovative "flag handle method of controlling four-way angulation but the pictures were a bit fuzzy".
  - But by 1980, American colonoscope production ceased.
- *Japanese fiberscope development:*
  - Forward viewing colonofiberscope was first made by Olympus for Niwa in 1965 but without any angulation mechanism, and hence, it was not very popular.
  - *Matsunaga and Tajima* designed an oblique view long colonofiberscope and had some success in reaching the right colon (8% cases in the year 1970).
  - *Yamagata and his coworkers* through Machida Company designed a 190 cm long scope with four-way angulation.
  - Later Olympus designed a colonoscope with a 140-degree angle of view and two different wheels with a good range of tip angulation. Later, similar products were designed by Fujinon and Pentax.

5. Birth of Polypectomy

- In 1969, *Hiromi Shinya* **(Fig. 14)** from Beth Israel Medical Institute, New York, and *Dr William Wolff*, a cardiothoracic surgeon, were both credited for popularizing snare polypectomy using diathermy.
- In 1973, *Deyhle* of Erlangen group described submucosal saline injection polypectomy

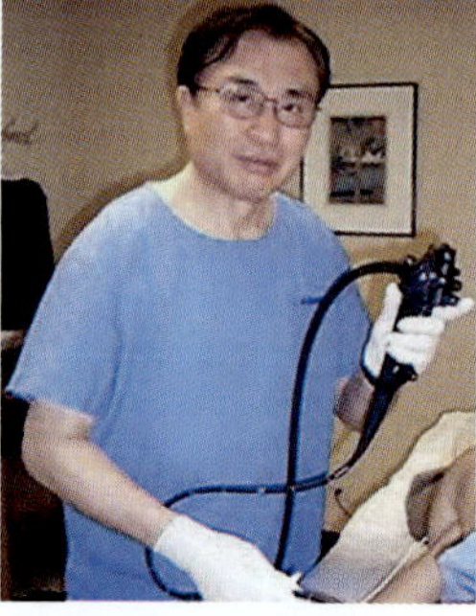

Fig. 14: Hiromi Shinya.

6. Era of Video Colonoscopy

- Fiberoptic colonoscope with "Lecture-scopes" (teaching attachments) were developed but with compromise in image quality.
- The video camera attached to the eyepiece was the next development (Keyed, London).
- Discovery of CCD allowed the birth of video colonoscopes
- *Welch Allyn Company*, USA, was the first to come out with video colonoscope in the year 1983 **(Fig. 15)**.

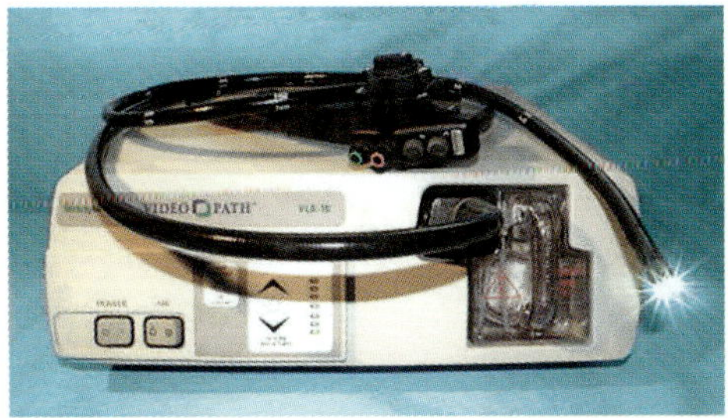

Fig. 15: Welch Allyn video colonoscope.

- Japanese companies subsequently joined the race and produced scopes with more and more advanced features
- After USA and Japan, Germany (Storz and Wolff), China, and Russia also started producing colonoscopes
- Image enhancement techniques and magnification improve the diagnostic potentials of video colonoscopes
- Variable stiffness colonoscopy helps to vary the shaft stiffness to aid easy navigation
- Imaging the shaft configuration was possible initially by fluoroscopy and now with magnetic imaging (ScopeGuide from Olympus) **(Figs. 16A and B)**.

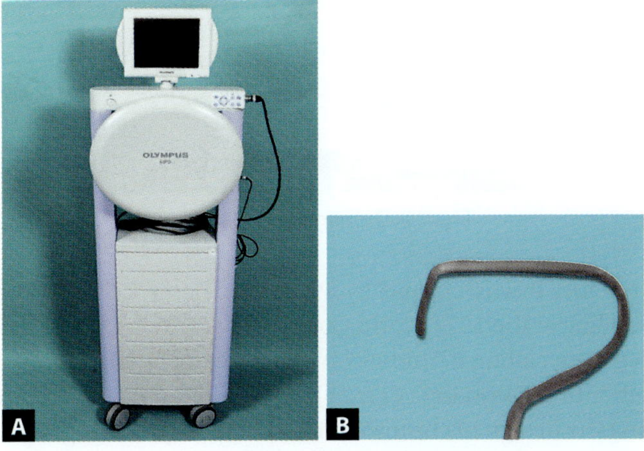

Figs. 16A and B: ScopeGuide (Olympus).

7. History of Endoscopic Retrograde Cholangiopancreatography

- In early 1970, Kasuri Ogoshi in the Niigata Cancer Center worked with Olympus and Itaru Oi in the Tokyo Women's Medical College worked with the Machida performed and reported cannulation of ampulla for diagnostic endoscopic retrograde cholangiopancreatography (ERCP) **(Figs. 17 and 18)**

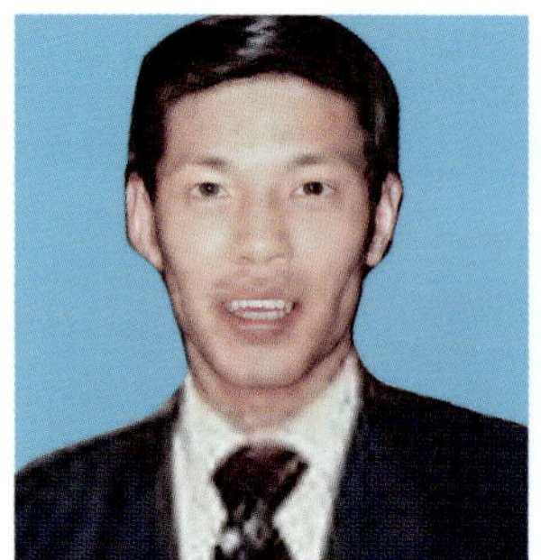

Fig. 17: Kasuri Ogoshi.

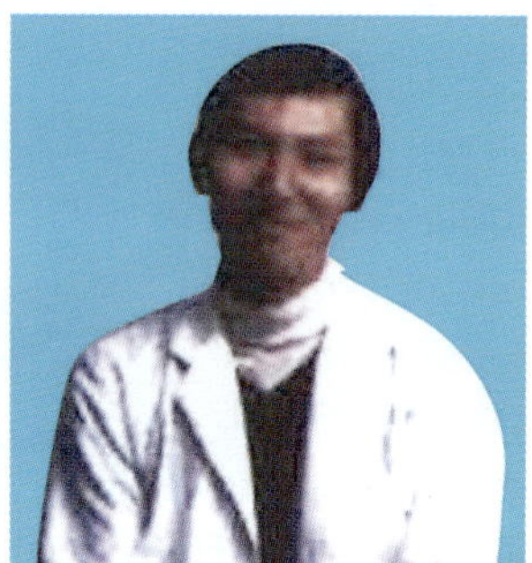

Fig. 18: Itaru Oi.

- Subsequently, Demling and Classen in Germany **(Fig. 19)** and Kawai, Nakajima, and their colleagues in Japan showed the world the technique of endoscopic sphincterotomy and bile duct stone removal.

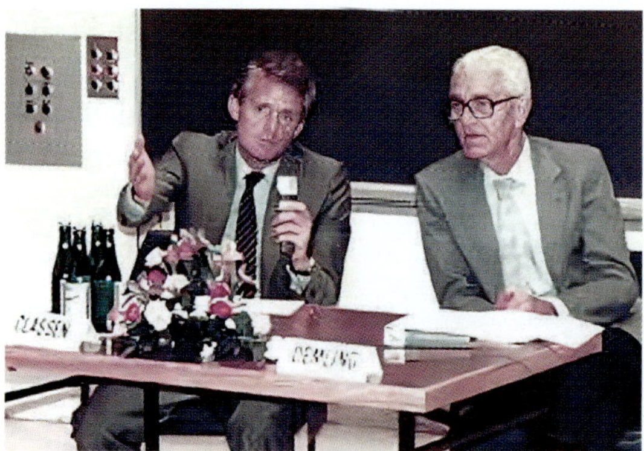

Fig. 19: Demling and Classen.

- The term ERCP was coined by Professor Peter Cotton **(Fig. 20)** and approved first at the 1974 World Congress in Mexico City. At that time, the Japanese were calling it "endoscopic pancreatocholangiography".
- Nib Soehendra, Germany **(Fig. 21)**, was credited for several innovations including the design of common bile duct (CBD) stenting.

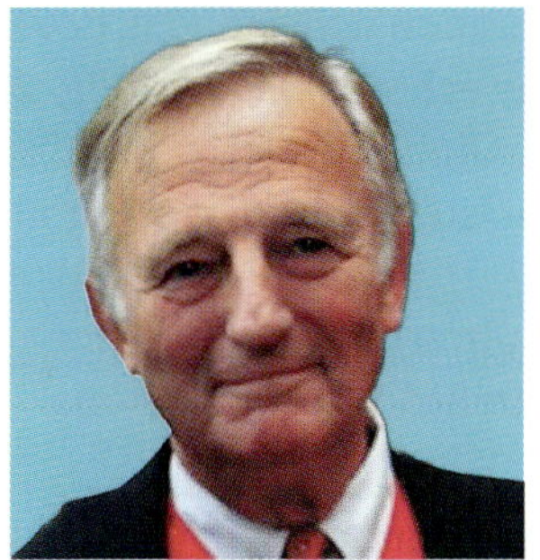

Fig. 20: Peter Cotton.

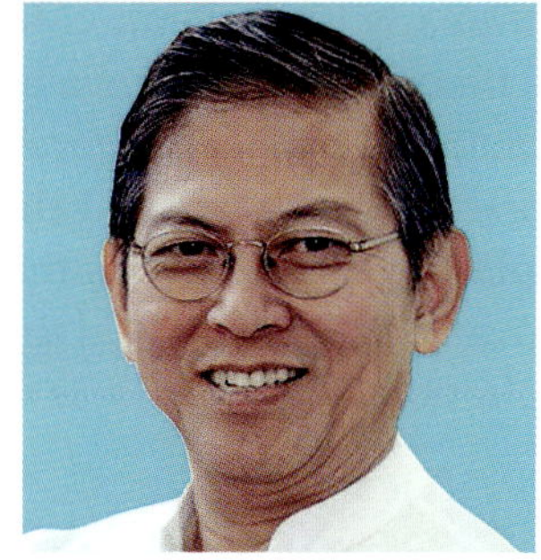

Fig. 21: Nib Soehendra.

8. History of Endoscopic Ultrasound

- It has been a remarkable journey for endoscopic ultrasound (EUS) over the past three decades. EUS has evolved from a technical curiosity into a procedure with a significant impact on gastrointestinal (GI) and pulmonary diseases. Thus, EUS has radically changed the ability to diagnose and stage GI cancers and to evaluate the pancreas.
- EUS was designed in the early 1980s in an attempt to improve US imaging of the pancreaticobiliary system. The addition of US probes to endoscopes allowed an improved visualization of the GI wall and its surrounding structures.
- The first radial echoendoscope was designed and provided by Olympus (Tokyo, Japan) in 1982 **(Fig. 22)**.

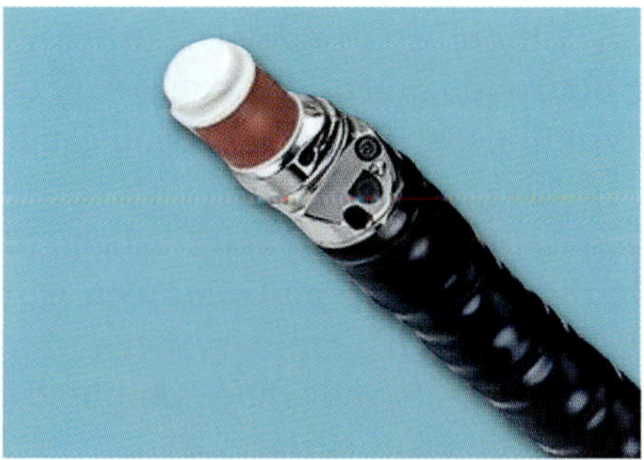

Fig. 22: Radial endoscopic ultrasound (EUS).

- In 1984, Tio and Tytgat depicted the possibility of using the biopsy channel for cytological puncture, which would increase the diagnostic value of EUS.
- Rösch and Classen presented the advantages of EUS along with its limitations, the most important being the lack of specificity in distinguishing between benign and malignant changes.

- In the early 1990s, Pentax Medical, in cooperation with Hitachi, developed the first commercially available linear-array echoendoscope **(Fig. 23)**.
- Vilmann et al., in collaboration with Medi-Globe GmbH, created special biopsy equipment, and this was a major step leading to the clinical application of the biopsy method.
- Giovannini et al. showed that endoscopic ultrasound-guided fine needle aspiration (EUS-FNA) was safe, with no significant complications.

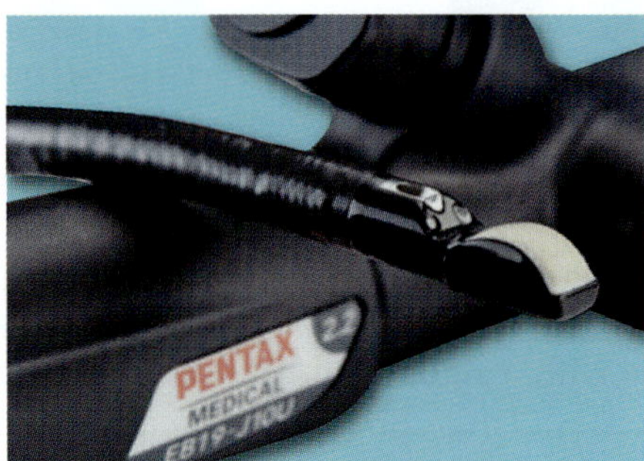

Fig. 23: Linear endoscopic ultrasound (EUS).

9. Recent Advances in the Development of Endoscopes

- *Magnification endoscopy:* Thanks to the optical zoom with movable lens and also digital zooming, we could now get magnification of images even up to 200 times. With better resolution and bigger images, now we can recognize even small mucosal lesions.
- *Chromoendoscopy:* Chromoendoscopy is a novel technique of staining mucosa to bring out subtle mucosal changes very well. With the added feature of magnification, even a tiny flat lesion can be easily recognized and tackled appropriately.
- *Narrow-band imaging (NBI):* Instead of white light, NBI uses two discrete bands of light: One blue at 415 nm and one green at 540 nm. Narrowband blue light displays superficial capillary networks, while green light displays subepithelial vessels and when combined offers an extremely high contrast image of the tissue surface.
- *Fluorescence spectroscopy:* It is the study of a characteristic pattern of light emission and absorption in the GI tract. Tissue has varying concentrations of fluorophores which emit light and chromophores which absorb light. The submucosa, with its high concentration of collagen and elastin, is the major fluorophore. Hemoglobin is the major chromophore in tissue. Autofluorescence is produced when tissue is excited by ultraviolet (<400 nm) or short visible wavelength light. Dysplastic tissue has more fluorophores, and hence emits more light, e.g., Barrett's esophagus.

Spectral endoscopy combines magnification, NBI, and fluorescence giving us images of the finest details.

- *Optical coherence tomography (OCT):* Unlike endoscopic ultrasound, OCT uses infrared light waves instead of sound waves and measures the optical reflectivity of tissue as a function of depth instead of acoustic reflectivity. After its successful application in the study of retina, now we start exploring its potential in gastroenterology. An OCT probe can be passed through the biopsy channel of an endoscope and can be kept in contact with the mucosa of interest which allows for a resolution of 7–10 micrometers and an imaging depth of 2–3 mm depending on the wavelength of light used and the type of tissue being imaged. This allows visualization of histologic morphology in real-time, especially the epithelial structures such as villi, crypts, and squamous and intestinal epithelium.
  It is useful in assessing cases of Barrett's esophagus, inflammatory bowel disease (IBD), and pancreatic and bile duct lesions.
- *Confocal endoscopy:* It is the fusion of endoscopy and confocal microscopy. Confocal microscopy uses a laser fiber as a pinhole, placed in-between the objective lens and the detector, to allow only the light that originates from within a tiny volume below the mucosal surface to be collected. All other sources of scattered light do not have the correct path to be detected and thus become "spatially filtered." This process creates a high-resolution image from a thin section within optically thick tissue and is known as optical sectioning.
  To create confocal images, blue laser light is focused on the desired tissue via the distal end. Applied fluorescent materials are excited by the laser light, and the special confocal optical unit exclusively detects the fluorescing light at an exactly defined horizontal level. Such optical slices of the mucosal surface give as real-time high-resolution imaging of cellular and subcellular tissue structures and are, hence, known as in vivo or virtual biopsy.
- *Endomicroscopy:* The endocytoscope is an ultra-high magnification (450–1,125 times) catheter-type endoscope that can be passed through the working channel of a colonoscope and used, in combination with chromo agents, to provide in vivo histological images.
  Unlike confocal endoscopy, endocytoscopic images are in color and have greater resolution. It allows us to obtain in vivo histological images.

10. Future of Endoscopy

- *Multiplex capsule endoscopy:*
  - We are sure to witness smarter capsules with better navigation ability and diagnostic capabilities with the help of artificial intelligence (AI).

- Could be armed with therapeutic modalities such as injection and biopsy modes

- *Endoscopic surgery:*
  - Natural orifice transluminal endoscopic surgery (NOTES) would develop further following the refinement of endoscopic hardware with more access channels and a stable platform to work with.
  - Cutting and suturing capabilities would improve.
- *Third-space endoscopy:*
  - "Third-space" endoscopy, also commonly referred to as submucosal endoscopy, is founded on the principle that the deeper layers of the GI tract can be accessed by tunneling in the submucosal space without compromising the integrity of the overlying mucosa.
  - Peroral endoscopic myotomy (POEM), endoscopic submucosal dissection (ESD), and submucosal tunneling endoscopic resection (STER) are innovative techniques within the field of third-space endoscopy in the management of esophageal disorders.
- *Robotic endoscopy **(Fig. 24)**:*
  - The EndoDrive (ECE Medical Products, Erlangen, Germany) is the first commercially available system for electromechanical support of shaft insertion of flexible endoscopes.
  - Kume et al. and Keeichiro et al. developed the master-slave endoscopic operation robot (EOR). It allows steering, advancing, rotating, and stabilizing of a standard colonoscope by two joysticks.
  - In 2017, Woo et al. in Korea also developed a master-slave robot with force feedback for colonoscopy
  - In 2017, Yang et al. developed a robotic system for holding a gastroscope, using a gastroscope intervention mechanism (GIM) with a pneumatic-driven clamping function.

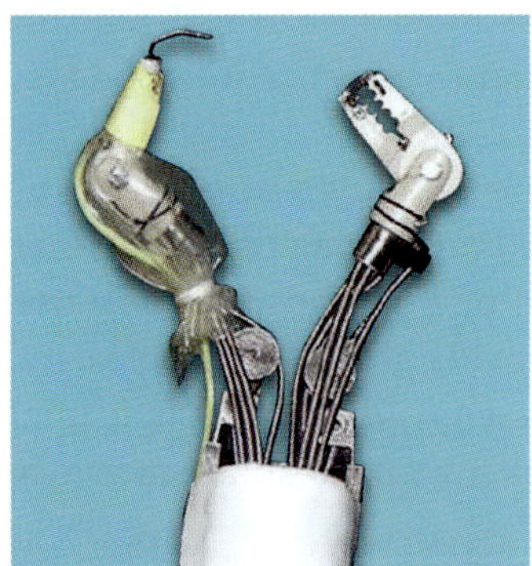

Fig. 24: Robotic endoscope.

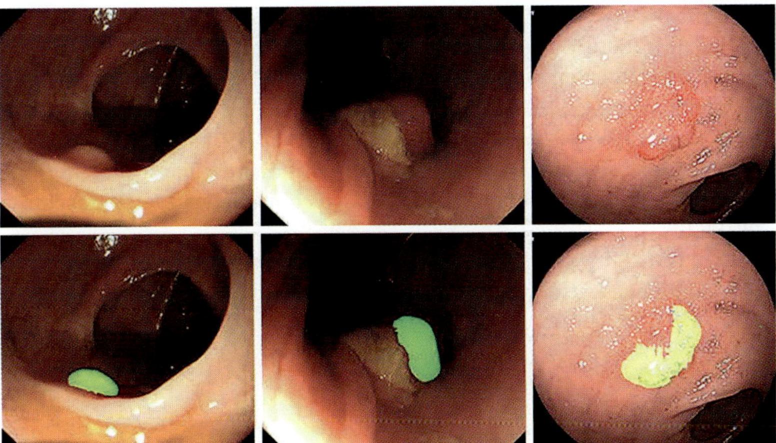

Fig. 25: Artificial intelligence (AI) in endoscopic diagnosis.

- Days are not far before we see autonomous robotic flexible endoscope for use in our clinical setting.

- *Computer-aided endoscopic diagnosis* ***(Fig. 25)****:* Pattern recognition with the help of AI would make it possible for the in vivo histological diagnosis of various colonic polyps hence helping in the subsequent therapeutic decisions.

Thanks to the monumental work and commitment of so many personalities and companies, we are now observing a real revolution in the field of gastroenterology. We are sure to see more exciting developments happening in the field of endoscopy in the coming days too.

SUGGESTED READING

1. Berci G, Forde KA. History of endoscopy: what lessons have we learned from the past? Surg Endosc. 2000;14:5-15.
2. Brown GJE, Saunders BP. Advances in colonic imaging: technical improvements in colonoscopy. Eur J Gastroenterol Hepatol. 2005;17(8):785-92.
3. Conio M, Ponchon T, Blanchi S, Filiberti R. Endoscopic mucosal resection. Am J Gastroenterol. 2006;101:653-63.
4. Edmonson JM. History of the instruments for gastrointestinal endoscopy. Gastrointest Endosc. 1991;37(2):S27-56.
5. Gross S, Kollenbrandt M. Technical evolution of medical endoscopy. Acta Polytechnica. 2009;49(2-3):15-9.
6. Katsanos K, Sabharwal T, Adam A. Stenting of the lower gastrointestinal tract: current status. Cardiovasc Intervent Radiol. 2011;34:462-73.
7. Middleton P, Suterland LM, Maddern GJ. Transanal endoscopic microsurgery: a systematic review. Dis Colon Rectum. 2005;48(2):270-84.

8. Mouton WG, Bessell JR, Maddern GJ. Looking back to the advent of modern endoscopy: 150th birthday of Maximilian Nitze. World J Surg. 1998;22(12):1256-8.
9. Rathert P, Lutzeyer W, Goddwin WE. Philipp Bozzini (1773-1809) and the Lichtleiter. Urology. 1974;3(1):113-8.
10. Tischendorf JJW, Wasmuth HE, Koch A, Hecker H, Trautwein C, Winograd R. Value of magnifying chromoendoscopy and narrow band imaging (NBI) in classifying colorectal polyps: a prospective controlled study. Endoscopy. 2007; 39:1092-6.
11. Wilcox CM. Fifty years of gastroenterology at the University of Alabama at Birmingham: a festschrift for Dr. Basil I. Hirschowitz. Am J Med Sci. 2009;338(2): 1-5.

Expert's Comment

Dear Friends,

Man's quest for discoveries is unquenchable. And so is the surgeon's desire to peer into the origins of disease is infinite. Thus began the incredible journey and voyage into the internal luminal organs, and this remarkable time travel is mind-boggling.

This treatise on the unravelling of endoscopic excellence and universal ubiquitous collateral contributions in the alleviation of human suffering has been extraordinarily expressed by the authors Dr Easwaramoorthy et al. and the pioneering works of the Father of Endoscopy in India, Professor B Krishna Rau.

I would also like to recollect the work of a few other famous personalities.

The field of endoscopy originally belonged to surgeons. Endoscopic variceal banding by Dr Steigman, biliary stenting by Dr Nib Sohendra, percutaneous endoscopic gastrostomy by Dr Ponsky, and peroral endoscopic myotomy (POEM) by Dr Inouye are some of the classic examples of how surgeons have been instrumental in developing many therapeutic endoscopic procedures.

Dr Jerome Waye at Mount Sinai Hospital was a prolific colonoscopic surgeon noted for his time and efforts in training all gastrointestinal surgeons in the art of colonoscopy. He has also written several articles and books on colonoscopy, and one of his masterpieces is the "Textbook of Colonoscopy" written along with Dr Christopher Williams from St Mark's Hospital, London.

Endoscopic sphincterotomy for bile duct stones by Professors McCune and Classen in Germany had prompted Dr Eric Muhe to invent the technique of laparoscopic cholecystectomy using parts of his bicycle.

Over the last two decades, we have witnessed a technological revolution with endoscopes getting slimmer and smarter with several added features. Image enhancement, magnification, variable stiffness, and scope guide are some of the more recent innovations. With the arrival of 330° colonoscopy, endomicroscopy, and colonoscopy with artificial intelligence (AI) (endo-brain) technology, we are now able to make more precise preprocedural diagnosis and plan an appropriate treatment strategy.

With its increasing diagnostic and therapeutic potentials, I am sure that the flexible endoscopic platform will soon become indispensable equipment in the hands of surgeons and enable them to perform various surgical procedures with ease and precision.

The future is bright for endoscopic surgeons.

Professor Dr A Zameer Pasha
Trichy

CHAPTER

Importance of Endoscopy for Surgeons

Chapter Outline

- Surgeons have been doing Endoscopies for Decades
- Surgeons are Needed to Provide Widespread Gastrointestinal Service
- Endoscopy Skillset would Help Surgeons with more Comprehensive Surgical Practice
- Surgeons are Capable of Swiftly Attaining the Endoscopy Skillset
- Surgeons' Perspectives are Different While Performing Preoperative Endoscopy
- The Era of Endoscopy Laparoscopy Cooperative Surgery
- Endoscopic Surveillance after Gastrointestinal Surgery
- Endoscopic Rescue for Postoperative Complications
- Natural Orifice Scarless Surgery is a More Attractive Option to our Patients
- Endotherapy is becoming a Better Alternative to Conventional Surgical Procedures

Keywords: Flexible endoscopy, therapeutic endoscopy, endoscopy rescue, intraoperative endoscopy

INTRODUCTION

Fewer surgeons are competent and keen to perform endoscopy at present. Ironically, surgeons with a flexible endoscopy skillset have more scope in their clinical practice. Let us explore the reasons why and how surgeons should be performing endoscopy in this era of laparoscopy.

SURGEONS HAVE BEEN DOING ENDOSCOPIES FOR DECADES

The field of flexible endoscopy originally belonged to surgeons. Endoscopic procedures like Colonoscopic polypectomy by Dr Shinya, Endoscopic variceal banding by Dr Steigman, Biliary stenting by Dr Nib Sohendra, Percutaneous Endoscopic Gastrostomy by Dr Ponsky, and Per Oral Endoscopic Myotomy by Dr Inouye are some of the classic examples of how surgeons have been instrumental in developing several therapeutic endoscopic procedures.

We should continue to do what our predecessors were good at and expand the scope of endotherapy with continued commitment and innovation.

SURGEONS ARE NEEDED TO PROVIDE WIDESPREAD GASTROINTESTINAL SERVICE

India with >1.4 billion people needs a huge number of doctors to provide gastrointestinal (GI) services such as screening of GI cancers, diagnosis, and management of various GI disorders such as advanced GI and hepatopancreaticobiliary (HPB) diseases. Relying on the service of gastroenterologists alone would be insufficient and unsustainable. General surgeons with basic flexible endoscopy skills could take up this huge task of providing nationwide GI service proficiently.

ENDOSCOPY SKILLSET WOULD HELP SURGEONS WITH MORE COMPREHENSIVE SURGICAL PRACTICE

Surgeons are usually called for rescue in case of complications following endoscopy, such as perforation and bleeding. Instead, he or she should take an active role in the comprehensive management of patients presenting with GI disorders.

Surgeons, gastroenterologists, and interventional radiologists should work as a team for the benefit and safety of the patients. All GI bleeding cases, and jaundiced patients can be discussed in their multidisciplinary team meetings to define the treatment protocol using minimal access to ensure maximum success. Given that many of the diseases identified at endoscopy are ultimately treated surgically, a surgeon's involvement from the early stage of management is reasonable and preferable.

SURGEONS ARE CAPABLE OF SWIFTLY ATTAINING THE ENDOSCOPY SKILLSET

Surgeons tend to have a shorter learning curve when it comes to achieving competence in performing endoscopic procedures. With open and laparoscopic surgical experience, and better hand-eye coordination, surgeons are quick at grasping endoscopic skills. Surgeons usually have a better understanding of two-dimensional and three-dimensional GI anatomy. Several studies have demonstrated that surgeons are very competent in performing screening colonoscopy and polypectomy even though the number of cases performed during their surgical residency was much less compared to gastroenterologists. The quality of endoscopic training is more important than the quantity of training duration. Structured simulation-based training courses followed by hands-on endoscopic training in clinical settings are enormously beneficial to endoscopic enthusiasts.

SURGEONS' PERSPECTIVES ARE DIFFERENT WHILE PERFORMING PREOPERATIVE ENDOSCOPY

Several studies have highlighted the importance of preoperative endoscopy done by the operating surgeons. The presence of hiatus hernia, severe esophagitis, and gastric pathologies would change the treatment algorithms for morbid obesity. Gastric bypass is better suited than sleeve gastrectomy in patients with severe acid reflux. A major portion of the stomach would be excluded from the food pathway in cases of gastric bypass. Hence, a detailed inspection of the whole upper GI tract is paramount. It will ensure prior management of any incidental gastric polyps or *H. pylori* gastritis before performing a gastric bypass.

In gastric tumors, preoperative endoscopy should ideally be done by operating surgeons, so that all the key details such as the exact location and size of the tumor, how much tumor extension along the lesser curve, and how close the upper limit of the tumor from cardia, can all be ascertained to enable in making ideal surgical strategy. The surgeon can then determine the best approach for the patient whether it is endotherapy, laparoscopy, or open surgery.

THE ERA OF ENDOSCOPY LAPAROSCOPY COOPERATIVE SURGERY

There have been many situations during surgery when flexible endoscopy could come to the surgeon's rescue. We could enumerate some classical situations.

In the case of redo laparoscopic Heller's myotomy, intraoperative upper GI endoscopy would help to confirm GE junction, adequacy of myotomy, and also exclude any inadvertent mucosal breach during the procedure.

During laparoscopic bile duct exploration for multiple bile duct stones, intraoperative choledochoscopy would ensure completeness of stone removal prior to closure of choledochotomy. Surgeons with endoscopy skills can handle the flexible choledochoscope more efficiently.

Intraoperative laparoscopy-assisted small bowel enteroscopy could help to locate the source of obscure GI bleeding from the small bowel.

In gastric gastrointestinal stromal tumor (GIST) tumors, endoscopic inspection and assistance during laparoscopic sleeve resection would be greatly rewarding. It would preserve gastric volume but ensure the adequacy of the resection margin. Endoscopic full-thickness resection of gastric polyps can be done with laparoscopic inspection more safely and efficiently. Serosal sutures can be done by laparoscopic surgeons if needed.

Large colonic polyps in the cecum can be safely removed by colonoscopic polypectomy with laparoscopic inspection or laparoscopic sleeve resection of the cecum can be done with colonoscopic inspection. Such mutual understanding and assistance would improve the scope of surgical practice and ensure the safety of surgical procedures.

ENDOSCOPIC SURVEILLANCE AFTER GASTROINTESTINAL SURGERY

Surveillance colonoscopy following a previous colectomy for a cancer colon or after a colonoscopic polypectomy can be better done by the surgical team themselves.

Following laparoscopic fundoplication, postoperative endoscopy can be done by the operating surgeon to look for adequacy of fundal wrap, any wrap migration, and resolution of esophagitis.

The status of Barrett's esophagus can be assessed by the surgical team performing the antireflux surgery.

ENDOSCOPIC RESCUE FOR POSTOPERATIVE COMPLICATIONS

Flexible endoscopy has immense therapeutic potential, during the postoperative period following many abdominal procedures. Some of the classical examples are discussed further.

Any bleeding from upper GI or colorectal anastomotic sites could be visualized and if needed appropriate endoscopic hemostatic procedures such as hemoclip application can be done to manage the complication efficiently.

In bariatric patients, endoscopic CRE balloon dilatation (controlled radial expansion balloon) for stricture at the gastric bypass site and endoscopy-assisted suture narrowing of wide RYGB anastomotic sites to prevent regain of weight are classical examples of endoscopic rescue for these postoperative challenges.

Endoscopic deployment of the fully covered metal stent, endoscopic sponge therapy, and septotomy are classic examples of endoscopic rescue in case of post-sleeve gastrectomy leaks.

NATURAL ORIFICE SCARLESS SURGERY IS A MORE ATTRACTIVE OPTION TO OUR PATIENTS

From the era of open surgery now we have moved on to an era of minimal access surgery. What was accomplished by a big incision can now be easily performed by small incision or even incision-less surgery. It is paramount that surgeons are now well versed in all facets of surgery so that surgeons can offer the ideal treatment modality as per the needs of the clinical scenario and expectation.

Surgery on a flexible endoscopy platform is the future as there is an increasing number of endoscopic treatment options available now for several surgical conditions. Hence this is obviously going to be an attractive choice once safety and efficacy are proved and ease of performance is improved.

Consider the management of pancreatic pseudocysts nowadays. Open surgery is replaced by laparoscopic cystogastrostomy. In recent times endoscopic cystogastrostomy using lumen apposing metal (LAM) stent has become the standard of care!

No incision surgery is always preferable to even keyhole surgeries. Beware!

ENDOTHERAPY IS BECOMING A BETTER ALTERNATIVE TO CONVENTIONAL SURGICAL PROCEDURES

With the arrival of technological innovations like HD endoscopy with image enhancement and magnification, various endoscopic accessories, and energy sources, several surgical procedures are now feasible on flexible endoscopic platforms.

POEM instead of Laparoscopic Heller's myotomy, Percutaneous endoscopic gastrostomy instead of open feeding gastrostomy, and endoscopic sleeve gastroplasty in place of laparoscopic sleeve gastrectomy are some classic examples. The list is endless **(Table 1)**.

Hence advanced therapeutic endoscopic procedures are within the purview of general surgeons with adequate training, appropriate tools, and a team approach.

TABLE 1: Various endotherapy solutions for conventional surgical management.

Indication	*Surgical option*	*Endoscopic solution*
Bleeding varices	Shunts	Banding/sclerotherapy
Achalasia cardia	Lap Heller's myotomy	POEM
Gastric outlet obstruction	Gastrojejunostomy	SEM stent
Enteral feeding	Feeding gastrostomy	PEG
Morbid obesity	Sleeve gastrectomy	Endo sleeve gastroplasty
GERD	Lap fundoplication	Esophyx/GERDx
Polyps	Lap colectomy	ESD/EMR
CBD stone	Choledocholithotomy	ERCP/lithotripsy
Pseudocyst of pancreas	Lap cystogastrostomy	Endoscopic drainage
Viscus perforation	Open/lap suturing	Endoscopic clips/Stitch

(CBD: common bile duct; EMR: endoscopic mucosal resection; ESD: endoscopic submucosal dissection; GERD: gastroesophageal reflux disease; POEM: per-oral endoscopic myotomy; PEG: polyethylene glycol; SEM: self-expanding metallic)

CONCLUSION

Endoscopy skills are very essential for every surgeon. Like a knife to cut and laparoscopy to visualize and operate, now endoscopy has become another important tool for surgeons to master. The surgical fraternity should continue to train themselves and their juniors in the art and science of endoscopy. Endoscopic surgeons have a better scope and a brighter future.

SUGGESTED READING

1. Achord JL. The History of Gastrointestinal Endoscopy. In: Ginsberg GG, Kochman ML, Norton ID, Gostout CJ (Eds). Clinical Gastrointestinal Endoscopy, 2nd edition. St Louis, Missouri: Elsevier Saunders; 2012. pp. 5-11.
2. Britt L, Richardson JD. Residency review committee for surgery: an update. Arch Surg. 2007;142(6):573-5.
3. Donahue PE, Sugitani A. Gastrointestinal endoscopy and general surgical practice. Surgical endoscopy versus surgeon endoscopists. Am Surg. 1991;57(5): 330-3.
4. Fanelli RD, Sultany MS. Surgeons performing endoscopy: why, how, and when? Ann Laparosc Endosc Surg. 2019;4.
5. Lee AHH, Lojanapiwat N, Balakrishnan V, Chandra R. Is there a difference in adenoma detection rates between gastroenterologists and surgeons? World J Gastrointest Endosc. 2018;10(6):109-16.
6. Reed WP, Kilkenny JW, Dias CE, Wexner SD; SAGES EGD Outcomes Study Group. A prospective analysis of 3525 esophagogastroduodenoscopies performed by surgeons. Surg Endosc. 2004;18(1):11-21.
7. Wexner SD, Garbus JE, Singh JJ; SAGES Colonoscopy Study Outcomes Group. A prospective analysis of 13,580 colonoscopies. Reevaluation of credentialing guidelines. Surg Endosc. 2001;15(3):251-61.

Expert's Comment

Traditionally, globally, surgeons have played a key role in introducing therapeutic procedures into the endoscopic domain. In India, too, surgeons were among the first to adopt endoscopy, particularly at a time when it was primarily used for diagnostic purposes. Over time, gastroenterologists gradually took the lead, and with the advancement in technology, the scope of endoscopy has significantly expanded to include complex therapeutic interventions.

Many of these advanced endoscopic procedures require a high level of technical expertise, including precise hand-eye coordination, tissue handling, an in-depth understanding of tissue behavior, and familiarity with surgical anatomy, which are integral to surgical training. Innovations such as endoscopic suturing and submucosal dissections further blur the lines between endoscopy and surgery. Surgeons, with their comprehensive anatomical and operative knowledge, are uniquely positioned to learn, master, and innovate in these areas.

Moreover, management of complications arising from endoscopic procedures often requires surgical intervention, reinforcing the need for surgeons to be well versed in both diagnostic and therapeutic endoscopy. Endoscopy also serves as a valuable tool for preoperative planning, intraoperative guidance, and postoperative evaluation, making it an essential extension of the surgical armamentarium.

Given the increasing demand for endoscopic expertise across the country, particularly in remote and underserved regions, it is vital to train a larger number of surgeons in endoscopic techniques. Doing so will ensure wider access to high-quality, modern, minimally invasive treatments and help maintain surgical leadership in the evolving landscape of gastrointestinal and general surgery. Considering these factors, it is imperative that surgeons actively engage in learning and practicing both diagnostic and therapeutic endoscopy to remain at the forefront of patient care and technological advancement.

Dr Pravin Suryawanshi
Chhatrapati Sambhajinagar

3

CHAPTER

Hardware of Upper Gastrointestinal Endoscope

Chapter Outline

- Surface Anatomy of the Endoscope
  - Control Head
  - Insertion Section
  - Umbilical Cord
- Instrument Checklist
- Inside Anatomy of an Endoscope (How it Looks and How it Functions)
  - Inside of Insertion Section
  - Inside of Endoscope Tip
  - Inside of Control Head
  - Principle of Image Conduction
- Advances in Endoscopy
  - Magnification Endoscopy
  - Chromoendoscopy
  - Narrow-band Imaging
  - Fluorescence Spectroscopy
  - Endoscopic Ultrasound
  - Optical Coherence Tomography
  - Confocal Endoscopy
  - Endocytoscopy
- Handling and Storage of the Endoscopy

Keywords: HD endoscopy, image enhancement, magnification endoscopy, NBI, videoendoscopy, endocytoscopy

INTRODUCTION

If you want to become a safe and efficient driver of your new Mercedes or BMW, then better get familiarized with all its gadgets and their function. Likewise, one should spend enough time learning the intricate design of each endoscope and understanding how it functions. As surgeons, we know the importance of anatomy.

SURFACE ANATOMY OF THE ENDOSCOPE

The basic design of all different endoscope makes and types are identical. Let us look at the videoendoscope and understand its various parts and functions. Videoendoscope has the following three main parts **(Fig. 1)**, namely:

1. Control head
2. Insertion section
3. Umbilical cord

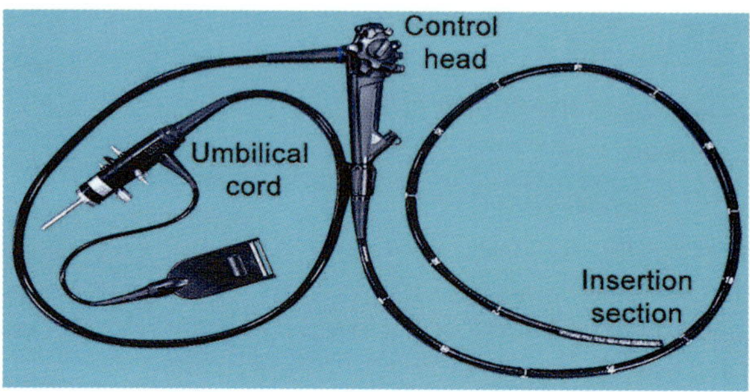

Fig. 1: Parts of videoendoscopy.

Control Head (Fig. 2)

- It is the heart of the endoscope
- It has all the wheels, locks, and buttons
- Hold the control unit in your left hand by docking it in the first web space between your thumb and index finger and gently embrace it with ring and littlc finger

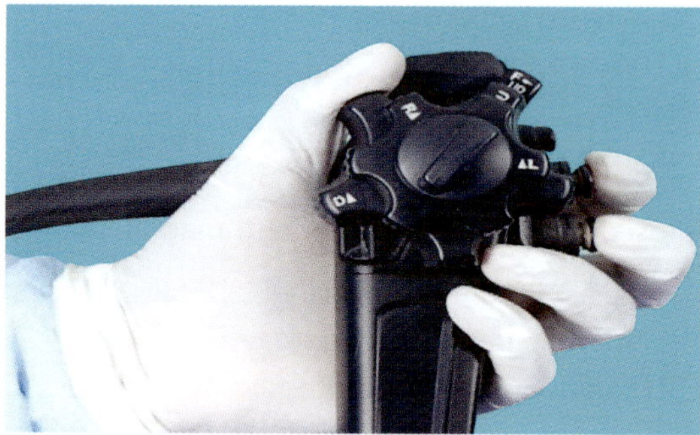

Fig. 2: Control head.

Familiarize yourself with the big and small wheels on the right side **(Figs. 3A and B)**. Like in a car, these are the steering wheels of the endoscope tip. The big wheel is for moving the scope tip up and down. The small wheel is for turning the scope tip right or left. Learn to control the wheels with your left

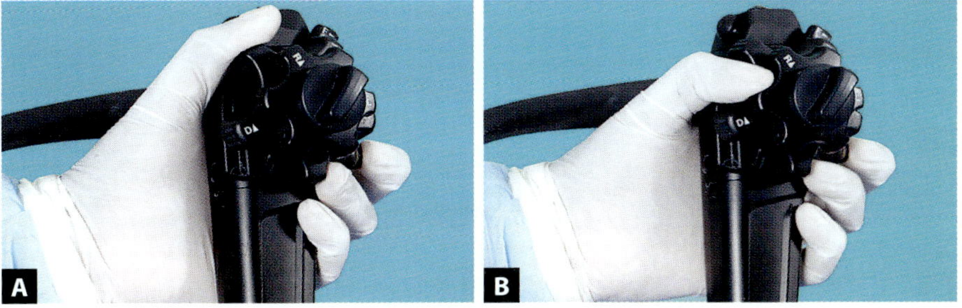

Figs. 3A and B: (A) Big wheel; and (B) Small wheel.

thumb. Each wheel is guarded by a latch like a hand brake **(Figs. 4A and B)**. Push the locking latch forward (away from you) to unlock or free the movement of the wheels and turn the latch backward (toward you) to lock the wheels. But remember to keep the endoscope in an unlocked position always. Only when you plan to do some therapeutic intervention you may want to lock a wheel to freeze the movement of the endoscope tip.

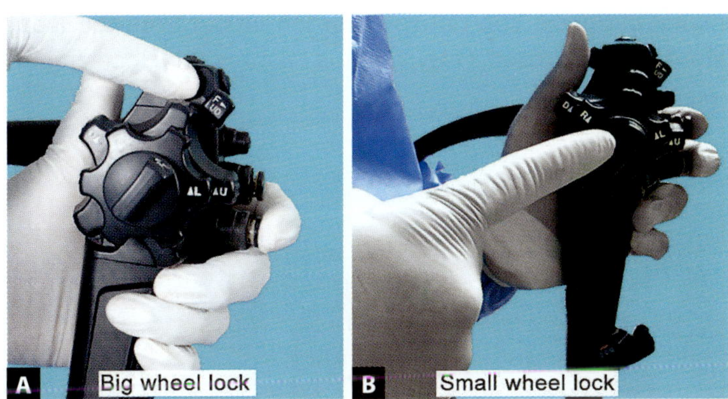

Figs. 4A and B: Pushing the locking latch away from you to unlock.

Next, familiarize yourself with the two big buttons in front of the control head **(Figs. 5A and B)**. The buttons are detachable and color-coded to ensure the correct button is docked in the correct place. The Superior button is for suction (remember S for S) and is coded red. It is activated by pressing it with your left index finger. Use suction intermittently and intelligently to remove saliva, residual gastric fluid, or food debris to ensure smooth conduct of endoscopy. For therapeutic endoscopies like banding, good suction is very essential. Suction determines success in such situations!

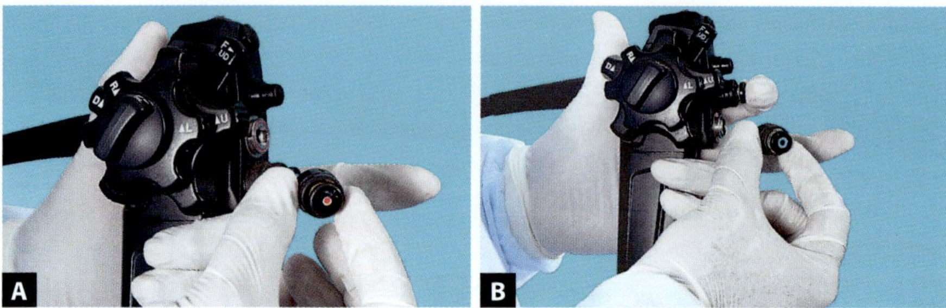

Figs. 5A and B: (A) Superior button; and (B) Inferior button.

The inferior button **(Figs. 5A and B)** is meant for two functions namely insufflation of air and instillation of water (Remember I for I). It is color-coded blue. Use your left middle finger to control it. Just place your finger to cover the hole over the button which will ensure a continuous flow of air as seen by dipping the scope tip in a basin of water **(Fig. 6)**. You will appreciate the continuous flow of big bubbles of air. This ensures adequate insufflation of the gut and aids in proper navigation of the scope tip. Now hold the scope tip out of the water basin, press the inferior button with your middle finger, and see what happens. You notice water jetting out from the scope tip like "an infant dribbling urine" **(Fig. 7)**. This ensures the cleansing of the lens

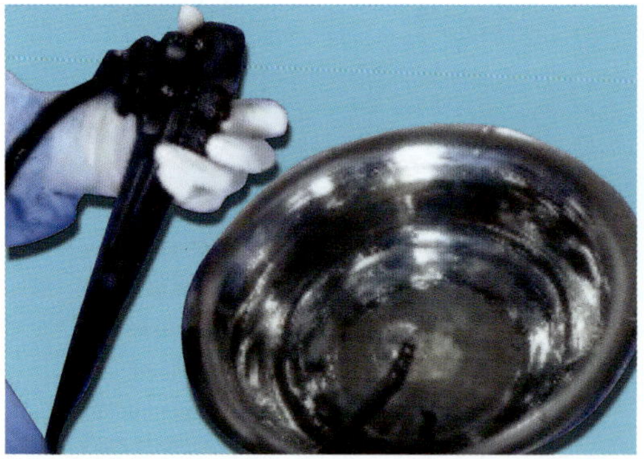

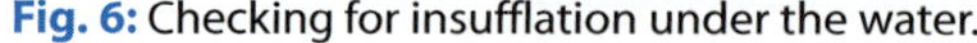

Fig. 6: Checking for insufflation under the water.

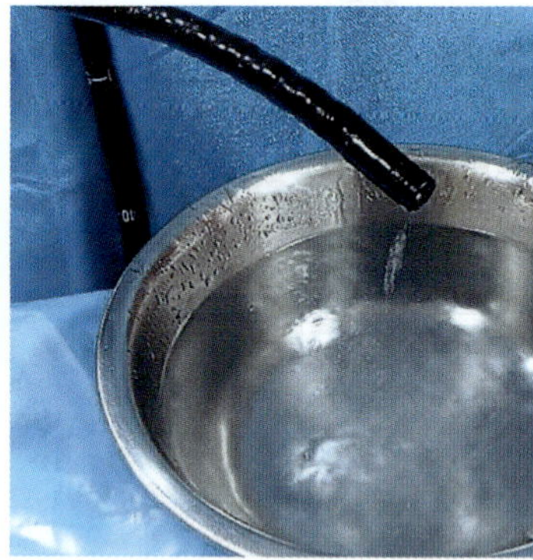

Fig. 7: Checking the irrigation.

at the endoscopy tip. While driving a car, we know how important it is to clean the windscreen with water to view the road clearly to drive safely. The same holds for driving the scope safely and swiftly. So, for smooth conduct of endoscopy, we need almost continuous insufflation, intermittent suction, and occasional instillation of water. Learn the art of controlling these function buttons appropriately.

In addition, we have additional two to four remote control function buttons depending on the make and type of the scope to zoom the image, freeze the image, or even give a print command to take a printout!

In fiberoptic endoscopy, the viewing eyepiece is normally located at the top of the control head.

The control head is connected to the light source and video processing unit (the brain of the endoscope) through the umbilical cord.

Notice the biopsy or access channel **(Fig. 8)** at the junction of the place where the control head is attached to the insertion section. Note the size of the channel and where it is exiting at the tip of the endoscope. It is usually 2.8–3.2 mm in diameter. When you pass a biopsy forceps through the access channel, see where it comes out in the picture seen on the monitor. Imagine the monitor like a big clock with the top middle of the monitor at 12 o'clock and the bottom middle at 6 o'clock. The biopsy forceps will be seen exiting either at 5 o'clock (Pentax) or 7 o'clock position (Olympus) **(Fig. 9)**. This is very important to understand for the successful conduct of various therapeutic interventions. So, treat the monitor like a clock!

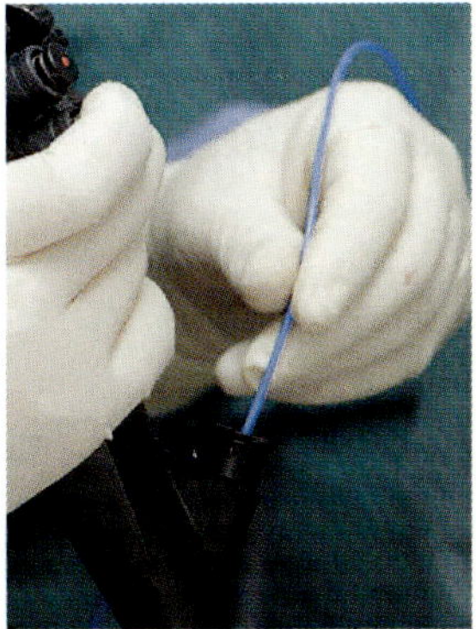

Fig. 8: Biopsy channel.

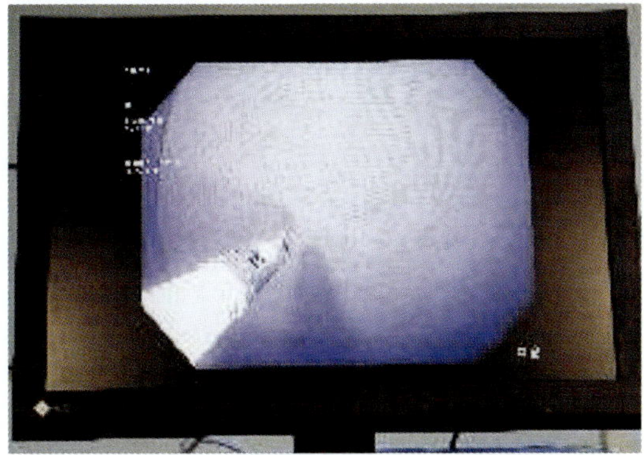

Fig. 9: Olympus monitor showing biopsy access at 7 o'clock position.

Insertion Section

The flexible insertion section is of a certain length, diameter, and stiffness depending on the type and make of the scope. It is about 110 cm for gastroscopes and >160 cm for colonoscopes. Newer scopes are slimmer with an excellent range of tip movements and a wide field of vision. Most of the gastroscopes are about 9.2 mm in diameter (ranging from 6 to 11 mm). Smaller or sleeker instruments inevitably involve some compromise in durability, image quality, and biopsy size.

Gastroscopes are available in standard adult, pediatric, and therapeutic models. Types of gastroscopes **(Figs. 10A to C)**. Some therapeutic

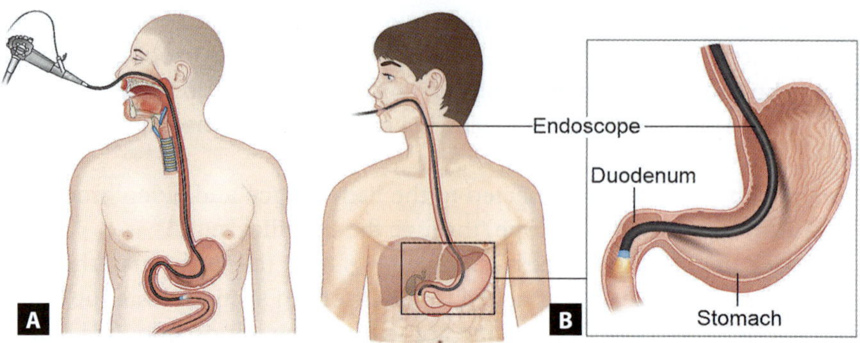

C

Types of gastroscopes	*Model number*	*Diameter of scope*	*Number of channels*
Trans nasal endoscopy	Olympus GIF-N180, GIF-XP170N	4.9 to 6 mm	1
Standard endoscopy	Olympus CV-170, Pentax EG29-i10	9.2 mm	1
Therapeutic endoscopy	Olympus GIF-2TH180, GIF-H290EC	9.8 to 13.2 mm	2

Figs. 10A to C: (A) Pediatric endoscopy; (B) Standard endoscopy; and (C) Therapeutic endoscopy.

gastroscopes have dual working channels for more complex interventions. Another type of gastroscope is an ultrathin variety in which the insertion tube diameter is 6 mm or less. These endoscopes may be used for unsedated peroral or transnasal esophagoscopy or to traverse tight strictures.

Distal most 15 cm is the "bending section" of the scope and has very critical parts. It is the face of the endoscope. It sees, breathes, sucks and turns! So, keep it clean and safe **(Fig. 11)**.

- Turn the big wheel toward you to turn the endoscope tip up and up till you make it like a hockey stick (like during the J maneuver) **(Figs. 12A and B)**.

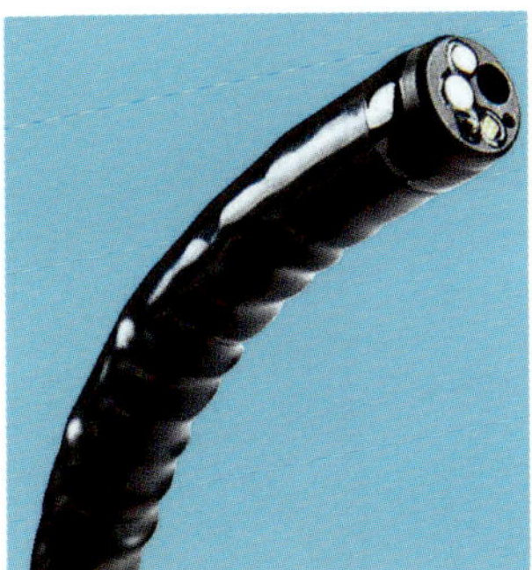

Fig. 11: The distal end of endoscopy.

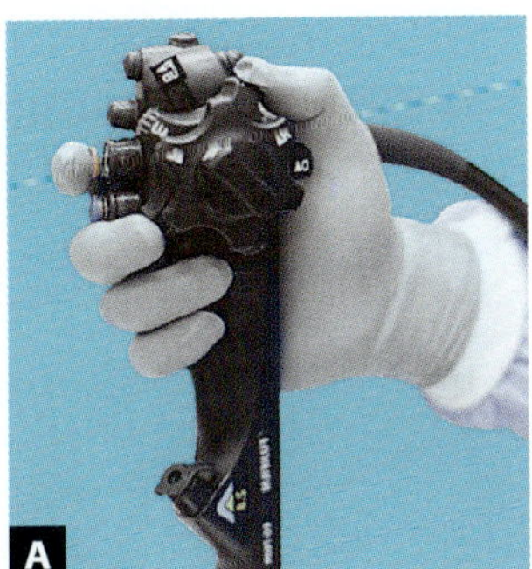

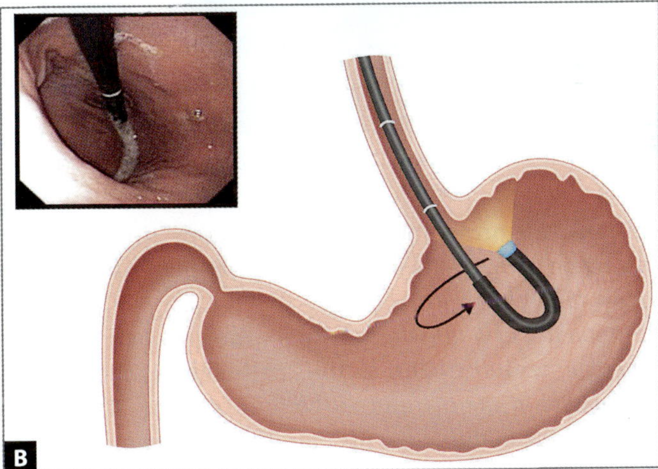

Figs. 12A and B: Big wheel fully toward you for J maneuver.

- Turn the small wheel away from you (clockwise turn) to move the scope tip to the right and vice versa **(Fig. 13)**.
- You could also torque or twist the shaft of the scope into clockwise direction to turn the tip to the right and torque it anticlockwise to turn it left **(Fig. 14)**.

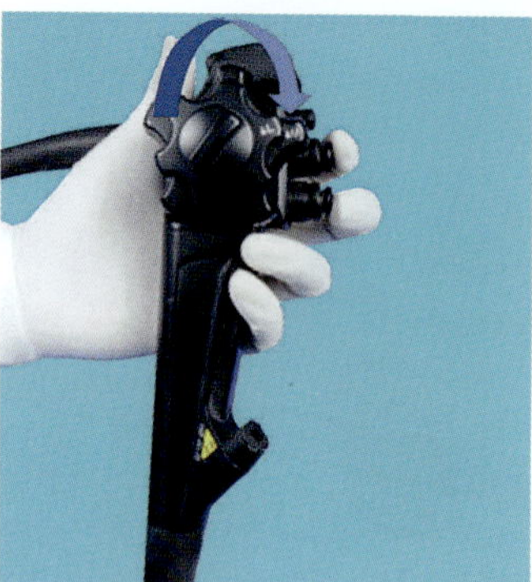

Fig. 13: Small wheel away from you.

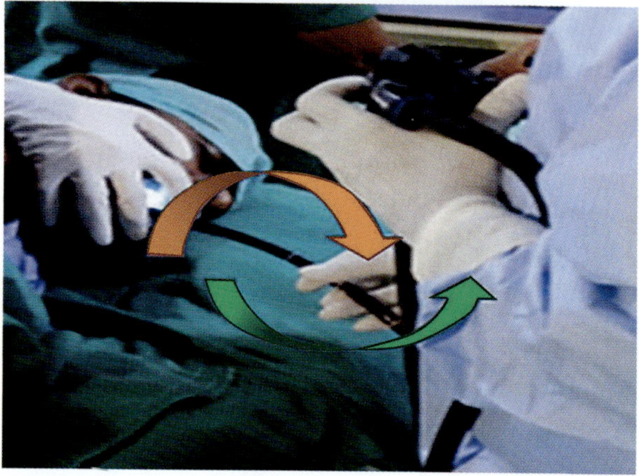

Fig. 14: Torquing the scope.

- Soon you will understand that endoscopy tip movement can be adjusted by turning the wheels, twisting the shaft of the scope, and even rotating your body!
- Take a magnifying glass and inspect the very end of the endoscope tip. As the name implies, in the "end viewing scope" the lens and channels are at the tip, and in the "side viewing scope" (ERCP) they are on the side of the scope tip. Familiarize yourself with the following pictures depicting various locations of key parts at the tip of the scope **(Figs. 15A and B)**.

Umbilical Cord (Fig. 16)

- The umbilical cord connects the baby (the endoscope) to the mother (processing unit).
- It carries the image guide cables, light guide bundle, suction channel, and water and air feeding channel between the scope and processing unit.

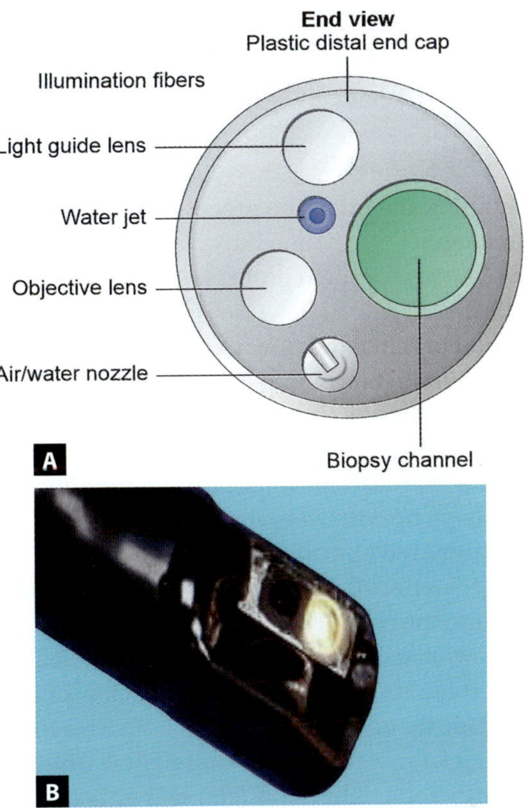

Figs. 15A and B: (A) End viewing scope; and (B) Side viewing scope.

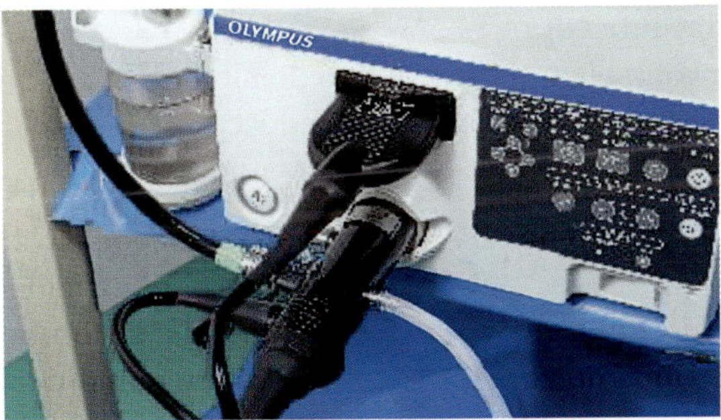

Fig. 16: Olympus CV-170.

- The supply plug connects the umbilical cord to the processing unit. It has a light guide and air feeder at the tip and the suction outlet and water jet outlet on either side as shown in the picture.
- Learn to understand how the supply plug has to be attached to the processing unit and light source.

- Familiarize yourself with the location of the suction outlet and air/water jet outlet to connect the suction unit and water bottle accordingly.
- Avoid undue bends or twist in the umbilical cord during endoscope handling.

INSTRUMENT CHECKLIST

- Connect the umbilical cord to the processing unit and attach the suction and air/water channel
- Turn the light source and video processing unit "ON"
- Turn the suction "ON."
- Ensure the water bottle is filled with distilled water (RO water) to the required level.
- Keep the locking latches on the wheels in the forward position to free the endoscope tip movement.
- Ensure you see a crystal-clear image on the monitor. White balance or wipe the endoscope tip with wet gauze or 70% alcohol, if needed.
- Press the superior (red) button with your left index finger to activate suction. Ensure suction is adequate by noticing a continuous flow of water pouring into the suction bottle.
- Check the airflow. Place your left middle finger to seal the hole over the inferior button (blue) to notice a "continuous flow of big bubbles" when you keep the scope tip underneath the water in a basin.
- Check the water jet. Press the inferior button now while holding the scope tip in midair with your right hand. You will notice a "water jet" like an infant passing urine.
  - Only when a scope is "cleaned and disinfected," "properly connected" and has undergone "all the above checks," we should start the endoscopy procedure.
  - So, train yourself and your staff to do all these rituals routinely, every day, and every time before doing endoscopy. This cockpit drill ensures seamless and successful conduct of endoscopy.

INSIDE ANATOMY OF AN ENDOSCOPE (HOW IT LOOKS AND HOW IT FUNCTIONS)

We have to spend long hours in the anatomy dissection hall during our medical career to learn and understand various parts of our body and their functions. Likewise, do not miss a rare opportunity to see the inside of an endoscopy with the help of the engineers during any structured endoscopy training course. Only then, you will appreciate the engineering marvel of endoscopy design and function. The compact endoscope we have today is the result of hard work and dedication by scores of scientists and doctors over several decades.

Look for and familiarize yourself with the following parts that are inside the scope.

Inside of Insertion Section

- Light guide bundle
- Image guide cable
- Suction/instrument channel
- Water jet and air feeding channel
- Pull wires for bending section

Inside of Endoscope Tip

- Lens
- Charge-coupled device (CCD) chip

Inside of Control Head

- Pulleys attaching the pull wires to the big and small wheels
- All cables and channels extend to the umbilical cord.

Principle of Image Conduction (Fig. 17)

- *Fiberoptic endoscope versus videoendoscope:*
  - The mechanical functional components such as wheels and buttons are similar in both video and fiberoptic endoscopes. However, the principle of image conduction is different.
  - A fiberoptic endoscope utilizes optical fibers to transmit both light and image. An optical fiber is composed of two layers of glass of different reflective values that trap the light inside the length of the fiber. The flexibility of the fibers enables the light to be bent around corners and curves. Thousands of fine optical fibers are carefully arranged in an orderly manner to obtain a coherent image guide bundle.

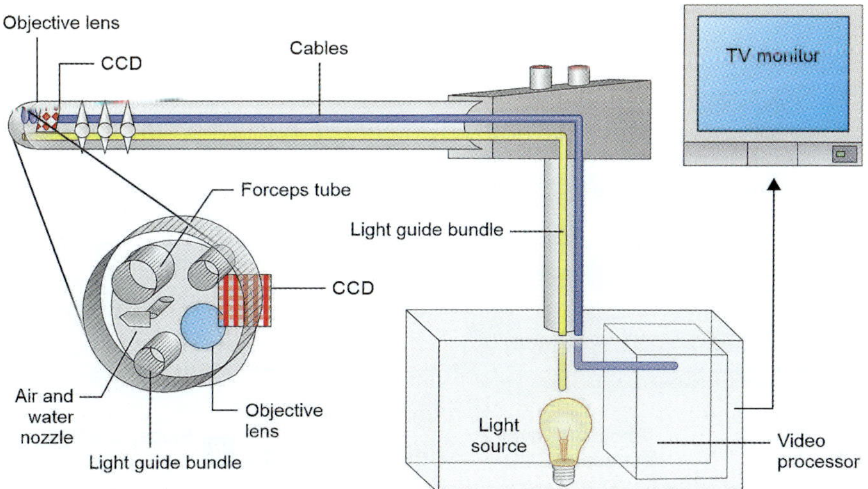

Fig. 17: Mechanism of electronic videoendoscope. (CCD: charge-coupled device)

Each tiny fiber (10 μm diameter) carries a small part of the image (like the compound eye of a cockroach!). The image is transmitted by total internal reflection. If any optical fiber is damaged, one may notice a black dot in the image corresponding to that damaged fiber. The more dots you see, it means more damage to the scope. So, it is easy to access the condition of a fiberoptic scope. Unlike the image conduct bundle, the light conduct fiberoptic bundle is composed of noncoherent optical fibers. It just transmits light from the light source to the scope tip through one or two bundles.

But a videoendoscope has light conduct bundles and image guide cables. Light from the xenon or halogen light source is carried by the light conduct bundle to the endoscope tip. The objective lens at the scope tip focuses the image onto the CCD chip (charged coupled device) which captures the image and sends the electrical signals through the image guide cables to the video processor.

- *About the CCD chips and image processing* ***(Figs. 18A and B)****:*
  - The CCD used in the videoendoscope, is a solid-state microchip used for image sensing. It is located near the tip of the endoscopy. The photosensitive surface of the chip is divided into an array (rows and columns) of cells, each able to directly convert the light (photons) focused upon it into electrical charges (electrons). These cells are more commonly called "pixels," a name derived from "picture element." A pixel represents the limit of image resolution and is the basic building block used to recreate an electronic image. By having greatly increased numbers of pixels we can increase the resolution of the image.
  - The electrical charge produced at each pixel corresponds to the intensity of the light falling on that particular pixel. By "reading" the charge developed at each pixel sequentially, the image focused on the CCD

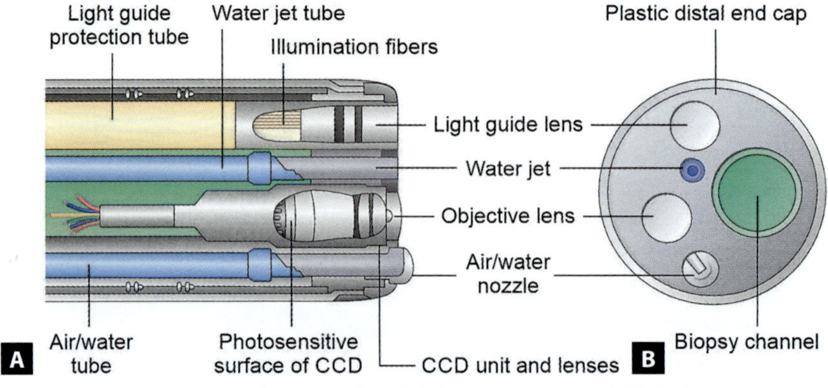

Figs. 18A and B: CCD chip. (A) Cross-section; and (B) End view. (CCD: charge-coupled device)

surface is turned into an electronic signal that can, after sophisticated processing, be accurately reproduced on a TV (video) monitor.

- This signal is converted to a color image by one of two systems: a red-green-blue (RGB) sequential system or a color CCD system.
- The RGB system uses a xenon lamp to arc white light through a rotating RGB filter
- Located between the lamp and the light guide; this results in bursts of red, green, and blue light to create a visual strobe effect. When tissue is illuminated, the reflected red, green, and blue images are sent through a CCD in the instrument tip and transmitted to the image processor.
- The color CCD system differs in that a micromosaic color filter is mounted over the CCD chip itself. White light illumination is provided by the xenon lamp and reflected color images on the CCD surface are processed by circuitry in the image processor.

▪ *Special features:*
  - *High definition (HD)*: HD endoscopes generate images with 850,000 to >1 million pixels compared with image signals of 100,000–400,000 pixels on standard endoscopes. They require HD-compatible image processors and monitors to produce true HD images.
  - *Image enhancement:* Some endoscopes are equipped with enhanced imaging capabilities including narrow-band imaging (NBI by Olympus Medical Systems) and multiband imaging (MBI) such as Fujinon intelligent color enhancement (FICE) technology by Fujinon and intelligent scan (I-SCAN by Pentax). NBI uses filters to illuminate the tissue at selected wavelengths of blue (415 nm) and green (540 nm), highlighting vascular detail from surrounding mucosa. MBI processes the white-light image digitally, reconstructing it through software rather than a filter to enhance the appearance of the mucosa. MBI can be combined with magnification. These image enhancement techniques are intended to assist in diagnosing and further characterizing lesions in the gastrointestinal (GI) tract **(Figs. 19A to C)**.

▪ *Light guide bundles:*
  - Xenon (300 watts) and halogen (150 watts) light sources are commonly used.
  - Xenon light is preferred in advanced versions given its intense pure white light. But it is rather expensive, and the bulb has a life span of about 500 light hours.
  - Light is focused by a parabolic mirror onto the face of the light guide bundle, and the transmitted intensity is controlled by filters and/or a mechanical diaphragm. Since these light bundles do not transmit a spatial image, the fibers within them need not be "coherent" and are randomly arranged. Because light intensity is reduced at any optical interface, light bundles run uninterruptedly from the tip of

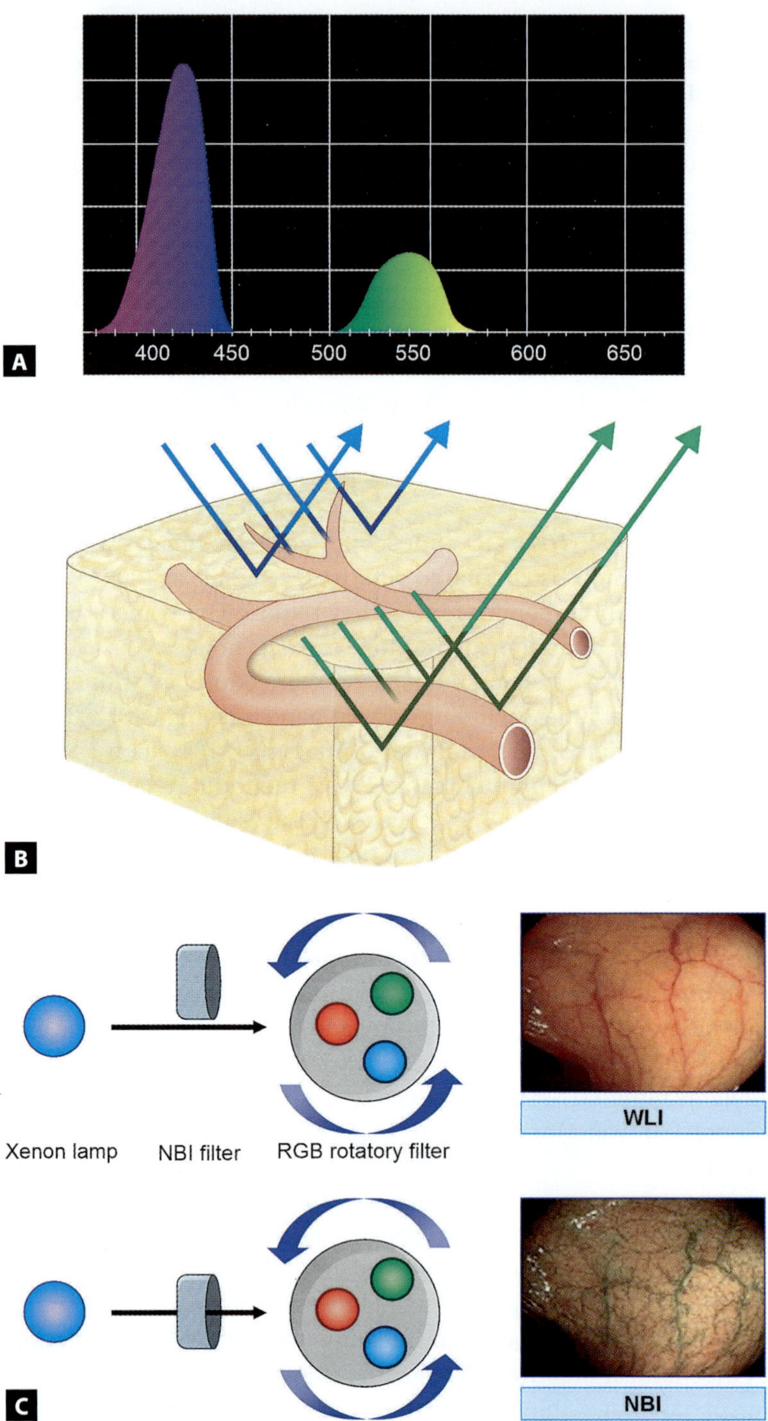

Figs. 19A to C: Narrow-band imaging (NBI) mechanism. (RGB: red-green-blue; WLI: white light imaging)

the instrument through its connecting "umbilical" cord directly to the point of focus of the lamp.

- The light sources made by different companies are not always interchangeable.

- *Instrument channels*:
  - *Biopsy and suction channels* ***(Fig. 20)***:
    - The biopsy or access channel allows the passage of different types of accessories (e.g., biopsy forceps, cytology brushes, sclerotherapy needles, and diathermy snares). The access channel joins the suction channel.
    - The suction/biopsy channel is basically a length of tubing running from one end of the endoscope to the other end with an on/off valve in the middle and attachments to stainless steel connectors at the ends. This tubing is required to be extremely flexible, pliable, and as well as strong.
    - The channel size varies from 2 to 6 mm. Bigger is better for therapeutic interventions, such as controlled radial expansion (CRE) balloon dilatation and stent deployment. Twin channel scopes are also available for endoscopic hemostasis.
    - In the endoscopic retrograde cholangiopancreatography (ERCP) scope, the tip of the channel incorporates a small deflectable elevator or bridge, which permits some directional control of the forceps and other accessories independent of the instrument tip.

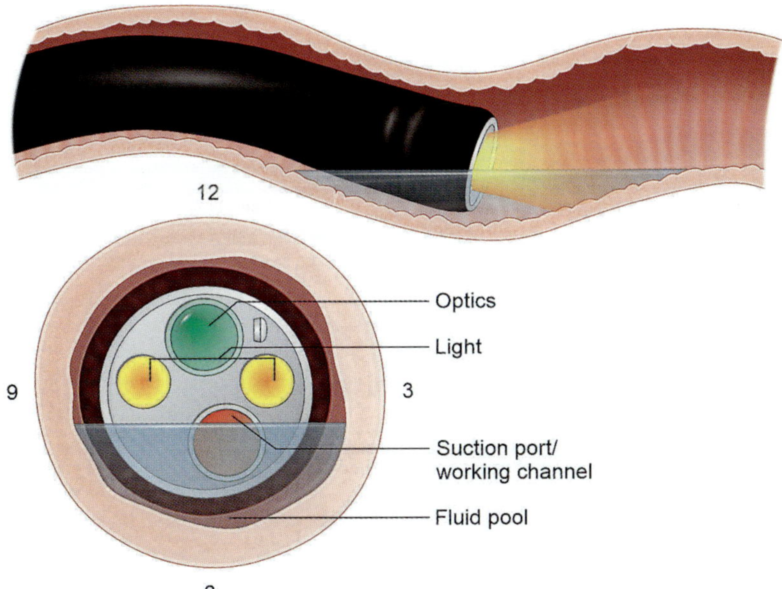

Fig. 20: Biopsy.

This elevator or bridge is controlled by an additional thumb lever located close to the wheels in the control head.
- The central or floor suction unit is connected to the supply plug in the "umbilical cord". Suction is initiated by pressing the superior red button. (Superior button for suction)
- Prompt cleaning of the endoscope after procedures and cautious insertion of any accessory into the suction/biopsy channels is the best way to ensure proper suction system operation. Avoid overflexing the umbilical cord and insertion section of an endoscope to prevent kinking or collapsing of the channel.

- *Air and water channels* **(Figs. 21 to 23)**:
    - An ancillary small channel transmits air to distend the organ being examined; the air is supplied from a pump in the light source and is controlled by the inferior blue button in the control head. The air system also pressurizes the water bottle so that a jet of water can be squirted across the distal lens to clean it. In colonoscopy, there is a separate proximal opening for the water channel, to allow high-pressure flushing with a syringe.
    - The air/water nozzle is the point of smallest inner diameter and can become obstructed with debris or crushed from an impact. Air infused into the gut during endoscopy may produce a luminal pressure high enough to force debris to back up several centimeters into the nozzle and the air and water channels. So, irrigate the channels immediately after each procedure to prevent clogging of the nozzles or channels.

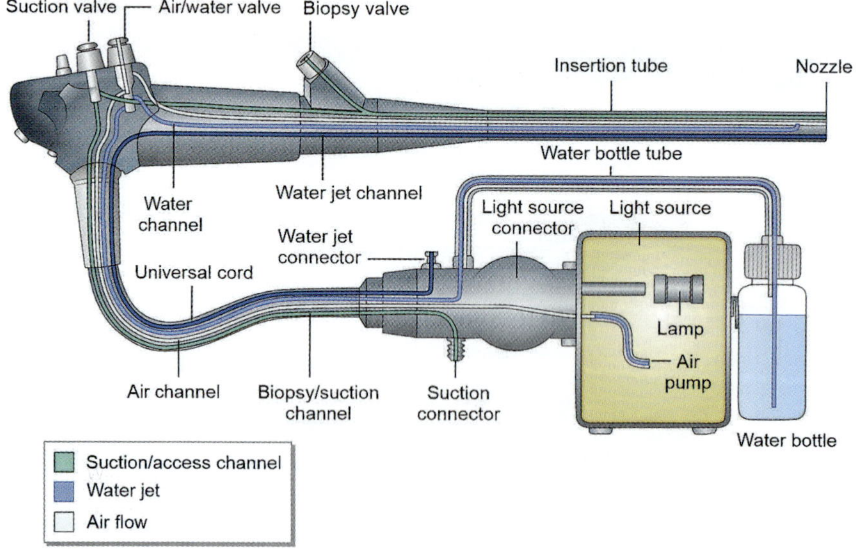

Fig. 21: Anatomy of air and water channel.

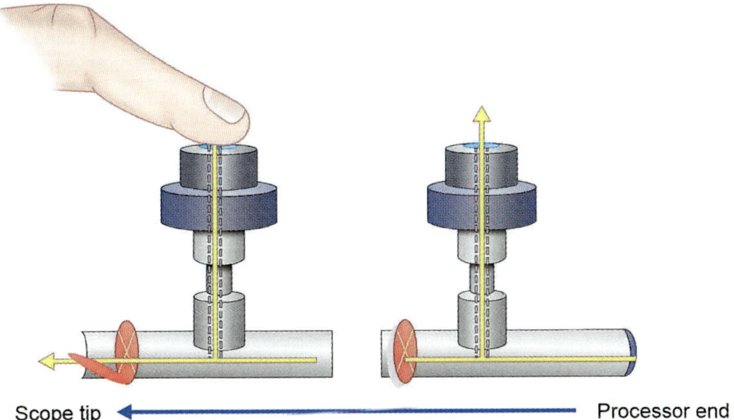

Fig. 22: Fundamentals of air feeding.

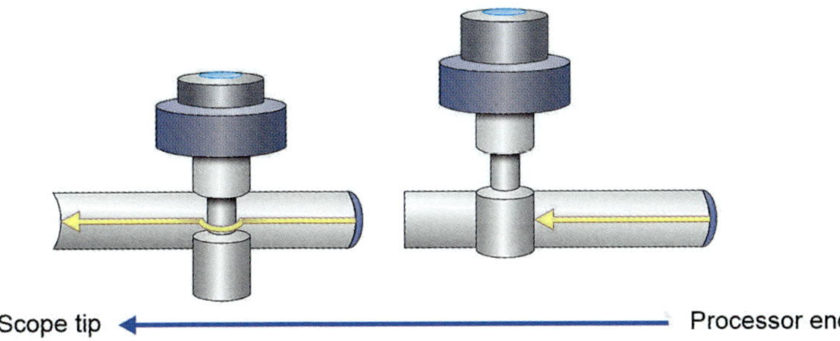

Fig. 23: Fundamentals of water feeding.

- Never probe the opening of the nozzle with a sharp object as it may damage or loosen the nozzle and could inadvertently scratch the image lens. A soft bristle brush should be used to clean the nozzle.

- *Angulation mechanism* ***(Figs. 24A and B)****:*
  - Either a wire pulley assembly or a chain drive can articulate endoscopes with the help of the big and small wheels in the control head.
  - Angulation wires from the endoscope tip pass through the insertion section onto the control wheels through a shaft.
  - A flexible metal coil covers the outer aspect of the scope, and this ensures protection and proper function of the angulation mechanism.

ADVANCES IN ENDOSCOPY

- Magnification endoscopy
- Chromoendoscopy
- Narrow-band imaging

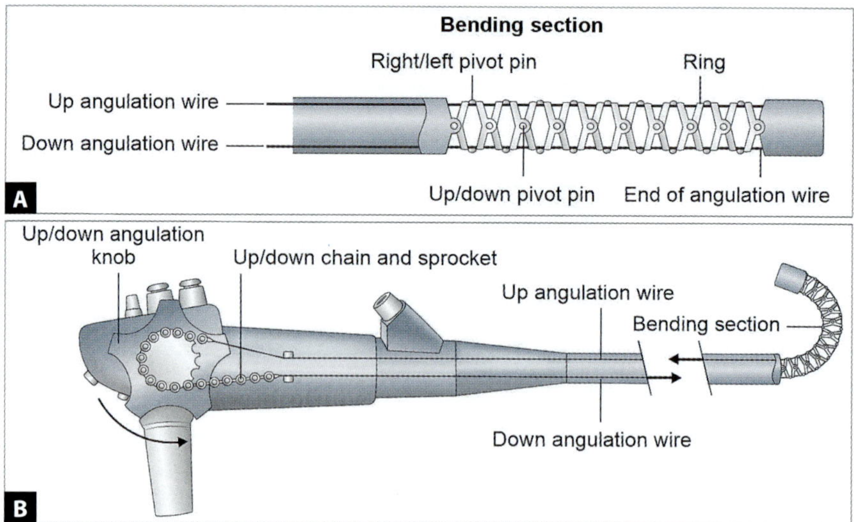

Figs. 24A and B: Angulation mechanism.

- Fluorescence endoscopy
- EUS
- Optical coherence tomography
- Confocal endoscopy
- Endocytoscopy

Magnification Endoscopy

Endoscopes can enlarge the view with digital and optical zooming. Standard endoscopes magnify the endoscopic image 30–35 times at baseline. Endoscopes with the ability to increase magnification further are also available. These "zoom" endoscopes optically magnify images up to 150 times using a movable optical lens in the endoscope tip to obtain a more detailed image of a target lesion while maintaining high resolution. A transparent distal cap may be used to stabilize the focal length between the lens and the mucosal surface to obtain a crisp image. In addition, we could also digitally enlarge an image but with a loss of resolution.

Chromoendoscopy

Chromoendoscopy is a novel technique of staining of mucosa to bring out subtle mucosal changes very well. With the added feature of magnification, even a tiny flat lesion can be easily recognized and tackled appropriately.

- Chromo endoscopy is of particular use in the following conditions, namely:
    - Barrett's esophagus
    - Gastric cancer

- Colorectal polyps
- Chronic ulcerative colitis (UC)

- There are three types of mucosal stains used in chromoendoscopy, namely:
  1. Absorptive stains
  2. Contrast stains
  3. Reactive stains

Absorptive stains **(Figs. 25A and B)** are taken up by specific epithelial cells of the GI tract giving the image contrast, e.g., Lugol's iodine, Methylene blue. Lugol's iodine solution is an absorptive stain that stains benign, glycogen-containing, non-keratinized squamous cells brown but does not stain dysplastic, inflamed, or malignant squamous cells or columnar mucosa.

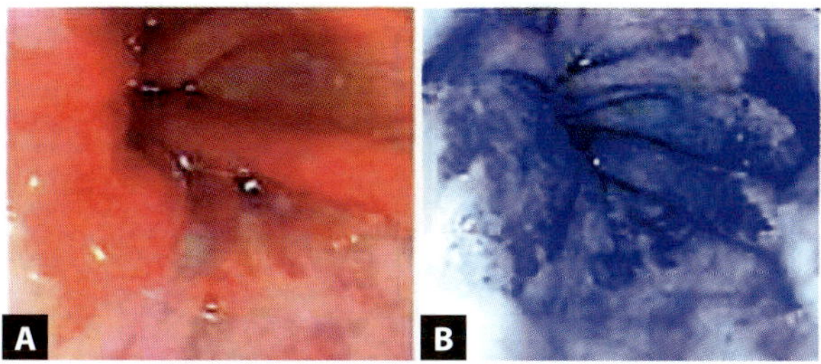

Figs. 25A and B: Chromoendoscopy.

A 1.5–4% solution is sprayed on the esophagus and within minutes the normal whitish squamous mucosa will change to dark brown as a result of binding of the iodine to glycogen within the non-keratinized squamous epithelium. Squamous cells that are inflamed, dysplastic, or malignant will not stain, and columnar epithelium remains pink and unstained. Methylene blue (MB) is an absorptive stain that stains actively absorbing intestinal-type cells but does not stain squamous and gastric cells or gastric-type metaplasia. It can help differentiate the specialized intestinal metaplasia (SIM) of BE from the gastric-type epithelium. MB stains SIM in BE with high accuracy with no side effects **(Fig. 26)**.

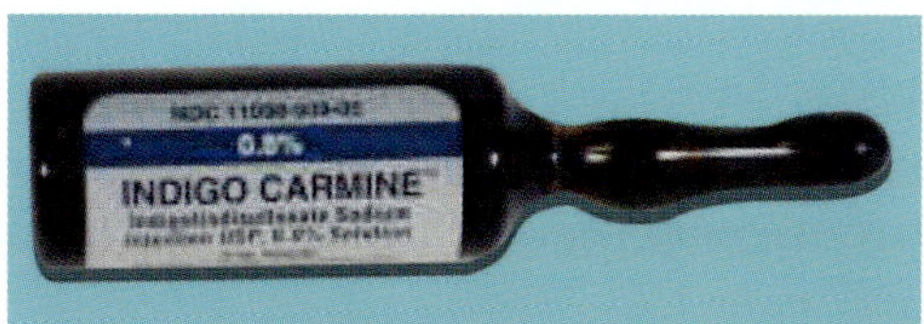

Fig. 26: Indocyanine green (ICG) ink.

Contrast stains just pool in the crevices of the mucosa (are not absorbed) to highlight the mucosal topography, e.g., Indigo carmine. A spray catheter is used to spray the selected stain followed by flushing with water and examining the area of interest with magnification endoscopy to look for subtle mucosal changes, e.g., pit patterns of colonic polyps.

Reactive STAINS chemically react with the tissue constituents to bring out distinct mucosal color and contrast, e.g., Congo red and phenol red.

Narrow-band Imaging (Figs. 27A and B)

- *Instead of white light, NBI uses two discrete bands of light:* One blue at 415 nm and one green at 540 nm. Narrow-band blue light displays superficial capillary networks, while green light displays subepithelial vessels and when combined offers an extremely high contrast image of the tissue surface.

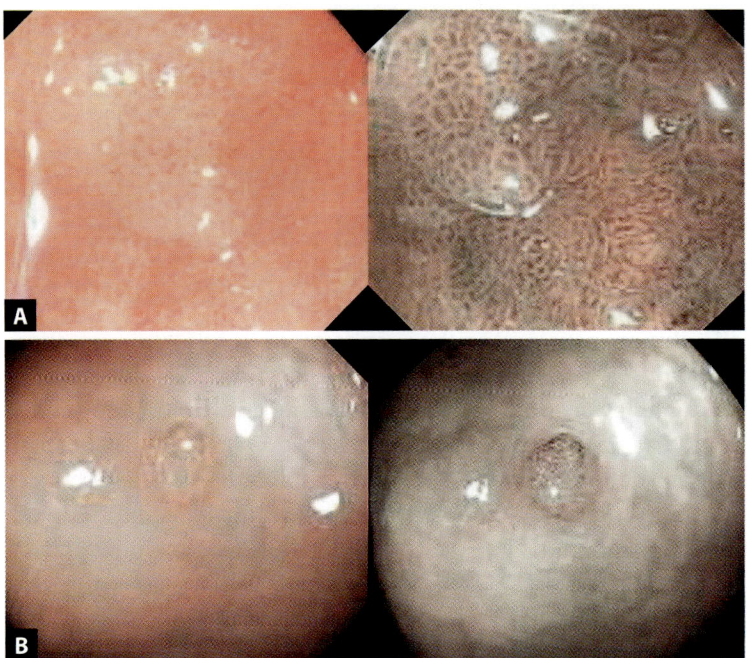

Figs. 27A and B: (A) White image versus; and (B) Narrow-band image.

- Like chromoendoscopy, NBI is also very useful in conditions, such as esophagitis, Barrett's esophagus, inflammatory bowel disease (IBD, and polyps).

Fluorescence Spectroscopy (Figs. 28A and B)

- It is the study of the characteristic pattern of light emission and absorption in the GI tract

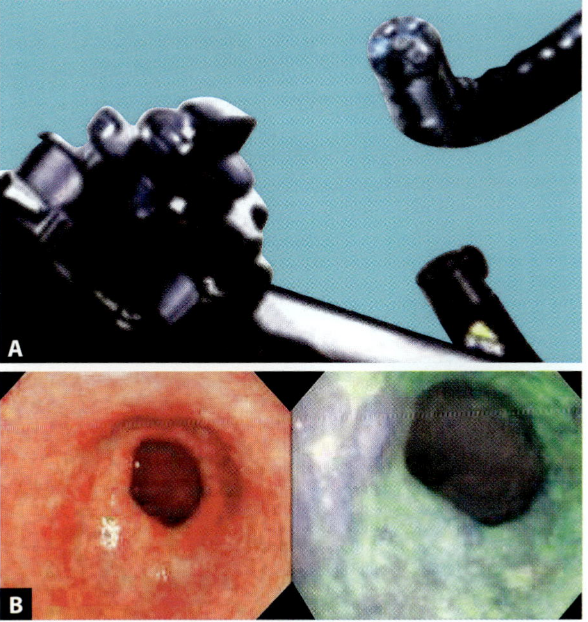

Figs. 28A and B: Fluoroendoscopy.

- Tissue has varying concentrations of fluorophores which emit light from varying wavelengths, and chromophores which absorb light. The submucosa, with its high concentration of collagen and elastin, is the major fluorophore.
- Hemoglobin is the major chromophore in tissue. Autofluorescence is produced when tissue is excited by ultraviolet (<400 nm) or short visible wavelength light.
- Dysplastic tissue has more fluorophores and hence emits more light, e.g., Barrett's esophagus
- Spectral endoscopy combines magnification, NBI, and fluorescence giving images of the finest details.

Endoscopic Ultrasound (Figs. 29A and B)

- Armed with ultrasound at the tip of the insertion section, this special endoscope allows one to get both endoscopic images of the GI tract and ultrasound images of the GI wall in great detail.
- Ultrasound image of the GI wall displays 5 distinct layers of GI wall as follows: The epithelium, lamina propria, submucosa, muscularis propria, and serosa (adventitia)
- There are two types of EUS, namely radial and linear.
- Linear EUS is preferred as this also allows one to perform various therapeutic interventions.

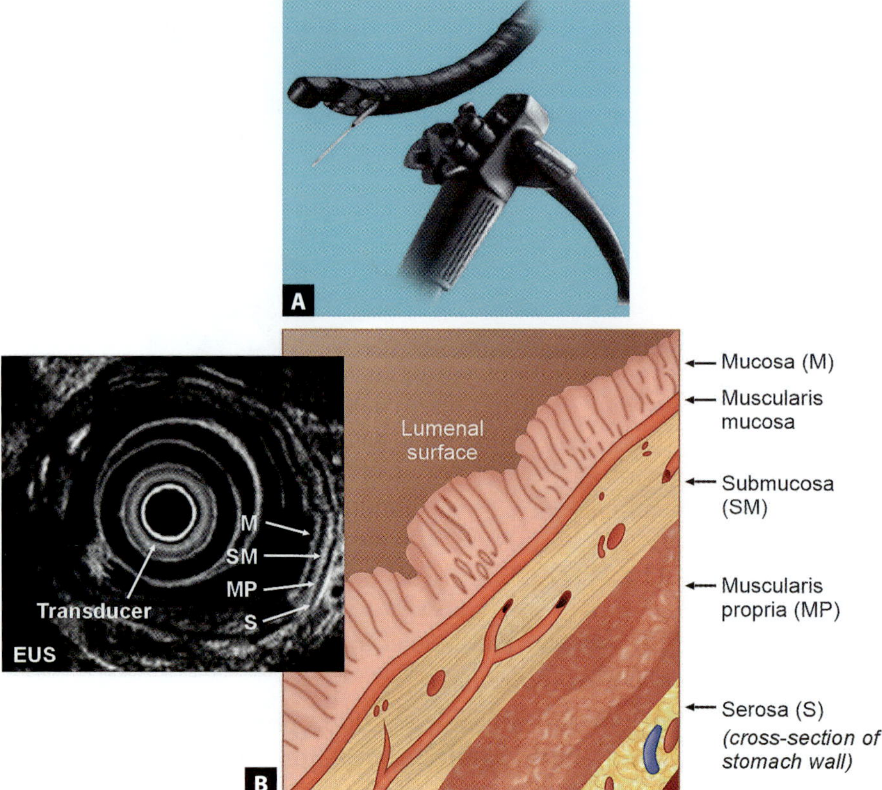

Figs. 29A and B: Endo ultrasound (EUS).

- Linear EUS creates ultrasound images parallel to the axis of the insertion tube. This orientation facilitates real-time ultrasonographic guidance of interventions such as fine needle aspiration (FNA) allowing us to view simultaneously the needle and the target area of interest on the video monitor. Real-time viewing allows us to proceed directly from observation to puncture, and with the addition of Doppler, we can also identify and avoid vascular structures, making it easier to select the optimum puncture position and direction.

Current Application and Benefits of Endoscopic Ultrasound

- For T and N staging of esophageal, rectal, and gastric tumors **(Fig. 30)**
- To evaluate cystic lesions of the pancreas and pancreatic tumors **(Fig. 31)**
- To diagnose bile duct stones
- To diagnose and grade chronic pancreatitis

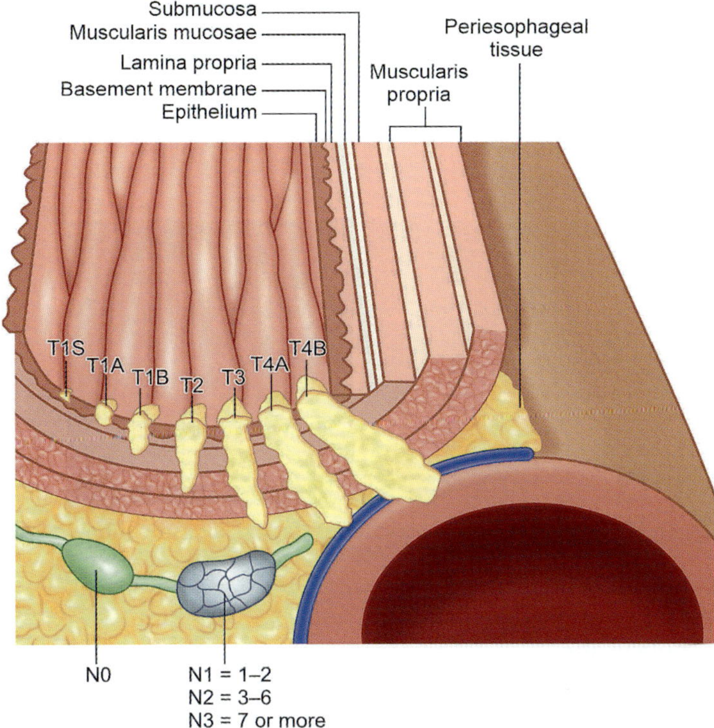

Fig. 30: Endoscopic ultrasound (EUS) staging T and N staging of esophageal or gastric tumor.

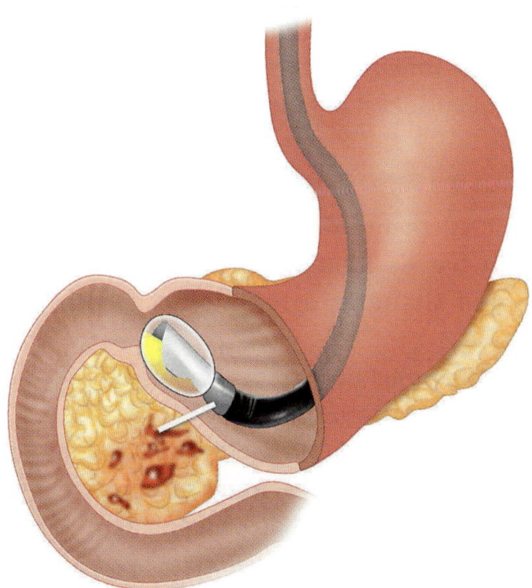

Fig. 31: Endoscopic ultrasound (EUS) staging in evaluating pancreatic neoplasm.

- For assessment of submucosal GI tumors **(Figs. 32A and B)**
    - *Identify both layers of lesion in the gut wall and its echo features:*
        - *Lipoma:* Hyperechoic
        - *GIST:* Hypoechoic
        - *Cyst:* Anechoic

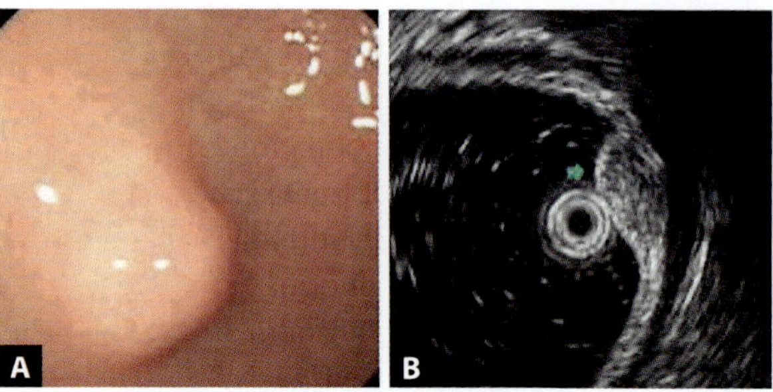

Figs. 32A and B: Endoscopic ultrasound (EUS) staging in gastric submucosal lesions.

- *To evaluate benign anorectal conditions:*
    - Fistula in ano
    - Incontinence
    - IBD
- *EUS-directed interventions:*
    - Fine needle and trucut biopsy
    - Coeliac plexus block
    - To guide access to the bile duct
    - To monitor glue injection of gastric varices
    - Drainage of pseudocyst of pancreas

Optical Coherence Tomography

Unlike endoscopic ultrasound, optical coherence tomography (OCT) uses infrared light waves instead of sound waves and measures the optical reflectivity of tissue as a function of depth instead of acoustic reflectivity.

After its successful application in the retina study, we now start exploring its potential in gastroenterology.

An OCT probe can be passed through the biopsy channel of an endoscope and can be kept in contact with the mucosa of interest which allows for a resolution of 7–10 micrometers and an imaging depth of 2–3 mm depending on the wavelength of light used and the type of tissue being imaged. This allows visualization of histologic morphology in real-time, especially the epithelial structures such as villi, crypts, and squamous and intestinal epithelium.

Useful in assessing cases of Barrett's esophagus, IBD, and pancreatic and bile duct lesions.

Confocal Endoscopy (Figs. 33A and B)

It is the fusion of endoscopy and confocal microscopy:

- Confocal microscopy uses a laser fiber as a pinhole, placed in between the objective lens and the detector, to allow only the light that originates from within a tiny volume below the mucosal surface to be collected. All other sources of scattered light do not have the correct path to be detected and thus become "spatially filtered." This process creates a high-resolution image from a thin section within optically thick tissue and is known as optical sectioning.
- To create confocal images, blue laser light is focused on the desired tissue via the distal end. Applied fluorescent materials are excited by the

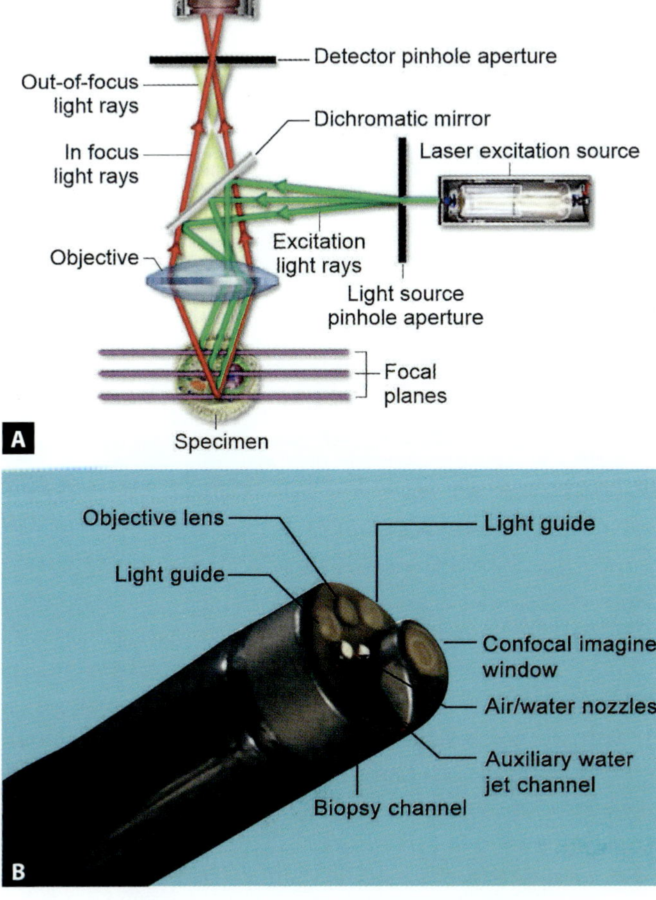

Figs. 33A and B: Confocal endoscopy.

laser light, and the special confocal optical unit exclusively detects the fluorescing light at an exactly defined horizontal level.

- Such optical slices of the mucosal surface give real-time high-resolution imaging of cellular and subcellular tissue structures and are hence known as in vivo or virtual biopsy.

Endocytoscopy (Figs. 34A and B)

- The endocytoscope is an ultra-high magnification (450–1,125 times) catheter-type endoscope that can be passed through the working channel of a colonoscope and used, in combination with chromo agents, to provide in vivo histological images.

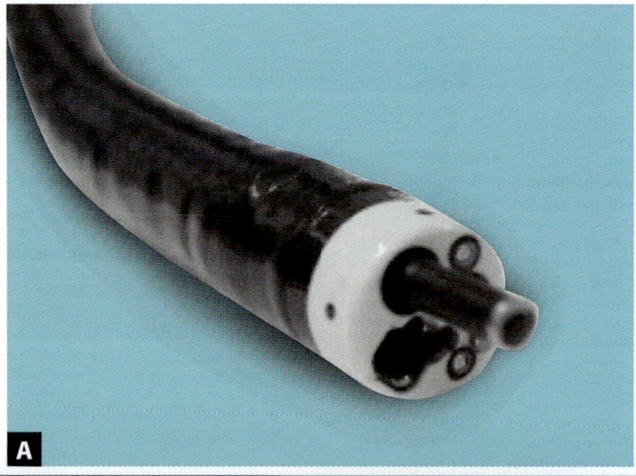

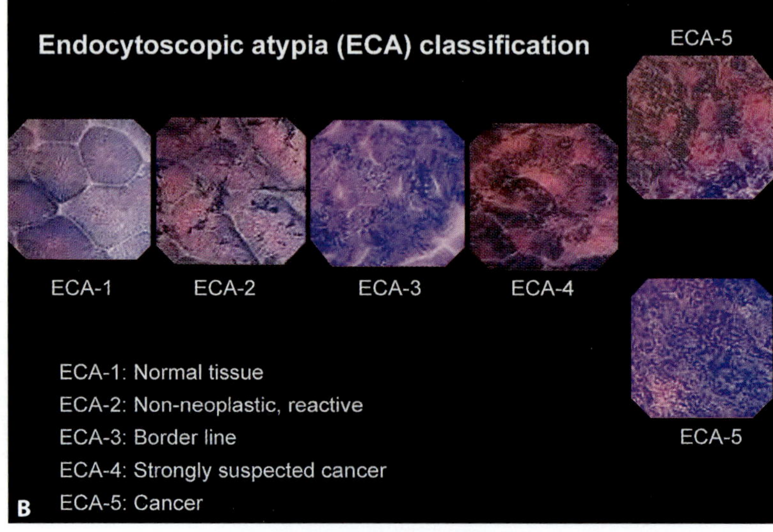

Figs. 34A and B: Endocytoscopy.

- Unlike confocal endoscopy, endocytoscopic images are in color and in greater resolution
- It allows us to obtain in vivo histological images!

The overall compact design of the scope: The endoscope has many delicate parts and electrical wires and is nicely wrapped up by three different layers of outer covers: coil metal pipes, metal mesh, and a Teflon sheath. This design of outer sheathing maintains flexibility while ensuring its stability and leak-proof nature.

Modern videoendoscopes are completely immersible in water.

HANDLING AND STORAGE OF THE ENDOSCOPY (FIG. 35)

- The control head, tip, and the supply plug of the umbilical cord should all be held while transporting a scope to avoid any damage.

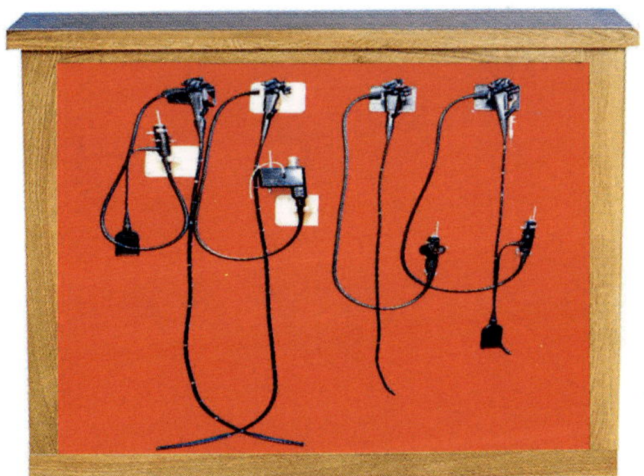

Fig. 35: Storage of endoscopy.

- Store the endoscope in a well-ventilating cupboard, hanging them vertically. Never store them in a closed suitcase. Moisture invites infection

CONCLUSION

Flexible videoendoscopes are a testament to engineering marvels. The compact and intricate design of endoscopy combined with flexibility, and stability allow us to perform both diagnostic and many therapeutic procedures with ease and efficiency. Careful usage and maintenance are paramount for the utility and longevity of the endoscopy.

SUGGESTED READING

1. Canto MI, Setrakian S, Willis J, Chak A, Petras R, Powe NR, Sivak MV Jr. Methylene blue-directed biopsies improve detection of intestinal metaplasia and dysplasia in Barrett's esophagus. Gastrointest Endosc. 2000; 51(5):560-8.

2. Cotton P, Williams CB (Eds). Practical Gastrointestinal Endoscopy, 4th edition, Oxford: Blackwell Science; 1996.
3. Inoue H, Rey JF, Lightdale C. Lugol chromoendoscopy for esophageal squamous cell cancer. Endoscopy. 2001;33(1):75-9.
4. Jung M, Kiesslich R. Chromoendoscopy and intravital staining techniques. Baillieres Best Pract Res Clin Gastroenterol. 1999;13(1):11-9.
5. Rijsbergen CJV (Ed). Gastrointestinal Endoscopy: Beyond the basics. Newton, MA: Butterworth Heinemann; 1997.
6. Sivak Jr MV, Kobayashi K, Izatt JA, Rollins AM, Ung-Runyawee R, Chak A, et al. High-resolution endoscopic imaging of the GI tract using optical coherence tomography. Gastrointest Endosc. 2000;51(4):474-9.
7. Soehendra N, Binmoeller KF, Seifert H, Schreiber HW (Eds). Therapeutic Endoscopy. Stuttgart: Thieme; 1998.
8. Technology Status Evaluation Report. Technology status evaluation report. High-resolution and high-magnification endoscopy. Gastrointest Endosc. 2000; 52(6):864-6.
9. Yoshida S, Tanaka S, Hirata M, Mouri R, Kaneko I, Oka S, et al. Optical biopsy of GI lesions by reflectance-type laser-scanning confocal microscopy. Gastrointest Endosc. 2007;66(1):144-9.

Expert's Comment

Knowledge of the intricate anatomy of various types of endoscopes and their functions is crucial for every endoscopic surgeon.

A modern upper gastrointestinal (GI) endoscope is just 9.2 mm in diameter and could easily be used in children as young as 1 year for the removal of foreign body from the esophagus, dilatation, etc.

The trajectory of the access channel is worth remembering. In Olympus gastroscopy, the endoscopic accessory exits at the 7 o'clock position, while it is at 5 o'clock position in Pentax and 6 o'clock position with Fujinon gastroscope. This is important to remember when we do any endotherapy. In case of hot snare polypectomy, we should bring the polyp to the lower left quadrant during gastroscopy, but to the lower right quadrant during colonoscopy for ease of the procedure.

It is also worth knowing the diameter of the biopsy channel, which is narrower in the gastroscope (2.8 mm) compared to the colonoscope (3.2 mm). Hence, suction will not be effective during any therapeutic gastroscopy, as the channel is almost blocked by the presence of an accessory.

While laparoscopes are chip-in-head technology, the flexible endoscopes are mostly chip-in-the-tip technology. In video endoscopes, charge-coupled device is kept in the bending section of the endoscope, which converts the endoscopic images to pixels and transfers the electrical signals to the processor.

Maintenance of the endoscopes should be done as per the manufacturer's instructions to safeguard the integrity and longevity of the endoscopes.

- The endoscope must be coiled into gentle curves, rather than folding it in acute angles.
- Never drop the endoscope, allow a wheeled cart to roll over it, or allow the patient to bite down on the endoscope.
- After each use, wash off any gross contamination and suction water through the endoscope.
- Do not allow blood, mucus, stool, or other foreign matter to dry on the endoscope or in the channels or valves.
- Be careful to follow the manufacturer's instructions for sterilization to avoid potentially severe damage to the endoscope.

We should not underestimate the importance of dedicated endoscope storage cabinets.

Endoscopes should be held gently, like handling newborn babies; only then can the safety of the scopes be ensured.

Modern high-definition video endoscopes have revolutionized the management of GI disorders.

Dr Satish Midha
Ranchi

CHAPTER 4

Steps of Upper Gastrointestinal Endoscopy

Chapter Outline

- Indication for Upper Gastrointestinal Endoscopy
  - Diagnostic Endoscopy
  - Surveillance Endoscopy
  - Screening Endoscopy
  - Therapeutic Endoscopy
- Contraindication for Endoscopy
- Caution
- Informed Consent for Upper Gastrointestinal Endoscopy
- Patient Information Leaflet
- Pre-endoscopic Check Lists
- 20 Key Steps of Diagnostic Endoscopy
- Postendoscopic Steps
- Top 10 Technical Tips for the Difficulty Experienced during Diagnostic Upper Gastrointestinal Endoscopy

Keywords: Indication for endoscopy, diagnostic endoscopy, surveillance endoscopy, technique of endoscopy, complications of endoscopy

INTRODUCTION

Considering the diagnostic and therapeutic potentials of endoscopy, training and expertise in the art of endoscopy is paramount for all gastrointestinal (GI) specialists. The advent of video endoscopy and subsequent advances such as image enhancement and magnification along with the development of novel therapeutic techniques have made a significant impact in the algorithm of management of gut diseases. This chapter describes the indication for endoscopy and technical tips for performing upper GI endoscopy with an outline of possible adverse events that might happen during the procedure.

INDICATION FOR UPPER GASTROINTESTINAL ENDOSCOPY

- Diagnostic endoscopy
- Surveillance endoscopy
- Screening endoscopy
- Therapeutic endoscopy

Diagnostic Endoscopy

- *Dyspepsia:* Discomfort in the upper abdomen present with nausea, vomiting, or postprandial fullness is one of the most common reasons for performing an endoscopy.
- Dysphagia is an ominous symptom and merits early endoscopy to exclude esophageal cancer.
- *Atypical chest pain:* Retrosternal or left-sided chest pain with normal treadmill test and Echo would require thorough evaluation to exclude any esophageal causes for pain such as gastroesophageal reflux disease (GERD) or motility disorders.
- Hematemesis and melena are the symptoms of upper GI bleeding and early endoscopy is warranted. Chronic anemia (microcytic and hypochromic) could be due to peptic ulcer, gastritis, or more sinister pathology like carcinoma stomach so consider endoscopy in your diagnostic algorithm.
- *Suspected cases of portal hypertension (HT):* In known cases of chronic liver diseases due to alcoholism, hepatitis B and C, or patients with splenomegaly and in patients presenting with massive hematemesis, endoscopy is warranted to look for esophageal and fundal varices.
- Anorexia, asthenia, and weight loss could be due to gastric malignancy and endoscopy is helpful in such individuals.
- Chronic diarrhea could be due to inflammatory bowel disease (IBD) or celiac disease. Gastroduodenal lesions are not unusual in Crohn's disease. Biopsy of the duodenum to look for villous atrophy is important in a suspected case of celiac disease in addition to serology to look for antigliadin antibody.
- Chronic cough and recurrent chest infection could be the atypical presentation of achalasia cardia or large hiatus hernia with reflux. Endoscopy could reveal the reason for the intractable cough.
- In the case of polyposis coli and IBD, endoscopy would aid us in assessing the extent of GI involvement by the disease process.

Surveillance Endoscopy

- Surveillance endoscopy is done in patients with already known pathology at planned intervals to look for any changes.
- In cases of Barrett's esophagus periodic endoscopy is warranted to look for any extension or changes suspicious of cancer. Multiple biopsies to look for Barrett's esophagus are essential to look for any dysplastic changes. In cases of low-grade dysplasia, we recommend 6–12 monthly endoscopies while cases of high-grade dysplasia warrant definitive treatment or at least 3 monthly close watch.

- In all cases of bleeding esophageal varices, monthly endoscopy and banding are done until all the varices are eradicated. Then 6–12 monthly surveillance is needed to watch out for any recurrent varices developing either in the esophagus or in the fundus of the stomach.
- Patients who had surgery for upper GI malignancy would require 3–6 monthly endoscopy reviews to look for any local recurrence.

Screening Endoscopy

Screening endoscopy is done for persons who are at high risk of developing lesions because of a family history of GI malignancy or polyposis coli, or who have a history of previous gastric bypass for ulcer disease >10 years before.

Therapeutic Endoscopy

- *Foreign body (FB) esophagus:* FB esophagus such as fish bone, food bolus, coin, or button battery merits early endoscopy within 24 hours to avoid risk of aspiration and perforation.
- *Stricture esophagus:* Malignant stricture would warrant biopsy and dilatation, and in selected cases like tracheoesophageal, fistula may even require self-expanding metal stent deployment.
- Big esophageal varices (grades 3 and 4) need banding while small varices (grades 1 and 2) benefit from sclerotherapy
- Fundal varices require glue injection (butyl cyanoacrylate)
- Portal gastropathy with blood loss may benefit from argon plasma coagulation.
- Polyps would require snare polypectomy, endoscopic mucosal resection (EMR), or endoscopic submucosal dissection (ESD).
- Peroral endoscopic myotomy (POEM) has been increasingly considered in cases of achalasia.

CONTRAINDICATION FOR ENDOSCOPY

- *Suspected bowel perforation:* In patients with severe upper abdominal pain with guarding or rigidity, it is better we first go for an X-ray chest erect and the abdomen supine or even CT abdomen to exclude bowel perforation.
- *Recent myocardial infarction (MI)/cardiac failure:* Inferior wall MI could present with epigastric discomfort. Hence in any such cases or in patients with previous cardiac ailments, better to wait till ECG, Echo, and proper cardiac evaluation are done before rushing in for endoscopy in such a dire situation.
- *Respiratory distress:* Patients with severe dyspnea or orthopnea are not going to tolerate endoscopy and a respiratory arrest is a distinct possibility and hence improves the respiratory status before any such heroics.

CAUTION

- *Zenker's diverticulum/postcricoid web:* In cases of dysphagia, wherein there is some difficulty proceeding beyond 15 cm, then be careful and look for the reasons for difficulty and proceed accordingly.
- *In patients with corrosive poisoning:* Early endoscopy within 24 hours by an experienced endoscopist is useful to evaluate the grade and extent of damage. Risks of perforation or bleeding are distinct possibilities. So do take care.
- In patients with gastric outlet obstruction with a history of projectile vomiting or undigested foul-smelling food residue, one has to be careful not to rush for endoscopy. There are risks of aspiration and unsatisfactory examination. In such cases, prior nasogastric decompression would be beneficial.
- Uncooperative or violent patients are a danger to the equipment and staff and so better prepare to abandon the procedure. One may decide to restrict and hold such persons with more staff around or by rational use of sedatives.
- Patients who are hemodynamically unstable due to massive GI bleeding are also high-risk individuals. We better consider proper resuscitation with fluids and blood and even do prior intubation to prevent aspiration. Endoscopy is often risky in such a patient with a stomach full of clotted blood. Consider pharmacotherapy such as IV terlipressin or Sengstaken tube insertion for cases of variceal bleeding before transferring to another institute for endoscopy.

INFORMED CONSENT FOR UPPER GASTROINTESTINAL ENDOSCOPY

- Written informed consent is paramount for moral and ethical reasons and also to prevent any medicolegal consequences.
- Consent should be ideally taken by the endoscopist himself/herself.
- Ensure that the patient is competent to give consent. Obtain consent from parents or spouses for young children and unconscious or mentally disturbed patients.
- Consent should be given voluntarily by the patient after receiving sufficient information regarding the endoscopy procedure namely why it is done, how it is done, what are the benefits and risks of the procedure, any alternatives to endoscopy, and the possibility of performing any additional procedures if needed.
- Give a "patient information leaflet" written in simple and easy-to-follow language with all the details regarding the endoscopy procedure.
- Patient should be encouraged to ask questions and clarify any doubt.
- Patient should sign with his name and address in bold letters with the date and time.

- The consent form should also have the name and signature of the endoscopist and a witness (next of kin).

PATIENT INFORMATION LEAFLET

What is an Upper GI Endoscopy?

Videoendoscope allows us to see inside of your food pipe, stomach and duodenum to look for abnormality. Patients with abdominal pain, indigestion, difficulty swallowing, vomiting, blood vomiting, passage of dark stools, unexplained weight loss, loss of appetite or family history of stomach cancer would require this novel investigation.

What is an Endoscope?

Endoscope is a long slim flexible tube with a tiny camera chip at its tip. This allows us to take video or pictures of interior of your gut in fine details and help us in making the diagnosis.

Why do I Need Endoscopy?

Obviously your symptoms suggest possibility of upper GI pathology and hence your doctor asked you to undergo upper GI endoscopy.

Alternatives to Endoscopy

Though US abdomen, CT abdomen and barium X-rays can be considered, they have several limitations. They won't be as sensitive and useful as endoscopy.

How is Endoscopy done?

Your will be asked to starve overnight or come fasted with nothing to eat or drink for at least 6 hours prior to the test.

Your BP and pulse and body weight will be checked, and nurse will ask you and note down your other medical illnesses, previous abdominal surgery, any medication and any history of allergy. Kindly bring all your medical prescription and investigation reports and films.

You will be changed to hospital gown and a venflon needle may be placed on the back of your hand if any injection to be given.

You will be asked to sign the informed consent form. You could ask any relevant questions.

Your will be administered oxygen by a nasal cannula and throat will be made numb by squirting xylocaine spray. A plastic guard will be kept in your mouth to protect your teeth and the endoscope.

Endoscopy usually takes about 10 minutes, and it is a safe and painless procedure. There won't be any trouble breathing. So, try to relax and concentrate on your breathing while the surgeon does the procedure.

The procedure is usually recorded and any abnormality noted will also be taken as still images for reporting and printing.

Additional procedure like biopsy or injection may be done as when required.

What Happens Next?

- Once endoscopy is over, you will be taken to recovery area to recuperate.
- You will be allowed to take liquids 30 minutes after and solids 1 hour after the procedure
- You may feel drowsy if sedation was given and, in that case, you will not be able to drive your car or ride a motorbike for a day.
- You may be asked to get admitted if any therapy was given.
- If any biopsy was done, then the specimen will be sent to histology lab and results would take few days

What are the Risks of the Procedure?

- Endoscopy is by far very safe procedure
- Mild throat discomfort is not unusual. You may feel bit bloated.
- If you have severe chest or stomach pain, kindly inform the medical personnel.
- Complications could happen due to your previous illnesses like IHD or COPD
- Some unexpected complications could rarely happen to 1 in 500 patients like heart or chest difficulties, bleeding, and perforation in the gut. If any of the problems happens, then you may have to stay in the hospital and even require surgery in rare instances.

When to Contact Us?

- If you have persisting chest or abdominal pain, blood vomiting or fever, then don't hesitate to contact the hospital or else call us on this phone no: 97900-28328
- You will be given appointment with doctor to discuss the result of the endoscopy and all other reports and decide about further therapy

PRE-ENDOSCOPIC CHECK LISTS

- *Equipment checklist:*
  - Endoscopy leak tested and disinfected and ready
  - Processor unit, and monitor turned on and working
  - Water bottle full and suction unit turned on and ready
  - Check suction, airflow, and water jet in the scope
  - Mouth guard

- *Patient checklist:*
  - Know the indication
  - Exclude any contraindication
  - Drug history and comorbidity known
  - Informed consent
  - Fasting for at least 6 hours
  - No denture or loose tooth

20 KEY STEPS OF DIAGNOSTIC ENDOSCOPY

Under local 10% xylocaine spray (conscious sedation using 2–5 mg of IV midazolam in selected patients)

1. *Position:* Patient is lying left lateral with head in the neutral position **(Fig. 1)**.
2. *Ergonomic position of surgeon, staffs, and monitors* ***(Fig. 2)****:* Ensure the table is of proper height and you stand comfortably about 1 foot from the table at the shoulder level of the patient facing the patient's head in line with the monitor (straight line principle as in laparoscopic surgery).

   One staff should be standing behind the patient's head with her/his right index and middle finger forming something like a victory sign and holding the mouth guard in the patient's mouth. Remove any loose tooth or denture. If mouth opening is inadequate due to malocclusion or micrognathia then consider a smaller mouth guard or a mouth retractor. A mouth guard ensures the patient is not biting and damaging the pricy scope. To maintain the neutral position of head and to avoid extension of the head during the procedure, the staff should keep her/his left hand behind the patient's occiput. She should be trained to observe the

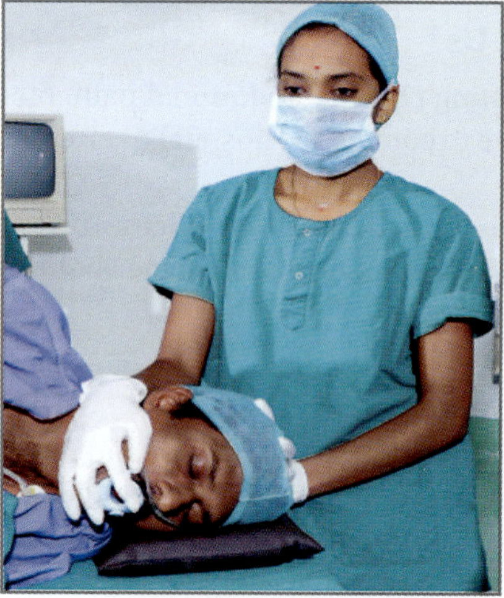

Fig. 1: Position of patient.

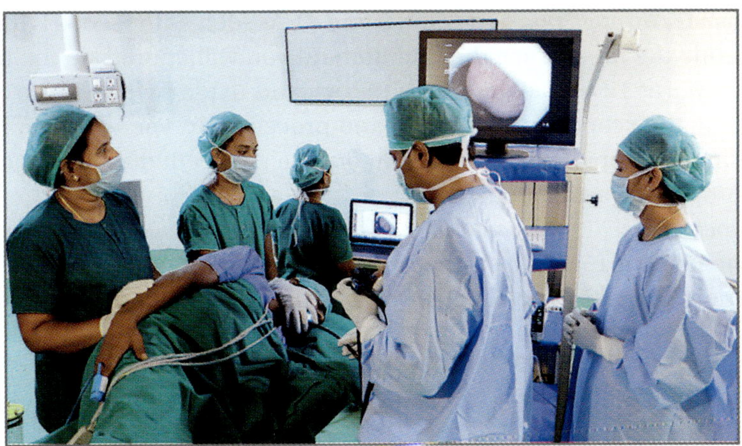

Fig. 2: Position of staffs and trolley.

patient for any distress or difficulty in breathing during the procedure and also constantly communicate and reassure the patient about the progress of the procedure. She should also keep a Yankauer suction and a kidney tray ready to keep the oral cavity free of secretion.

In addition, we need two more staffs for the procedure. One person should stand behind the patient next to the staff at the head end. In addition to restraining the patient, she/he will also monitor the vitals shown in the monitor. She/he should be responsible for administering drugs during the procedure.

One experienced staff should stand next to the surgeon to assist during endoscopy. Flushing the channel, taking a biopsy, and assisting in various therapeutic interventions are her/his duties. He/she should anticipate and keep the required accessories well in advance to be ready for use.

Often there is a monitor in the instrument trolley by the side of the endoscopist. But for ergonomic reason and to avoid neck strain, it is preferable to have the main monitor kept behind the patient's back (straight line principle).

Perform all the instrument checklist and patient checklist as mentioned earlier. Reassure the patient once again that the procedure would take only a few minutes and painless and would not affect his/her breathing.

3. *Grip and hold the scope comfortably at 20 cm level:* Hold the control body in your left hand with your index finger and middle finger over the suction button and insufflation button, respectively. Your right hand should be gently holding the insertion section of the scope like a pen (not like a sword) at a level of 20 cm. Ensure the tip of the scope maintains a gentle curve by turning the big wheel slightly toward you. Thus, it takes the shape of the gentle curve of the tongue.

4. *Journey through pharynx* **(Figs. 3 and 4)**: As soon as the scope is inserted inside the mouth, see the monitor and you will appreciate the tongue above (at 12 o'clock on the monitor), and uvula below (at 6 o'clock). Keep the scope in the midline and proceed and you will then have a glimpse of epiglottis. One should not see any teeth during this journey through the oropharynx.
5. *Dock and wait at cricopharynx* **(Fig. 5)**: Once the scope is inserted to the level of 15 cm from the incisor teeth, then take a few seconds to orient yourself. The vocal cords and the windpipe are in front at the

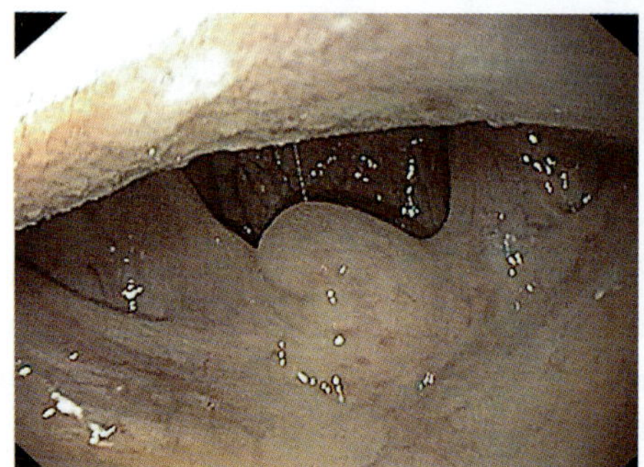

Fig. 3: Tongue at 12 o'clock position.

Fig. 4: Glimpse of epiglottis.

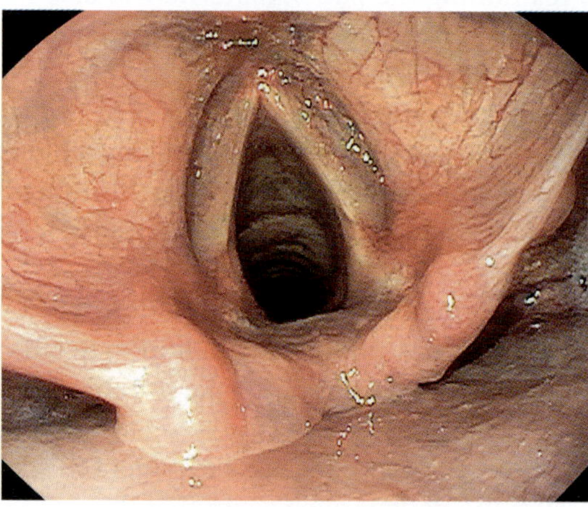

Fig. 5: Cricopharynx at 15 cm.

12 o'clock position and you will appreciate both pyriform fossa (right at the 3 o'clock position and the left at the 9 o'clock position) in the monitor and the posterior pharyngeal wall at 6 o'clock.

Look for the momentary opening of the cricopharynx and enter the esophagus under vision without using any undue force. Beware of postcricoid web or Zenker's diverticulum or postcricoid growth in any case of any resistance observed.

It is always preferable to reach the cricopharynx under vision as mentioned above. But in case of any difficulty, one may choose the finger-guided blind technique. You put your left index finger inside the patient's mouth beside the mouth guard to steady the tongue and guide the scope tip to enter the laryngopharynx.

6. *Sneak down the cricopharynx as patient takes a swallow* **(Fig. 6)**: Encourage the patient to take a swallow of saliva while you gently pass the scope into the esophagus. If the patient struggles or coughs, stop and retreat as you may be entering the trachea as evidenced by seeing the tracheal rings and classical bifurcation of bronchi.

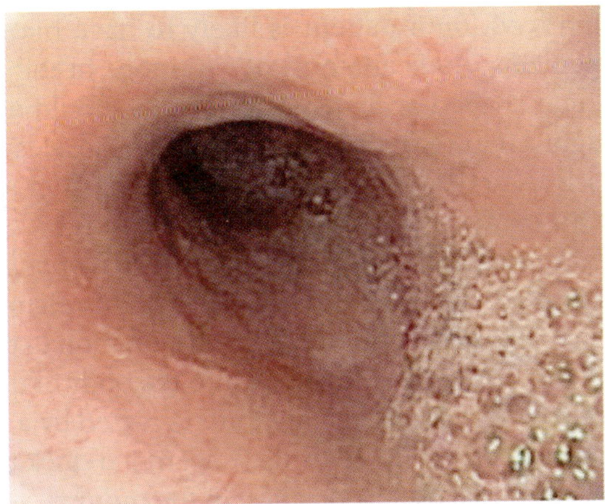

Fig. 6: Mid esophagus.

7. *Navigate straight till you to see the Z-line at 40 cm* **(Fig. 7)**: The esophageal journey is like traveling in a straight motorway. One may notice indentations of the spine posteriorly in thin individuals. At 25–27 cm

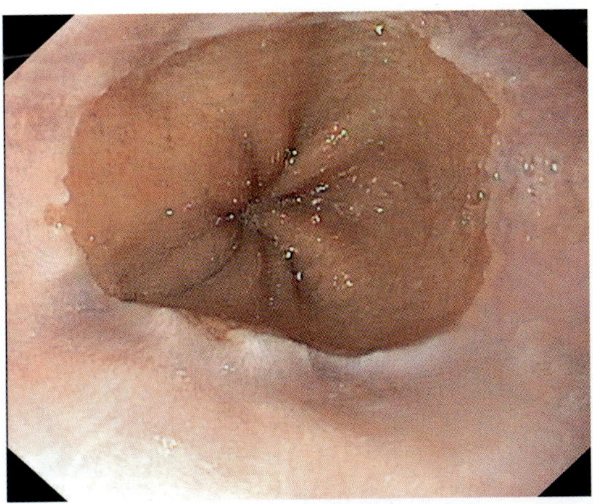

Fig. 7: Reaching Z-line at 40 cm.

level, one may notice indentation due to arch of the aorta and crossing left main bronchus anteriorly. Just below these landmarks, one often observes the beating heart (left atrium).

Usually, esophagus is empty. If there is any fluid or food residue in the esophagus, it always signifies some pathology such as achalasia or stricture.

Notice the squamocolumnar junction (Z-line) at 40 cm level. The pale esophageal mucosa changes to pinkish gastric mucosa beyond this line. Z-line is usually at or just above the diaphragmatic hiatus level. Ask the patient to sniff or say "Ah" to know the level of hiatal opening. If the Z-line is >2 cm above the hiatus and patulous or prolapsing gastric mucosa is noticed, then patient is likely to have hiatus hernia. One should recognize various anatomical variations in the appearances of Z-line (e.g., star shaped or flame shaped) and should not misdiagnose it as esophagitis. If lower esophageal sphincter (LES) is spastic and not letting the scope go through easily, and then consider achalasia cardia or tumor at the cardia (known as pseudoachalasia)

8. *Little anticlockwise rotation helps to slip through esophagus-gastric (OG) junction and enter stomach:* Sometimes slight anticlockwise twist of shaft of the scope is needed to bring the OG junction to the center of the monitor and this will aid easy passage into the body of the stomach.

   We enter the body of stomach and often greeted by a puddle of fluid. Fundus of stomach is on the left side (toward 9 o'clock of monitor) and the antrum is toward 3 o'clock position in the monitor.
9. *Inspect/suck any residue and insufflate and orient yourself* ***(Figs. 8 and 9)****:* Remember the clock:
   - *Lesser curve:* 12 o'clock
   - *Greater curve:* 6 o'clock
   - *Anterior wall:* 9 o'clock
   - *Posterior wall:* 3 o'clock

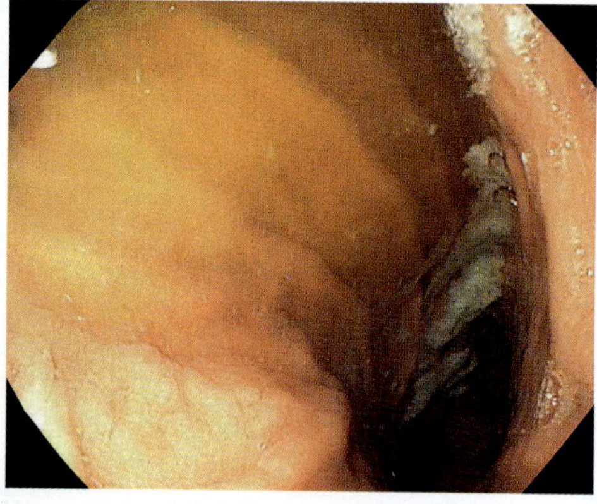

Fig. 8: Puddle of fluid at fundus.

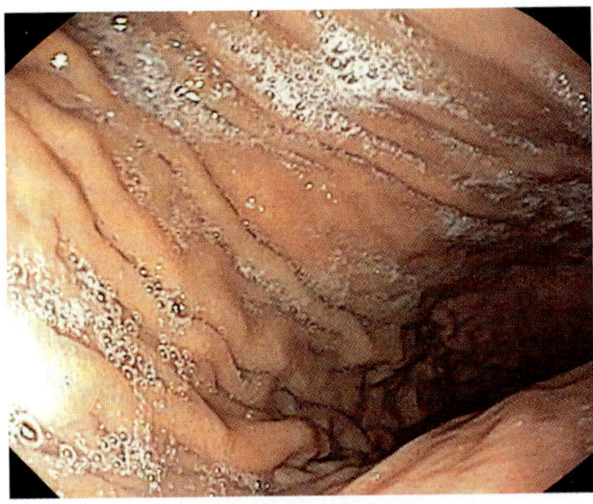

Fig. 9: Body of stomach.

Our aim is now to proceed toward antrum and pylorus. It is advisable to take the long route of traveling along the greater curve that will guarantee you reach the pylorus. If you follow the lesser curve often you may get lost. We should aim to swim along the greatest curve which is at 6 o'clock in the monitor. So, swim along the floor. Let us visit the lesser curve during our return journey.

10. *Proceed to pylorus* ***(Fig. 10)****:* Remember the three important maneuvers to navigate toward the pylorus:
    i. Turn the big wheel toward you
    ii. Twist the shaft of the scope clockwise to take right turn
    iii. Push the shaft of the scope at increments of 5 cm for 2–3 times

    Soon you will see the pylorus appearing in the horizon. Do not over insufflate. Reach near the pylorus (remember the incisura is at 12 o'clock position but not visible in the monitor at this moment).

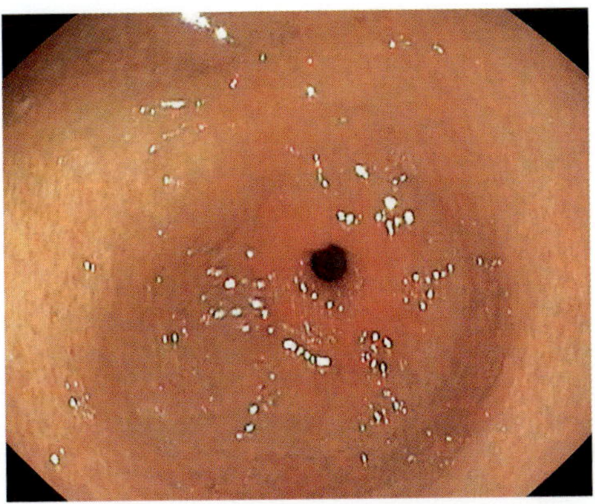

Fig. 10: Reaching pylorus.

11. *Enter the pylorus* ***(Fig. 11)****:* Wait until the pyloric spasm goes off and it is wide open and at the center of monitor. Ensure that the scope tip is also straight. So, enter the pylorus only when it is at the center and scope tip is straight and end-facing. Do not target a dancing pylorus or side facing pylorus. Do not traumatize pylorus and make it angry.

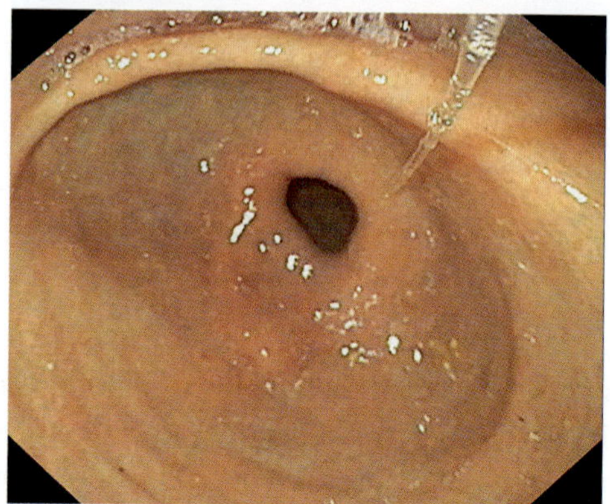

Fig. 11: Pylorus at center.

12. *See the bulbar part* ***(Fig. 12)****:* First part of the duodenum has the bulbar and postbulbar part and ends at the superior duodenal angle. The bulbar part is featureless and is the most common site for ulcers. Look for the size, site, and number of ulcers or extent of inflammation.
    - *Anterior wall*: 9 o'clock on the monitor
    - *Posterior wall*: 3 o'clock on the monitor

    Postbulbar region leads to the superior duodenal angle wherein we need to do the following maneuvers to enter the descending or second part of the duodenum.

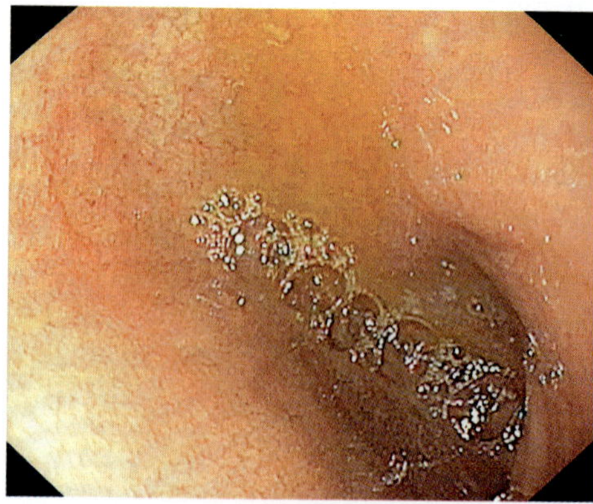

Fig. 12: Duodenal bulb.

13. *Entering second part of duodenum* ***(Fig. 13)***: Turn the big wheel toward you and turn your body toward the monitor and torque the scope clockwise to turn the scope tip to the right. Then pull and shorten the scope. You will notice the scope is now diving into the descending duodenum.

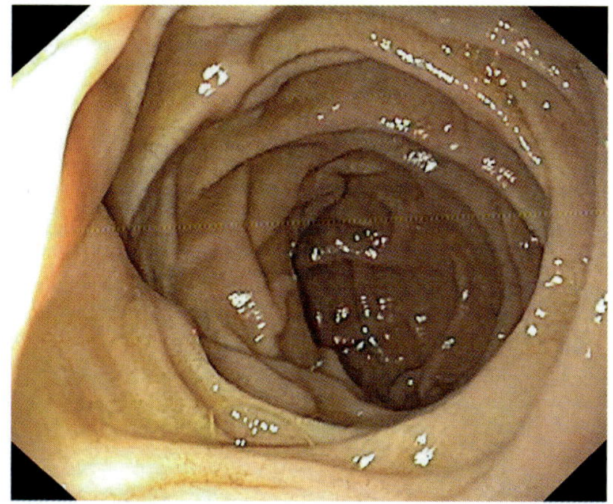

Fig. 13: Second part of duodenum.

- Granular looking duodenal mucosa with circular mucosal folds is characteristic of descending duodenum.
- One may notice the ampulla of Vater at 9 o'clock in the monitor typically when the scope is shortened to 60 cm. But, it may not be visible in all cases when we use end viewing scope.
- Understand that the scope is now taking the short route along the lesser curve.

14. *Retreat back to stomach and retroflex* ***(Figs. 14 to 16)***: Turn the big wheel gradually toward you to see incisura and then fundus.

    Incisura is an important endoscopic landmark seen as a fold or ridge along the lesser curve extending from 8 o'clock in the monitor to 2 o'clock position dividing the stomach to two halves. The bottom part below the incisura is the antrum and the part above the incisura is the body and fundus. Incisura is the common site of gastric ulcers.

    When the big wheel is fully turned toward you, the scope takes the shape of a "hockey stick" and you start looking at the roof. The fundus of stomach is seen using this J-maneuver.

    Pull the scope gently while either twisting the scope both clockwise and anticlockwise or turning your body sideways (dancing with the scope!) you will examine the fundus and cardia thoroughly.

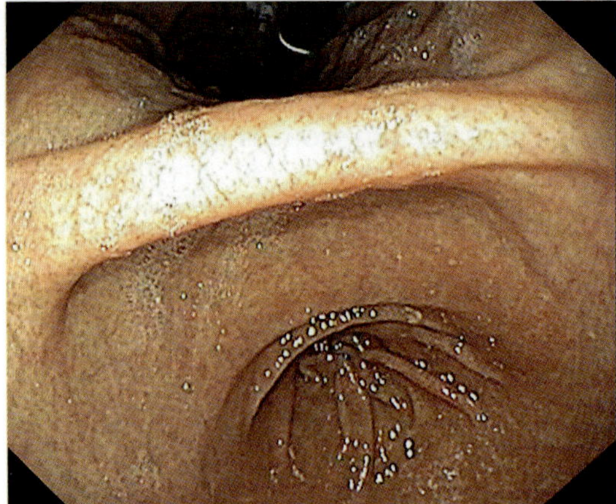

Fig. 14: Incisura.

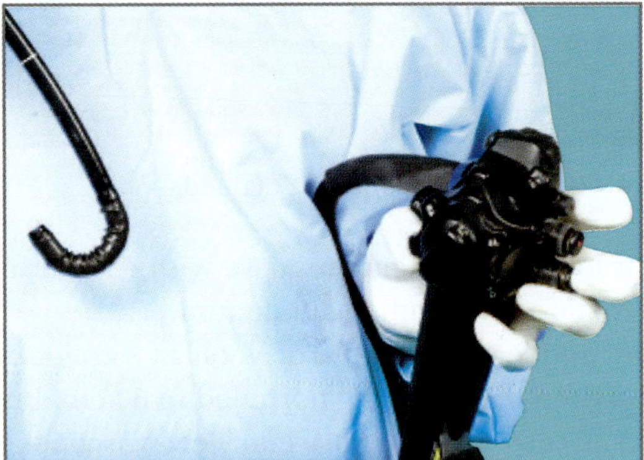

Fig. 15: Retroflexion.

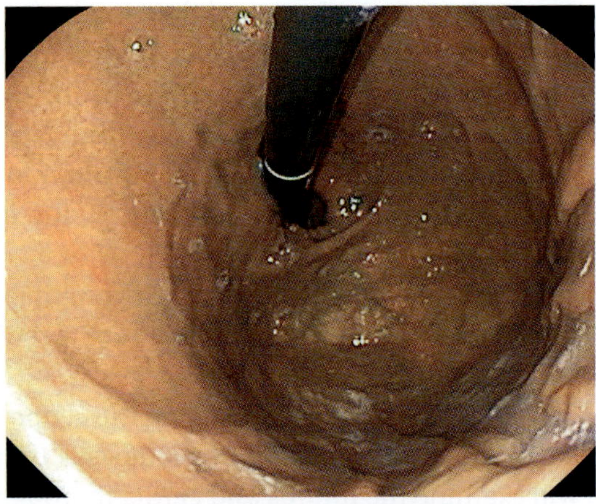

Fig. 16: Fundus and cardia.

Note the scope is firmly gripped by the diaphragmatic crus and the lesser curve is the part very close to the scope. If there is any laxity of hiatal opening, then it suggests the diagnosis of reflux disease.

But remember not to pull the scope beyond 50 cm level during J-maneuver or else you will damage the cardia.

You may appreciate the indentation or bluish discoloration at the fundus due to spleen and also cardiac pulsation.

15. *Straighten the scope and gently withdraw the scope:* Remember the landmarks once again:
    - Lesser curve at 12 o'clock position on the monitor
    - Greater curve at 6 o'clock position
    - Posterior wall of stomach at 3 o'clock
    - Anterior wall of stomach at 9 o'clock

    Appreciate the relationship of anterior abdominal wall to the stomach. Do finger indentation of abdominal wall to see the point in the anterior wall of the stomach (usually at 9 o'clock in the monitor). This is important for placing percutaneous gastrostomy tube. Also, one may appreciate transillumination through the abdominal wall during this step if you put off the lights in the endoscopy suite.

    One may notice the impression by the body of pancreas on the posterior wall of stomach.
16. *Test distensibility of stomach:* Insufflate the stomach with air and you see flattening of all rugal folds. Then apply suction to appreciate how fast the stomach contracts and you start noticing reemergence of rugal folds. In case of linitis plastica, it will be difficult to distend the stomach (leather bottle stomach).
17. *Revisit the Z-line and carefully examine the esophagus on the way out:* Look for the change of pinkish gastric mucosa changing to pale esophageal mucosa at the Z-line

    For any lesion in the esophagus, note the level and extent of lesion.
    - Cervical esophagus:
        - Hypopharynx to the thoracic inlet, which is at the level of the sternal notch.
        - By endoscopy, 15–20 cm from the incisors
    - Upper thoracic esophagus:
        - Thoracic inlet to lower border of the azygos vein
        - By endoscopy, 20–25 cm
    - Middle thoracic esophagus:
        - Lower border of the azygos vein to the inferior pulmonary veins
        - By endoscopy, 25–30 cm
    - Lower thoracic esophagus and OG junction:
        - Inferior pulmonary veins to the stomach; includes the intra-abdominal portion of the esophagus
        - By endoscopy, 30–40 cm

18. *Carefully evaluate the cricopharynx during retreat:* Examine piriform recess, postcricoid region, vocal cords, and vallecula.
19. *Document and print the endoscopy report*: Save important videos and pictures.
20. *Cleaning and disinfection of endoscopy:* Clean the endoscope and do a leak test. Disinfect the endoscopy as per the guidelines and store it in a dry ventilated cub board.

In summary, look for the following six sets of rule of three for successful navigation:

1. *Oral cavity:*
   - *Look for three structures:*
     i. Tongue at 12 o'clock
     ii. Soft palate at 6 o'clock
     iii. Glimpse of epiglottis
2. *Cricopharynx at 15 cm from incisor teeth*:
   - *Identify three structures:* Vocal cord, arytenoid folds, piriform fossa
3. *Esophagus:*
   - *Recognize three levels of narrowing:* 15 cm/25 cm/40 cm
4. *Stomach navigation: Three key steps to reach pylorus*:
   - Big wheel toward you, clockwise twist, and push/three times
5. *Duodenum:*
   - *Three key steps to enter D2:* (i) Big wheel toward you, (ii) clockwise twist, and (iii) turn body to right
6. *During scope withdrawal and on J-maneuver:*
   - *Look for three structures:* Incisura, fundus, and cardia

Abandon the procedure, if:

- The patient is uncooperative/restless
- Any indication of cardiorespiratory distress
- *Any indication of major complication:* Perforation/false passage/aspiration, etc.

POSTENDOSCOPIC STEPS

Endoscopy:

- Cleaning and disinfection

Patient:

- Discuss the findings and their implications
- Advice regarding further management
- Give a written report

TOP 10 TECHNICAL TIPS FOR THE DIFFICULTY EXPERIENCED DURING DIAGNOSTIC UPPER GASTROINTESTINAL ENDOSCOPY

The beginners may find various challenges during the upper GI endoscopy in navigation, interpretation of lesions, or challenges during attempts at therapeutic procedures. The following 10 tips will help the endoscopist with any navigational challenges.

1. *Not able to go beyond the oropharynx:* At times, you may find it difficult to go beyond the oropharynx due to a big or unsteady tongue, and large tonsils in an anxious patient. In such a frustrating moment, try the following steps:
   - Reassure the patient
   - Ensure the head is in a neutral position on a small pillow and slightly flexed.
   - Consider giving a small dose of sedative (2 mg of IV midazolam)
   - *Finger-guided intubation* **(*Fig. 17*)***:* Insert your left index finger on the side of the mouth guard and steady and depress the tongue while you pass the endoscope with your right hand

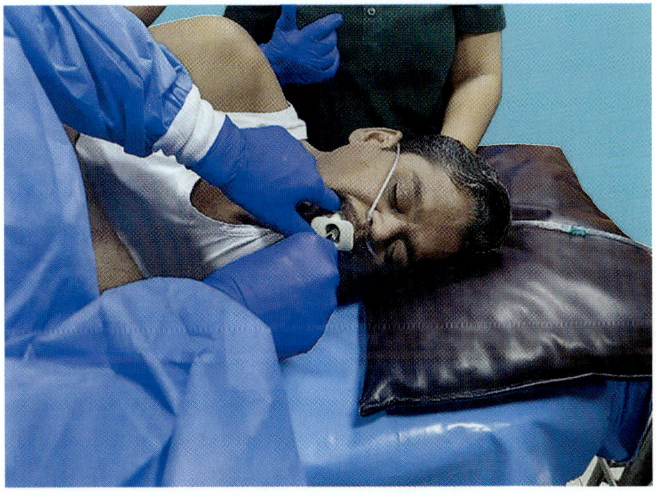

Fig. 17: Finger-guided intubation.

2. *Getting stuck at the cricopharynx:* Once you reach the level of the cricopharynx (15 cm from incisor teeth), recognize the vocal cords and piriform fossa. Normally without undue force, we should be able to pass the endoscope through the left piriform fossa seen at the 9 o'clock in the monitor.

   If there is any resistance felt at that time, it could be due to the postcricoid web, Zenker's diverticulum, or postcricoid stricture.

Using undue force blindly at this stage is one of the reasons for perforation. So, beware **(Fig. 18)**.

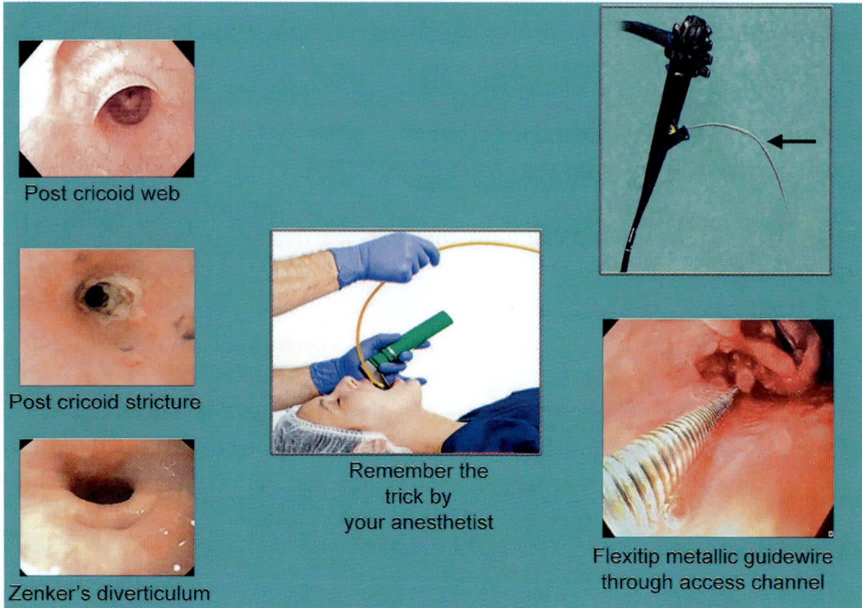

Fig. 18: Reason and how to approach during stucking at cricopharynx.

Remember what our anesthetic colleagues do when they have difficulty with endotracheal intubation. Bougie-guided intubation has often come to their rescue. Similarly, you could pass either a flexitip metallic guidewire or a biopsy forceps through the access channel and pass it through the cricopharynx without any resistance. Then you can pass the endoscopy down over the guidewire. Often this trick helps and is worth considering preferably with C-arm control if available.

3. *Getting stuck in the middle of the esophagus:* At times, you will not find the esophageal lumen if the patient has advanced carcinoma esophagus. Though one could consider guidewire-directed passage of endoscopy with the help of image intensifier screening, the safest thing to do in such a situation is to biopsy the lesion at the upper end and abandon the procedure. Plan CT thorax to assess the tumor and plan for further treatment later and avoid blind navigation (**Figs. 19A and B**). Avoid the disaster of iatrogenic trachea esophageal fistula or mediastinal perforations.
4. *Getting lost in the roomy stomach* ***(Figs. 20A and B)****:* Another common mistake for beginners could be the loss of direction inside the spacious stomach. A simple way to remember your path toward pylorus is as follows:

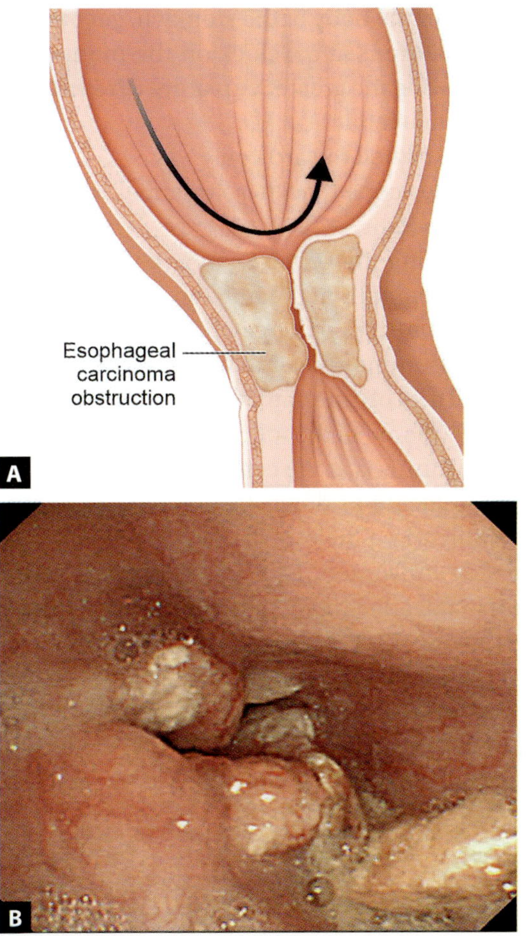

Figs. 19A and B: Esophageal tumor causing obstruction.

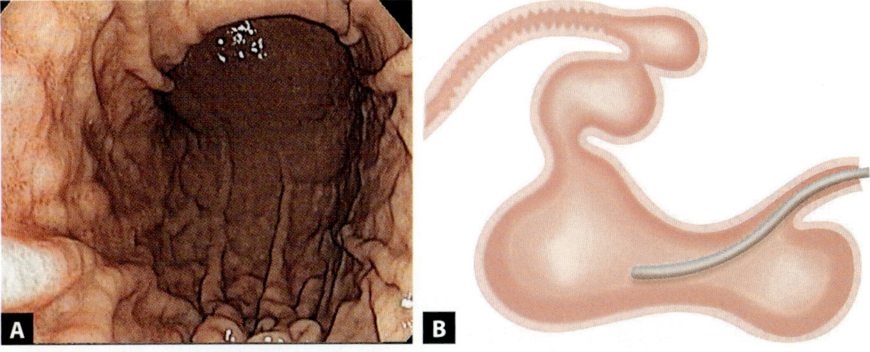

Figs. 20A and B: Going along greater curvature.

- Once you enter the body of the stomach, get oriented with anatomy. Greater curvature is at 6 o'clock on the monitor. So, take this long route of following the greater curvature to reach the pylorus by doing three key maneuvers:
    i. Big wheel turned toward you
    ii. Torque the scope clockwise or small wheel slightly away from you to turn right
    iii. Keep pushing the scope 5 cm at a time, three times to see the pylorus eventually at the horizon.

5. *Pylorus is not permitting passage of the scope* ***(Fig. 21)****:* Often due to pyloric spasm or undue movement of the pylorus (dancing pylorus), beginners spend a lot of time entering the duodenum. In such a situation, you may consider some of the following tips:
    - Ensure the pylorus is at the center of the monitor and facing directly to you. Side-facing or down-facing pylorus is impossible to cross. So, enter only when the pylorus is at the center.
    - Side-to-side movement of your body could help to synchronize with horizontal adjustment and big wheel adjustment will help with pylorus moving up and down. Also, avoid patient's hyperventilating by taking care of the airway.
    - Avoid too much distention of the stomach by sucking all the air so avoid peristalsis
    - You may consider using 20 mg of Buscopan as a last measure.

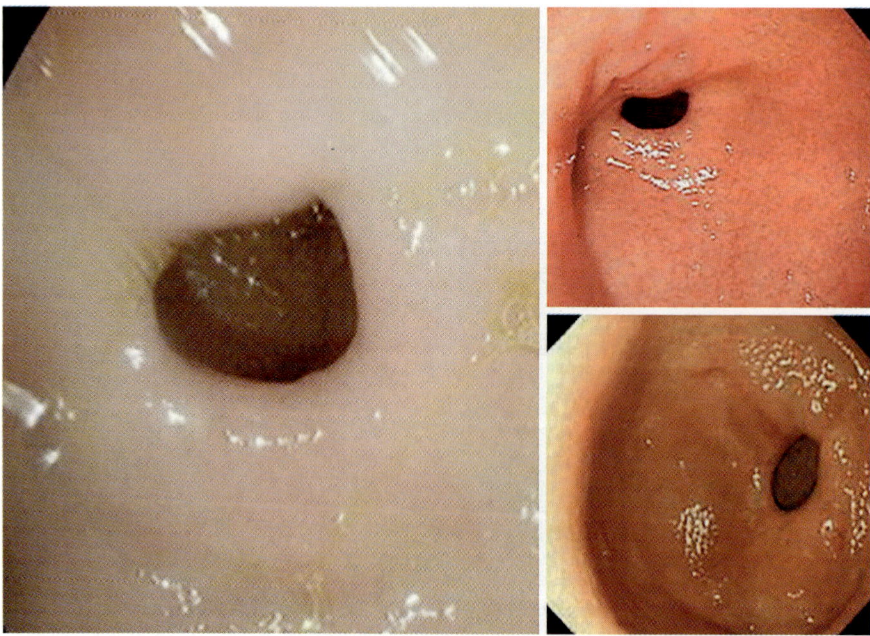

Fig. 21: Various looking of pylorus.

6. *Not able to see the posterior wall of the duodenum:* Unlike the stomach, the duodenum has narrow space, and visualizing all parts of it could be tricky. Gentle body movement or wheel movement will aid you. Once you are in the duodenal bulb, gently turn your body to the right and withdraw the scope gently. You will see a glimpse of the posterior wall of the duodenal bulb. Or, else turn the small wheel away from you to visualize the posterior duodenal ulcer.
7. *Diving deep into D2:* At times, you may find difficulty reaching deep into second part of the duodenum. Remember the following steps:
   - Turn the small wheel away
   - Turn your body to the right away from the patient and start looking at the monitor
   - Turn the big wheel toward you
   - Start pulling the scope back and you will find the scope diving deep into D2 paradoxically (short route).
8. *Importance of retroflexion of endoscope*: Several fundal lesions such as fundal varix, gastrointestinal stromal tumor (GIST), or even a small tumor at the fundus could be easily missed if the fundus is covered with fluid or blood clots.
   - Carefully suction at the fluid or blood clots to visualize the fundus
   - Consider gently raising the head-end of the patient by 45° to shift the fluid toward the antrum. Look up when the patient's head is up **(Fig. 22)**.

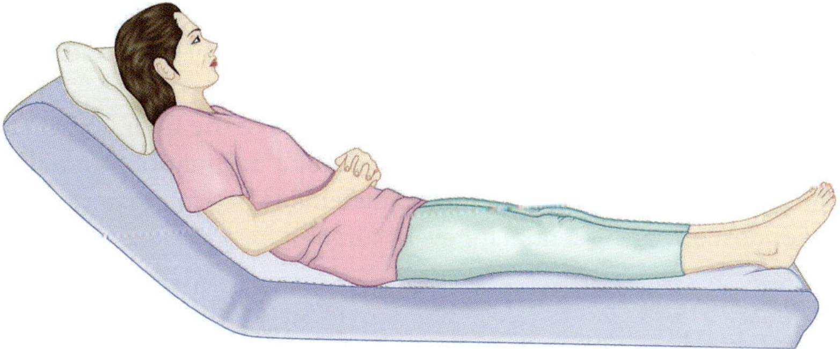

Fig. 22: Raising head end of patient to shift the fundal fluid.

9. *Biopsy of lesion in the fundus is not easy* ***(Fig. 23)****:* As the endoscopy is in retroflexion, the accessories will not traverse the acute bend and could endanger the integrity of the scope. So, consider the following six steps for a biopsy of a fundic lesion:
   i. Keep the scope in a straight position toward the antrum
   ii. Take the biopsy forceps very near the scope tip
   iii. Then do retroflexion of endoscopy

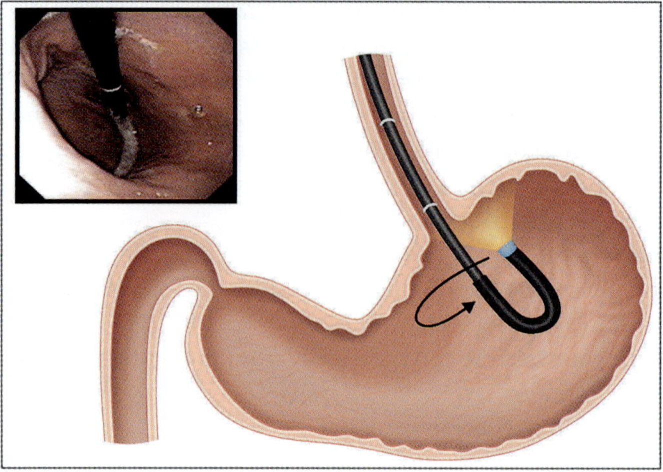

Fig. 23: Approaching the fundal lesions.

iv. Bring out the biopsy forceps and take the biopsy and wait
v. Straighten the bending section of the endoscope
vi. Then, only then, pull the biopsy forceps out of the access channel to retrieve the specimen

10. *Beware of impaled FB and adherent clots on the ulcer base:* Impaled FB-like fish bone could be penetrating the nearby vital organs such as the aorta or pericardium. So, CT scan of the chest is preferable before the removal.

    Forceful dislodgment of clots from the surface of the ulcer could restart bleeding again hence beware. Have the right tools and keep the team very alert for such eventuality.

    Structured endoscopy training is the need of the hour. Competence in the art and science of endoscopy is not a destination but a lifelong journey. Constant practice and unquenchable passion to perfect the art of endoscopy are essential for every surgeon.

CONCLUSION

- Before endoscopy, ensure the endoscopy checklist and patient checklist are completed.
- Vigilance and monitoring of vital signs during endoscopy are paramount.
- Meticulous examination of the gut warrants adequate training and expertise in the art of endoscopy

SUGGESTED READING

1. ASGE guidelines for clinical application. Statement on role of short courses in endoscopic training. American Society for Gastrointestinal Endoscopy. Gastrointest Endosc. 1999;50:913-4.

2. Catalano MF. Training in upper gastrointestinal endoscopy. Gastrointest Endosc Clin N Am. 1994;4:623-38.
3. Chun JH, Yoon YS, Oh SW, Lee ES, Kim MG, Kim YS, et al. Current State and Demand of Esophagogastroduodenoscopy Training in Family Practice Residency Programs. J Korean Acad Fam Med. 2003;24:1092-8.
4. Coleman WH. Gastroscopy: a primary diagnostic procedure. Prim Care. 1988;15:1-11.
5. Ende A, Zopf Y, Konturek P, Naegel A, Hahn EG, Matthes K, et al. Strategies for training in diagnostic upper endoscopy: a prospective, randomized trial. Gastrointest Endosc. 2012;75:254-60.
6. Kang SH, Hyun JJ. Preparation and patient evaluation for safe gastrointestinal endoscopy. Clin Endosc. 2013;46:212-8.
7. Koo JS, Choi JH. Conscious Sedation During Gastrointestinal Endoscopy: Midazolam vs Propofol. Korean J Gastrointest Endosc. 2011;42:67-73.
8. Lee KM, Choi SR, Jang BI, Kim SH, Kang CD, Kim YD, et al. Education and Training Guidelines for the Board of the Korean Society of Gastrointestinal Endoscopy. Korean J Gastrointest Endosc. 2011;42:207-14.
9. Park KH, Sung NJ, Lee DW, Jeong HS. Technical Competency of the Esophagogastroduodenoscopy (EGD) during the First 50 EGDs: The Training Result of Family Medicine Residents in a University Hospital. Korean J Fam Med. 2010;31:595-9.
10. Ponich T, Enns R, Romagnuolo J, Springer J, Armstrong D, Barkun AN. Canadian credentialing guidelines for esophagogastroduodenoscopy. Can J Gastroenterol. 2008;22:349-54.
11. Xiong X, Barkun AN, Waschke K, Martel M. Current status of core and advanced adult gastrointestinal endoscopy training in Canada: Survey of existing accredited programs. Can J Gastroenterol. 2013;27:267-72.

Expert's Comment

The chapter is exhaustive, well illustrated, and precise.

I have the following five points for consideration:

1. *Difficult intubation across the cricopharynx:* Sprinkle a few drops of water from the endoscope using the air-water button. This will start the peristaltic contraction of swallowing and relax the cricopharyngeal sphincter.
2. Follow the gastric mucosal folds along the greater curvature to reach the antrum and the pylorus.
3. For persistent pyloric spasm, pass a guidewire or a flexible metallic probe. Use biopsy forceps across the pyloric orifice and railroad the endoscope into the first part of the duodenum. There will be a small mucosal bleed.
4. In history, check if the patient is on anticoagulants before taking multiple biopsies.
5. While withdrawing the scope across the cricopharynx or oropharynx, apply suction in the scope to suck out any fluid in the oropharynx to prevent aspiration.

I greatly appreciate the efforts made by the author and the IAGES endoscopy board in bringing this practical book to all endoscopic surgeons.

Professor (Dr) B Krishna Rau
Chennai

CHAPTER 5

Endoscopic Atlas of Upper Gastrointestinal Pathology

Keywords: Upper GI pathology, Savary–Miller, Los Angeles classification, Borrmann's classification, Forrest classification, and grades of varices

INTRODUCTION

There are vast numbers of pathological lesions to watch for and recognize while performing upper gastrointestinal (GI) endoscopy. We could adopt a symptom-based approach in all endoscopic procedures to aid us in making a pathological diagnosis. At the outset, we should take a detailed clinical history to note down the key symptoms and duration, the history of any comorbid illnesses, drug history, allergies, any previous abdominal surgery, a habit of smoking or alcohol, and family history of GI tumor. Then perform a thorough clinical examination before endoscopic examination.

For each of the following key upper GI symptoms, there are several pathological conditions we need to consider and look for. Let us discuss each symptom followed by the pathology noticed in such a group of patients. The following are the key symptoms in patients requiring endoscopy **(Box 1)**.

DIAGNOSTIC ENDOSCOPY

Approach to a Case of Dyspepsia

Discomfort, dull aching pain, or burning sensation in the upper abdomen is a common symptom of upper GI pathology.

BOX 1: Key symptoms in patients requiring endoscopy.

- *Diagnostic endoscopy:*
  - Dyspepsia
  - Dysphagia
  - Upper gastrointestinal (GI) bleeding
  - Chest pain
  - Vomiting/regurgitation
  - Anemia/weight loss
- *Surveillance endoscopy:*
  - Barrett's esophagus
  - Varices
  - Postoperative cases
- *Screening endoscopy:* Family history of polyps/cancer
- Therapeutic endoscopy

You may find any of the following disorders in patients presenting with dyspepsia:

- Nonulcer dyspepsia (NUD)
- Esophagitis
- Gastritis
- Gastric ulcer
- Duodenal ulcer
- Carcinoma stomach

A Case of Nonulcer Dyspepsia (Functional Dyspepsia)

Endoscopy shows normal esophagus, stomach, and duodenum. We could perform an ultrasound of the abdomen in all cases to exclude any hepatobiliary or pancreatic pathology. NUD could be classified into three types: (1) Ulcer type, (2) dysmotility type, or (3) reflux type. An ulcer-type patient has typical ulcer-like pain related to food with nausea or vomiting but with normal endoscopy. A dysmotility-type patient often complains of early satiety and postprandial fullness. Nausea, vomiting, or belching may be present. Diabetic gastroparesis could present as a dysmotility type of NUD. Reflux type of patient often has retrosternal or epigastric burning sensation along with acid reflux or belching. We should consider doing a 24-hour pH study and manometry in the reflux type of NUD. Gastric motility study may be needed in some cases of dysmotility type of NUD.

Gastroesophageal Reflux Disease with Esophagitis

It will present as erythema, erosions with fibrin deposits, or ulceration over the crests of mucosal folds predominantly in the lower esophagus just above the Z-line. Look for and document the following findings namely:

- Level of Z-line
- Level of hiatus

- Any hiatus hernia
- Site and severity of esophagitis

Savary–Miller and or Los Angeles classification can be used to grade the severity of esophagitis.

Savary–Miller classification ***(Figs. 1 to 4)***:

- *Grade 1 esophagitis:* Linear column of erosion in the lower esophagus
- *Grade 2 esophagitis:* Confluent columns of erosions in the lower esophagus
- *Grade 3 esophagitis:* Circumferential erosions in the lower esophagus
- *Grade 4 esophagitis:* Peptic stricture, ulcers, and Barrett's esophagus (BE)

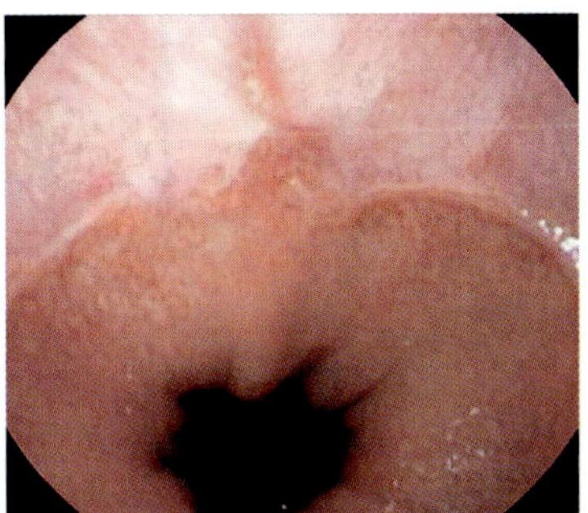

Fig. 1: Grade 1 esophagitis.

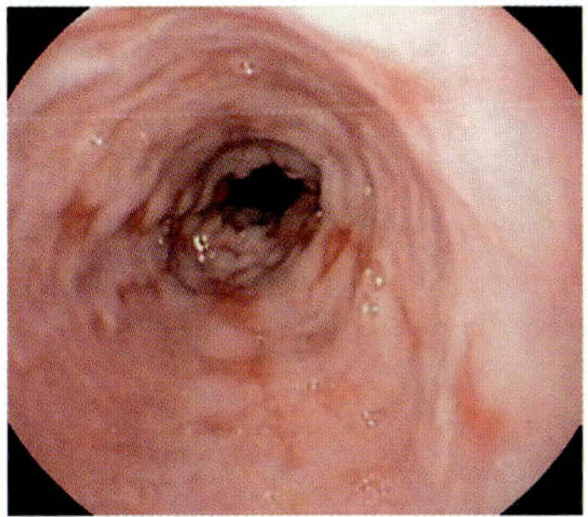

Fig. 2: Grade 2 esophagitis.

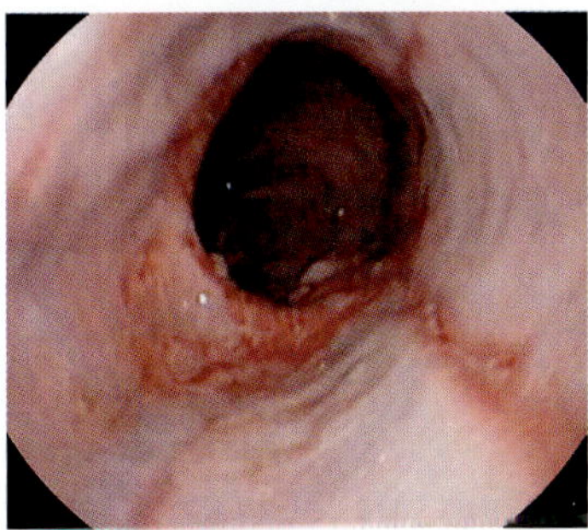

Fig. 3: Grade 3 esophagitis.

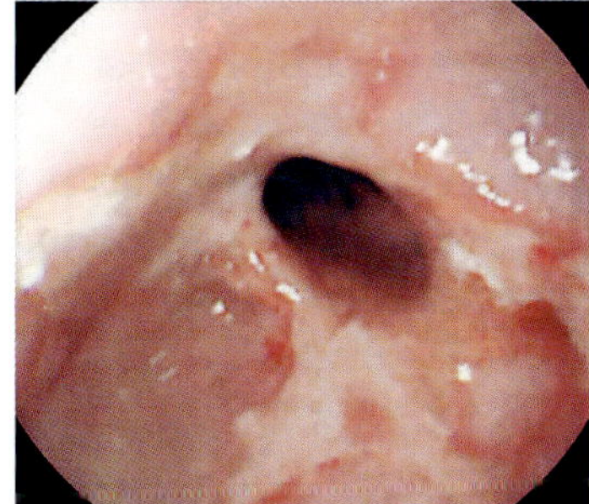

Fig. 4: Peptic stricture.

Los Angeles classification ***(Figs. 5 to 8)***:

- *Grade A esophagitis:* Linear column of erosions <5 mm in length
- *Grade B esophagitis:* Linear columns of erosions >5 mm in length
- Grade *C esophagitis:* Confluent esophageal erosions <75% circumference
- *Grade D esophagitis:* Circumferential esophageal erosions

We should also do a biopsy in cases of ulcer, stricture, or BE to look for any dysplasia. We consider evaluating with the use of narrow-band imaging (NBI) or chromoendoscopy. Consider pH study and manometry in all cases before contemplating any surgery. Following are the six components of 24-hour esophageal pH monitoring (DeMeester score):

1. Percent total time pH <4
2. Percent upright time pH <4

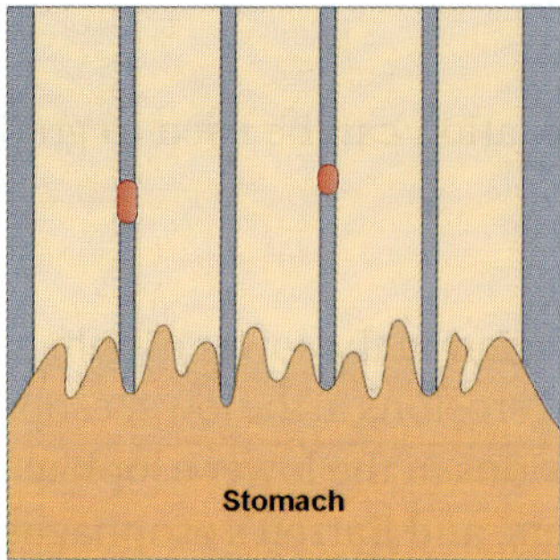

Fig. 5: Grade A esophagitis.

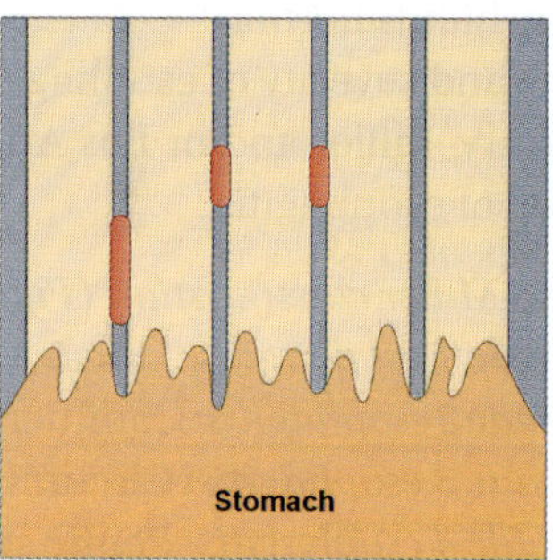

Fig. 6: Grade B esophagitis.

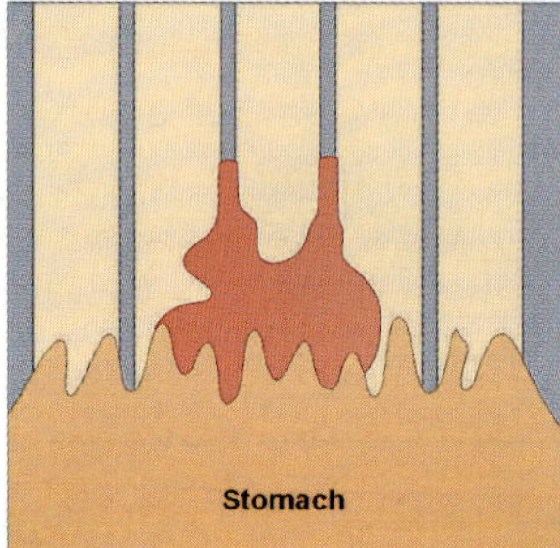

Fig. 7: Grade C esophagitis.

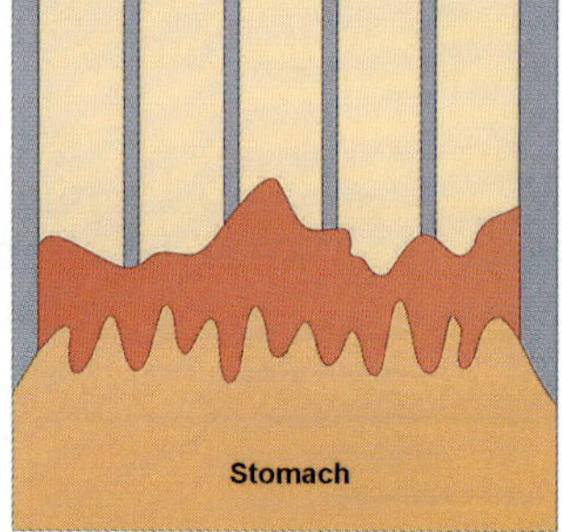

Fig. 8: Grade D esophagitis.

3. Percent supine time pH <4
4. Number of reflux episodes
5. Number of reflux episodes ≥5 minutes
6. Longest reflux episode (minutes)

Gastritis

It is a common finding noticed in the case of dyspepsia. It can be an acute or chronic type of gastritis. Acute gastritis is often due to *Helicobacter pylori* infection, alcohol, or drug intake [nonsteroidal anti-inflammatory drug (NSAID)]. We should be able to distinguish type A and type B of chronic atrophic gastritis.

- *Type A:* Found in pernicious anemia and affects mainly the fundus and body.
- *Type B:* Seen in *H. pylori* infection and involves mainly antrum of the stomach

  Note the site, severity, and extent of gastritis and describe it accordingly.
- *Site involved:*
  - Involving whole stomach (total or pangastritis)
  - Only fundus of the stomach (fundal gastritis)
  - Fundus and body of the stomach (proximal gastritis)
  - Mainly body of the stomach (corporal gastritis)

- Antrum of the stomach (antral gastritis)
- Antrum and body of the stomach (distal gastritis)

■ *Severity:*
- Mild
- Moderately severe
- Severe

■ *Extent of involvement could be:*
- Patchy
- Diffuse

Describe the nature of pathology as edematous gastritis, erythematous gastritis, hemorrhagic gastritis, or erosive gastritis.

■ *Edematous gastritis:* It appears as cobblestone-like mucosa **(Fig. 9)**
■ *Erythematous gastritis:* It appears with reddish streaks on the mucosa especially over the rugal folds **(Fig. 10)**
■ *Hemorrhagic gastritis:* It appears as areas of mucosal contusion or bleeding **(Fig. 11)**

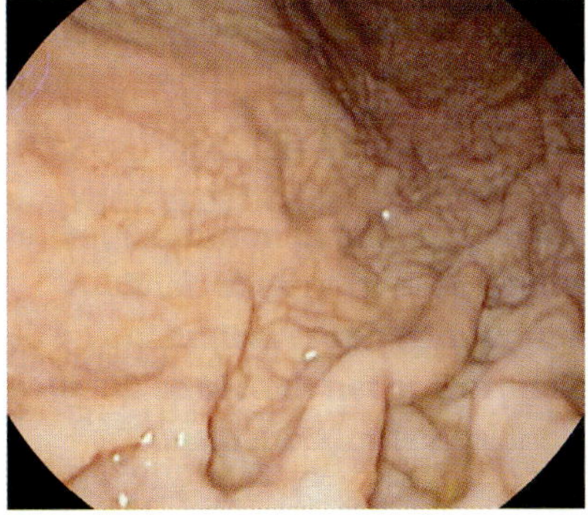

Fig. 9: Edematous gastritis.

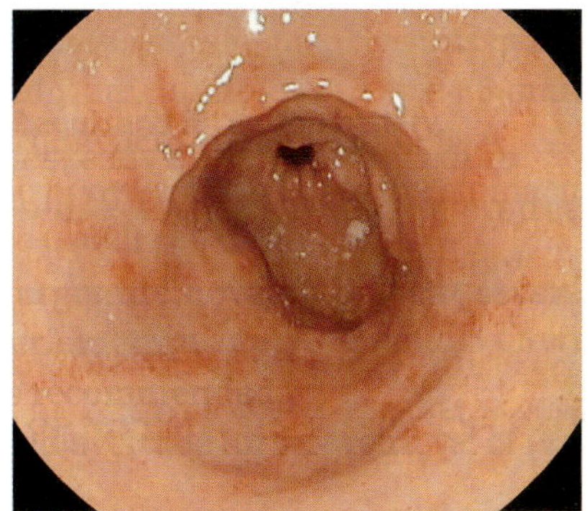

Fig. 10: Erythematous gastritis.

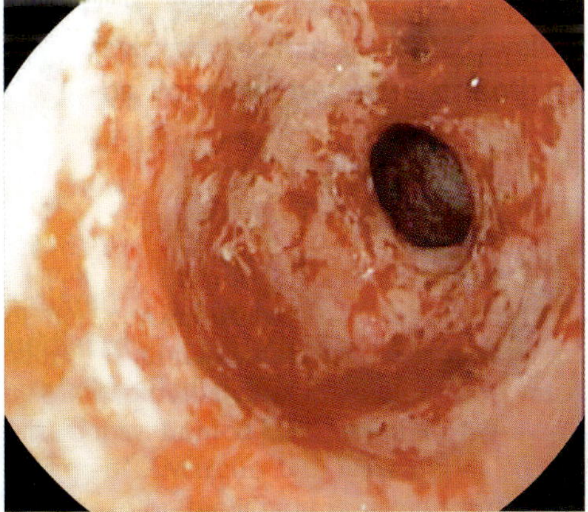

Fig. 11: Hemorrhagic gastritis.

- *Erosive gastritis:* It is characterized by the presence of superficial pin head mucosal defects covered by specks of yellowish slough **(Fig. 12)**.

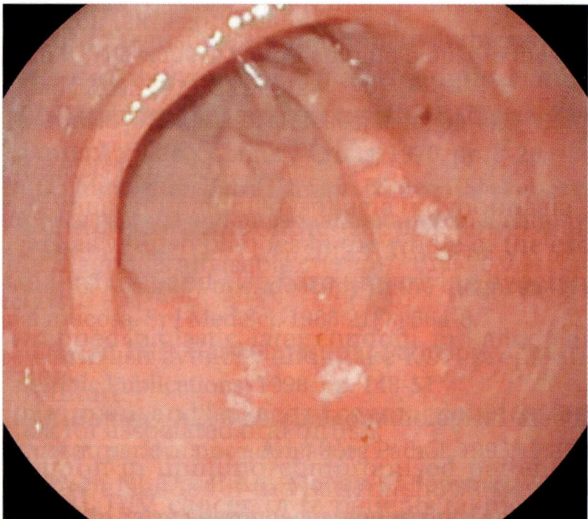

Fig. 12: Erosive gastritis.

Summarize the findings using all the above standard terminology, e.g., severe patchy erythematous antral gastritis, mild diffuse edematous proximal gastritis, and so on.

We need to perform *H. pylori* test in all cases of gastritis. Send a biopsy in cases of chronic gastritis to look for any intestinal metaplasia. We should recognize congestive gastropathy as a separate entity. In the case of portal hypertension, the stomach mucosa appears edematous and looks like snake or crocodile skin due to venous congestion of gastric mucosa **(Fig. 13)**.

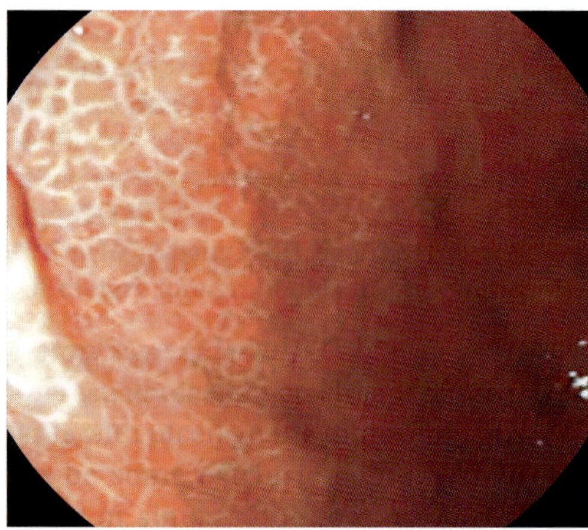

Fig. 13: Congestive gastropathy.

There is no inflammatory cell infiltrate in such a condition. Unwarranted biopsy only invites troublesome bleeding. Antral mucosa may appear as the surface of a cut watermelon due to streaks of edematous congestive mucosa. It is also known as gastric antral vascular ectasia (GAVE) syndrome **(Fig. 14)**.

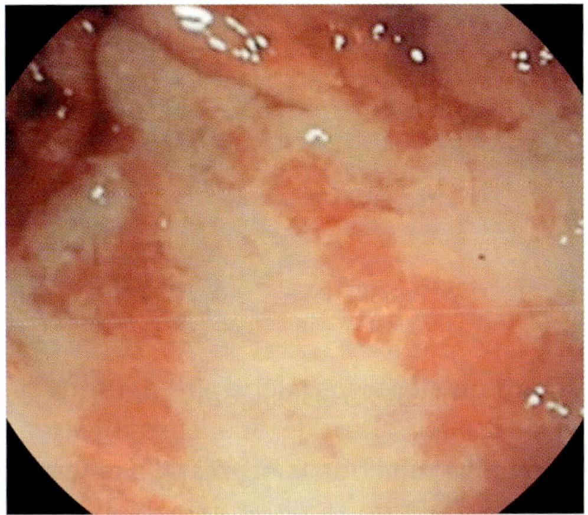

Fig. 14: Gastric antral vascular ectasia (GAVE) syndrome.

Gastric Ulcer (Fig. 15)

- Note the site, size, surface, and margin of the ulcer and see the surrounding mucosa and rugal folds
- Acute benign gastric ulcers are small (<1 cm) superficial lesions mainly in the prepyloric region. Perform the *H. pylori* test by taking a biopsy of the antral mucosa.
- Chronic benign gastric ulcers appear like a whitish crater with sloppy margins and converging rugal folds. It usually measures <2 cm and is

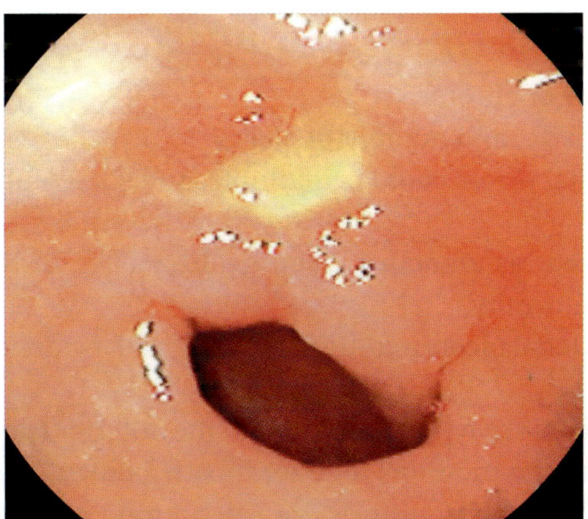

Fig. 15: Benign gastric ulcer.

located predominantly in the antral region or over the incisura. Take multiple biopsies from the margins and send for histopathological examination to exclude malignancy.

Duodenitis (Fig. 16)

- It appears as diffuse or patchy areas of redness with multiple pin head erosions are common.
- We should describe it as mild, moderately severe, or severe duodenitis.
- It can often be associated with gastritis (gastroduodenitis). So, perform the *H. pylori* test also.

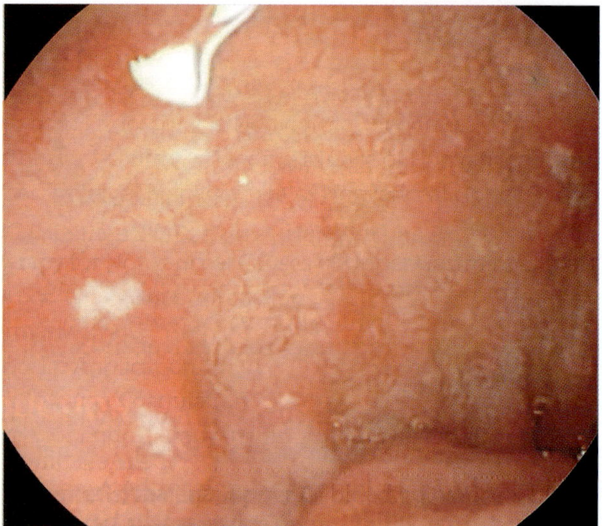

Fig. 16: Duodenal erosions.

Duodenal Ulcer (Fig. 17)

- It can be acute or chronic.
- Note the site, size, and number of ulcers
- Often duodenal ulcers could be multiple, and size could vary from 2 mm to 2 cm.
- It could present as an active ulcer, healing ulcer, or healed ulcer with scarring or deformity.
- Chronic duodenal ulcers may be presenting with evidence of some gastric stasis.

Duodenal ulcers are typically located in the anterior wall of the duodenal bulb (9 o'clock in the monitor) and are mostly benign. Posterior duodenal ulcers (3 o'clock in the monitor!) are uncommon and often overlooked. It has the risk of serious bleeding due to erosion of the gastroduodenal

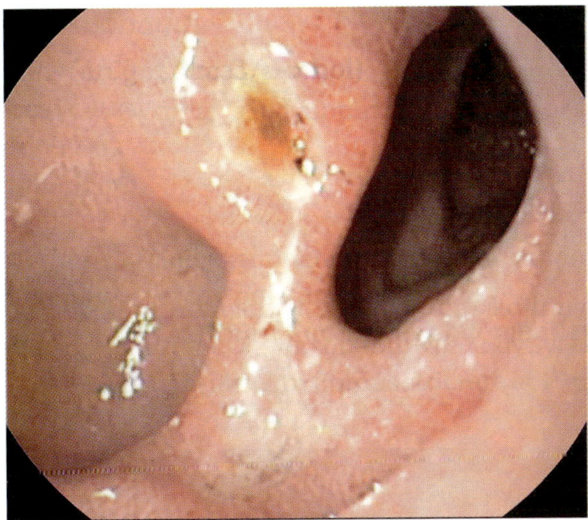

Fig. 17: Acute duodenal ulcer.

artery. Sometimes, both anterior and posterior ulcers coexist (kissing ulcers). Let us remember that the anterior ulcer perforates while the posterior ulcer bleeds. Postbulbar duodenal ulcers are unusual lesions and we should think of Zollinger–Ellison syndrome. Look for any stigmata for bleeding such as oozing, clots on the surface, or visible vessels. A clean-based ulcer is unlikely to bleed. Do antral biopsy in all cases of duodenitis and duodenal ulcers and look for *H. pylori* infection.

Basis of Rapid Urease Test

Helicobacter pylori is a gram-negative motile bacillus that can thrive in the hostile gastric acid media due to the presence of urease enzyme which can convert urea to ammonia and hence create a micro-alkali environment around each bacterium protecting it like armor from the onslaught of gastric acid. No other bacteria on this planet have this unique property. *H. pylori* thrives predominantly in the antral gastric mucosa. Hence in all cases of distal gastritis, duodenitis and duodenal ulcer take a biopsy of gastric antral mucosa and place it in a slide or bottle containing urea and phenolphthalein indicator. Change from yellow color to pink color indicates a positive rapid urease test (RUT) and usually, it takes just a few minutes. So, it is a very rapid, sensitive, and specific test for *H. pylori* infection.

Carcinoma Stomach (Fig. 18)

It usually presents as dyspepsia, weight loss, and anorexia. Hence early endoscopy is indicated in the following cases of dyspepsia namely:

- New dyspepsia after age of 45 years
- Dyspepsia with a family history of gastric cancer

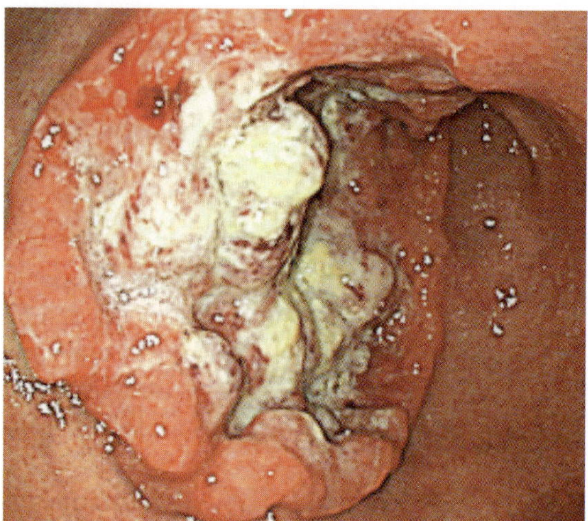

Fig. 18: Carcinoma stomach.

- *Dyspepsia with alarm symptoms (red flag symptoms):*
  - Weight loss
  - Anemia
  - Hematemesis or melena
  - Vomiting

Note the site, size, and nature of the lesion and describe it according to Borrmann's classification.

Borrmann's classification of gastric cancer is as follows **(Figs. 19 to 22)**:

- *Type 1:* Polypoidal tumor
- *Type 2:* Ulceroproliferative tumor
- *Type 3:* Ulceroinfiltrative tumor
- *Type 4:* Infiltrative type tumor

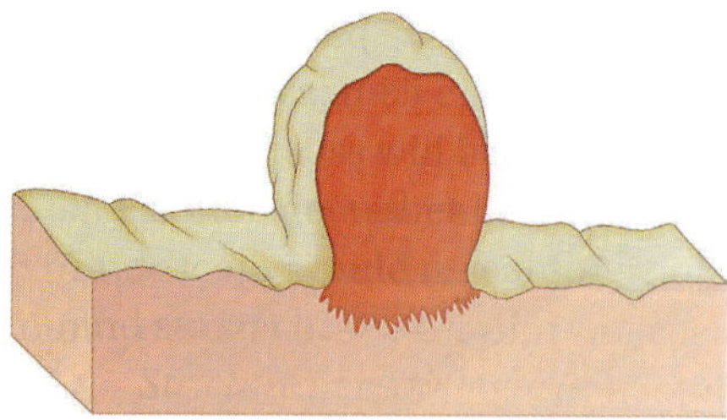

Fig. 19: Polypoidal carcinoma.

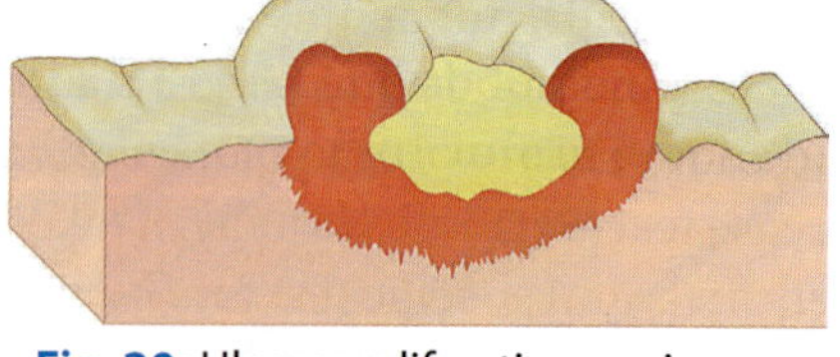

Fig. 20: Ulceroproliferative carcinoma.

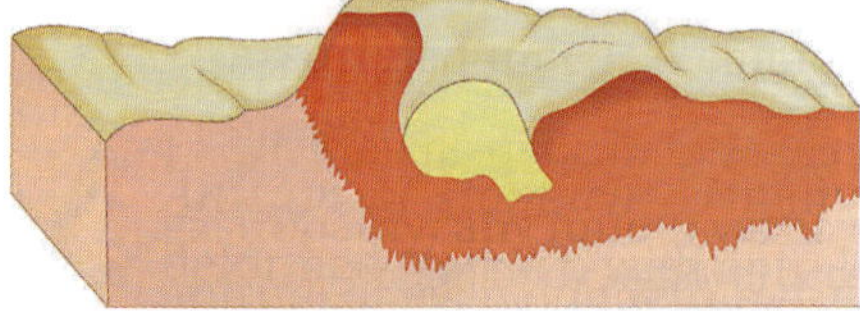

Fig. 21: Ulceroinfiltrative carcinoma.

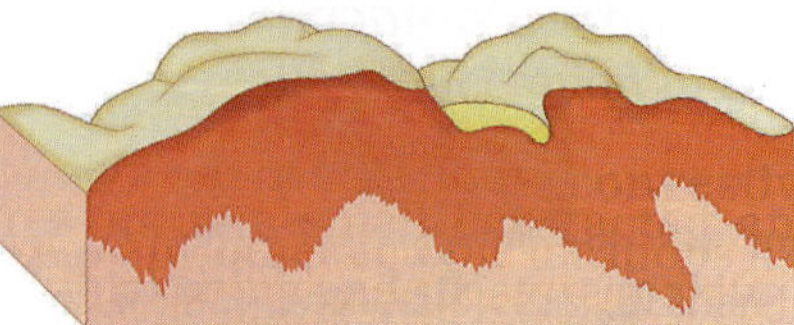

Fig. 22: Linitis plastica.

Take multiple bits for biopsy. Endoscopic US may give additional information on the T and N stage of the tumor. We should plan for a contrast CT scan for TNM (tumor, node, and metastasis) staging in all cases before any therapy. Early gastric cancers are unusual findings but to be remembered as a cause of dyspepsia. So, consider biopsy in all odd-looking lesions. Magnification endoscopy, chromoendoscopy, or NBI improves diagnostic accuracy. Early gastric cancer confines itself to the mucosa and is hence amenable to curative resection.

Types of early gastric cancer are as follows ***(Figs. 23 to 25)****:*

- *Type 1:* Protuberant lesions
- *Type 2:* Flat lesions
- *Type 3:* Excavated lesion

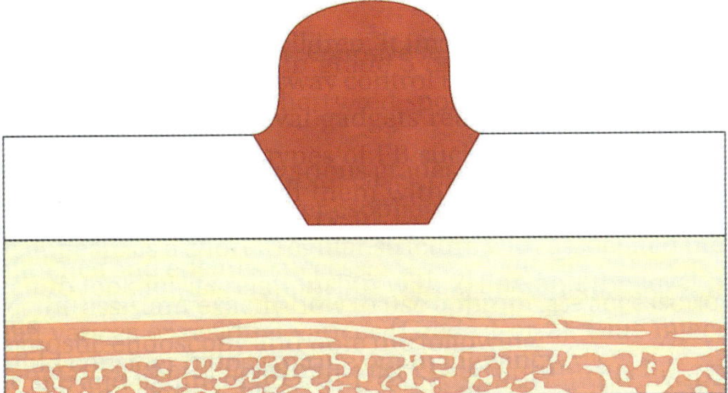

Fig. 23: Protuberant lesion.

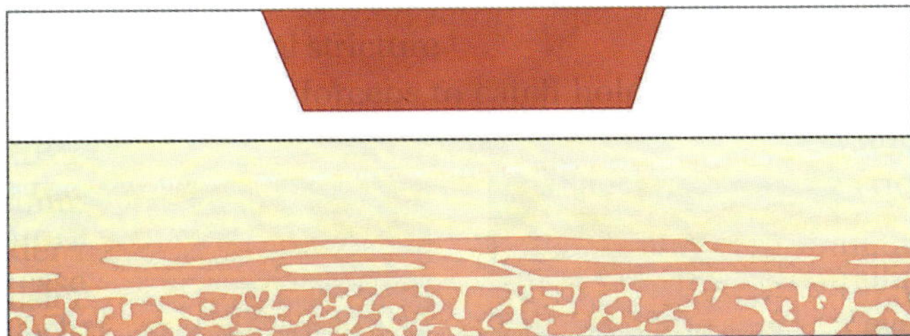

Fig. 24: Flat tumor.

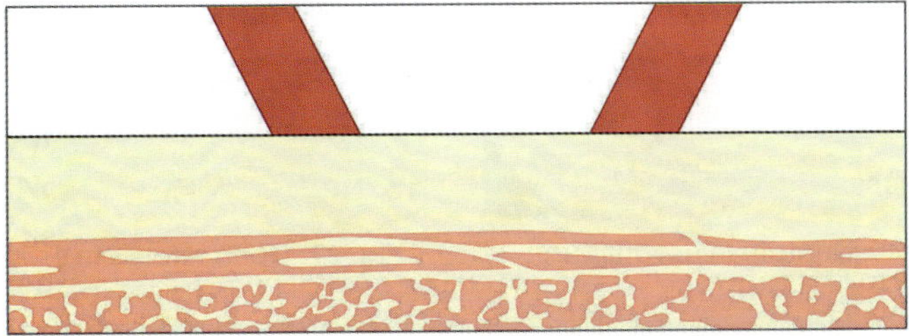

Fig. 25: Excavated lesion.

Approach to Cases of Dysphagia

- Take good history of onset and progress of dysphagia
- For solids or liquids or both
- Pain during swallowing (odynophagia)
- Associated with other symptoms such as vomiting, hematemesis, cough, and weight loss

We need to consider the following causes in patient presenting with dysphagia:

- *Intraluminal:* Food bolus/FB
- *In the wall:*
  - Various types of esophagitis
  - Benign stricture:
    - Postcricoid stricture
    - Corrosive stricture
    - Peptic stricture
    - Achalasia
  - Malignant stricture
- *Outside the wall:*
  - Zenker's diverticulum
  - Mediastinal mass
  - Enlarged left atrium
  - Aortic aneurysm

Foreign Body Esophagus (Figs. 26 and 27)

- Present as acute dysphagia and odynophagia
- Common in children
- Coins, pins, small toys, and button batteries are the usual swallowed objects.
- X-rays neck and chest are helpful.

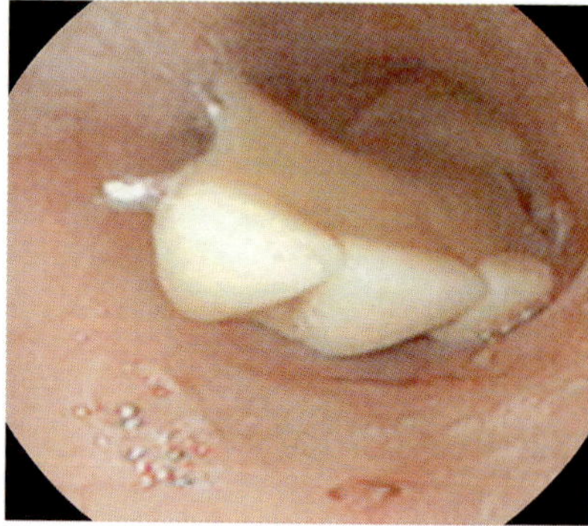

Fig. 26: Denture in esophagus.

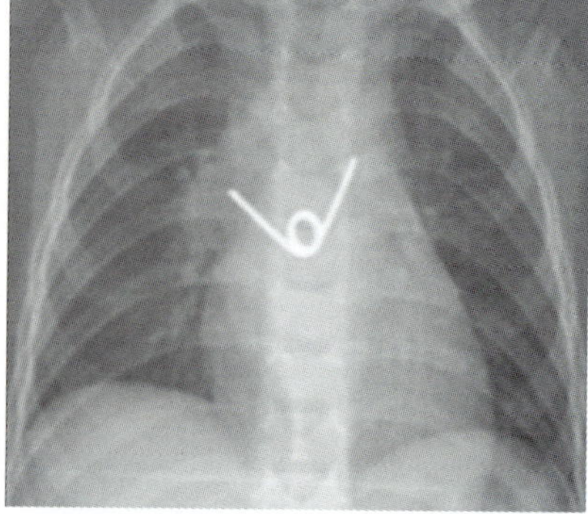

Fig. 27: Open safety pin esophagus.

- Plan for endoscopy within a few hours and keep all necessary accessories for FB removal.
- Locate the nature of FB and note its level in the esophagus
- Look for any local mucosal impaction and ulceration or even penetration
- FB with sharp edges or metal projections needs careful assessment and removal
- You may notice severe chemical esophagitis if button batteries are overlooked for a long duration. Hence, this situation merits urgent endoscopy under short general anesthesia (GA).

Food Bolus Obstruction

- Common in elderly and edentulous patients
- Chunk of meat, vegetable parts, chicken bone, and fish bone are often the culprit.
- Look for any local impaction or penetration of the esophagus by sharp objects
- Underlying stricture has to be considered and addressed.
- Radiological imaging may be needed including CT neck and chest in selected cases if impaction or perforation is suspected.
- Keep all different FB removal accessories ready during the procedure
- Your experience, expertise, common sense, and luck would determine the outcome.

Esophagitis

- Usually presents with acute onset of retrosternal discomfort and odynophagia
- Various grades of esophagitis due to gastroesophageal reflux disease (GERD) are commonly found.
- Also consider various types of esophagitis
- Common causes for esophagitis are as follows:
    - GERD
    - Infective
        - Viral
        - Bacterial
        - Fungal
    - Immune mediated
    - Chemical mediated
        - *Corrosives:* Acid/alkali
        - Drug induced
        - Alkaline reflux

Viral esophagitis:

- It is due to herpes simplex or cytomegalovirus (CMV) infection [as in an human immunodeficiency virus (HIV)-infected patient]
- It usually presents as vesicles, hyperemia, or ulcers predominantly in the mid and lower esophagus. We should consider a biopsy.
- It is usually treated with acyclovir (for H simplex) and ganciclovir or foscovir (for CMV) and repeat endoscopy after 10 days to see the response.

*Esophageal candidiasis **(Fig. 28)**:*

- It is a common cause for painful dysphagia (odynophagia).
- It often appears as whitish plaques in the whole of the esophagus which are difficult to flush out and also have underlying hyperemic esophageal mucosa.
- Take a biopsy or brush cytology and make KOH preparation and see for hyphae or do culture
- We should look for associated oral thrush.
- It is very common in immuno-compromised patients with diabetes, tuberculosis (TB), HIV, cancer, or in patients taking steroid inhalers or cancer chemotherapy.
- Two weeks of oral fluconazole is the therapy of choice.

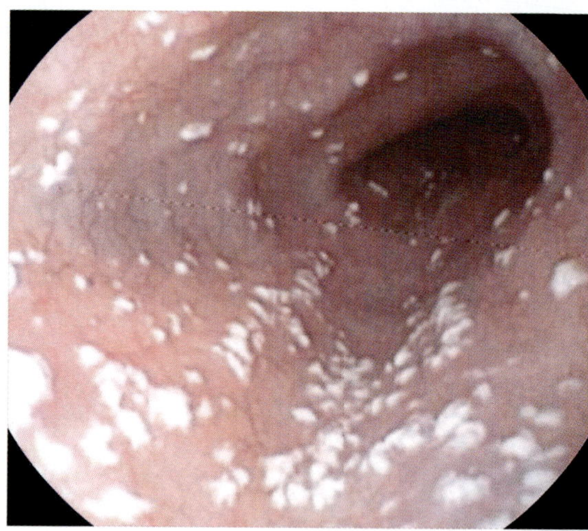

Fig. 28: Esophageal candidiasis.

*Tuberculosis of the esophagus **(Fig. 29)**:*

- It is very rare and usually seen in an already-known case of TB.
- It usually presents with ulcers in the midesophagus
- There may also be some extrinsic compression of midesophagus or penetrating ulcers or sinuses due to erosion of mediastinal caseating nodes into esophagus.
- Rarely, it could also present as traction diverticulum in midesophagus.

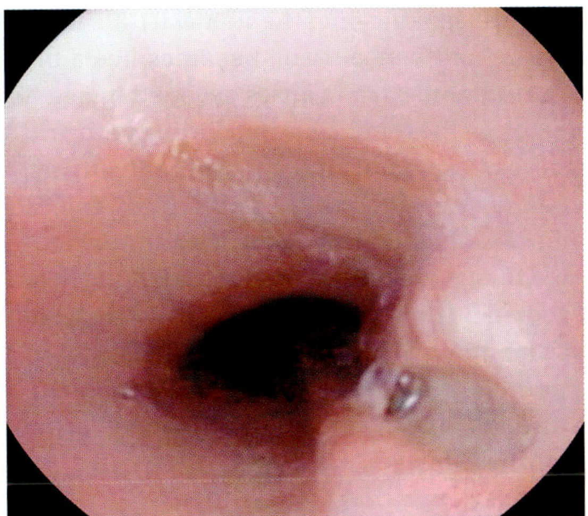

Fig. 29: Esophageal tuberculosis.

Corrosive esophagitis ***(Fig. 30)****:*

- *Common acids:* Battery acid, bathroom cleaners, or sulfuric acid and nitric acid in the laboratory or workplace
- *Common alkali:* Kitchen and bathroom cleaners
- It is due to accidental intake or with suicidal/homicidal intent in some cases.
- Acid has a pungent odor and burning taste and hence difficult to take large quantities while alkali is odorless and tasteless and one tends to gulp large quantities without realizing the consequences.
- Acid causes coagulation necrosis of affected tissue and often spares the esophagus but causes damage primarily to the antrum of the stomach

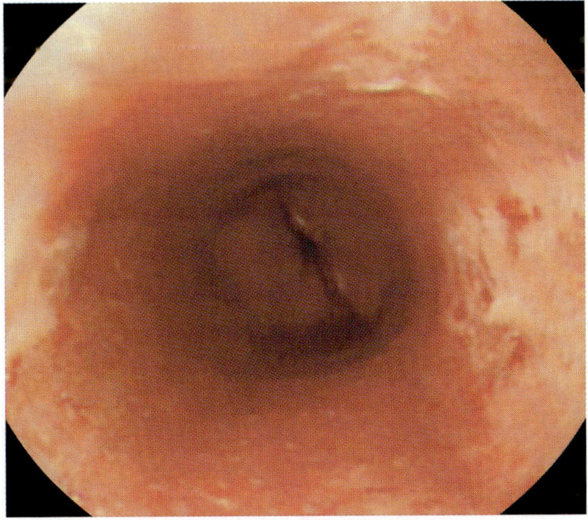

Fig. 30: Corrosive esophagitis.

(acid licks the esophagus but bites the stomach). Alkali causes liquefaction necrosis of tissue and hence tissue becomes like a blotting paper and is prone to perforation. Alkali causes severe damage to the esophagus (alkali is a demon to the esophagus but darling to gastric mucosa).

- In all cases of corrosive poisoning, assess the airway, breathing, and circulation before any endoscopic examination. Typically, they present with drooling of saliva, dyspnea, chest pain, odynophagia, and even hematemesis. Often patients could have stridor due to laryngeal edema.
- Endoscopy should be done early (within 24–48 hours) by an experienced endoscopist with minimal insufflation. Take measures to avoid retching.
- We should gently examine the oral cavity, esophagus, stomach, and duodenum and look for the type and severity of lesions and grade the degree of corrosive damage.
- *Grades of corrosive damage:*
  - *Grade 1:* Hyperemia of mucosa (heals well in few days)
  - *Grade 2:* Ulcers (prone to fibrosis and stricture)
  - *Grade 3:* Grayish appearance due to necrosis (risk of perforation)
  - Endoscopy is usually repeated 3 or 4 weeks later preferably following a barium study or CT chest and upper abdomen.

Pill-induced esophagitis **(*Fig. 31*)**:

- It usually presents with retrosternal pain on eating and drinking
- It often appears as short linear or punched-out ulcers typically in the midesophagus
- History of intake of drugs such as tetracycline, erythromycin, iron tablets, KCl, and some NSAIDs
- Advise liquid diet and oral anesthetic antacid gel (Mucaine gel)
- Consider repeat endoscopy and biopsy if symptoms persist for >1 week

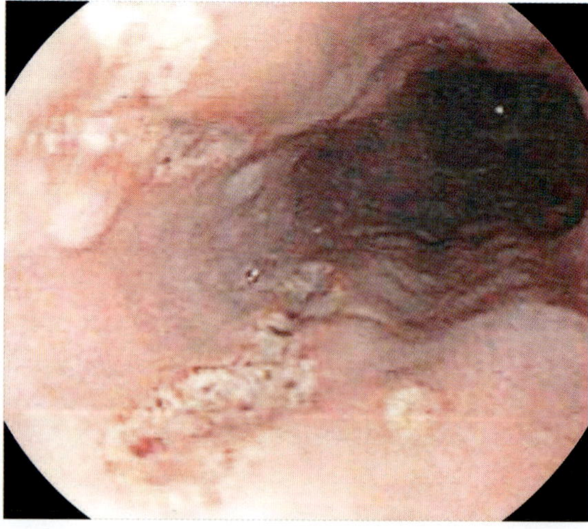

Fig. 31: Pill esophagitis.

Benign Stricture Esophagus

- Postcricoid web
- Zenker's diverticulum
- Corrosive stricture
- Peptic stricture
- Achalasia cardia

Postcricoid web ***(Fig. 32)****:*

- In case of severe iron deficiency anemia with koilonychia, glossitis (Plummer-Vinson syndrome/Patterson-Brown-Kelly syndrome)
- You may notice diaphragm-like thin fibrous stricture at 15 cm from incisor teeth.
- It is a premalignant condition.
- Bleeding or perforation could result if we use undue force during intubation of the esophagus.
- Consider endoscopy over a metal guidewire with a flexible tip or consider doing endoscopic dilatation under C-arm control
- We should investigate and treat anemia to prevent recurrence.

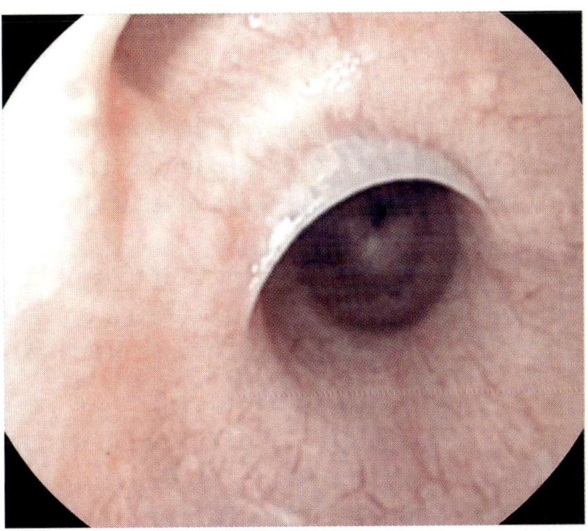

Fig. 32: Postcricoid web.

Zenker's diverticulum ***(Fig. 33)****:*

- Consider this entity in all cases of difficulty in intubation of the esophagus in elderly
- It is a type of pulsion diverticulum noted at a 15 cm level from the incisor between the transverse and oblique fibers of the inferior pharyngeal constrictor muscle.
- It may appear as a small pouch at a 15 cm level in early cases (but rare).

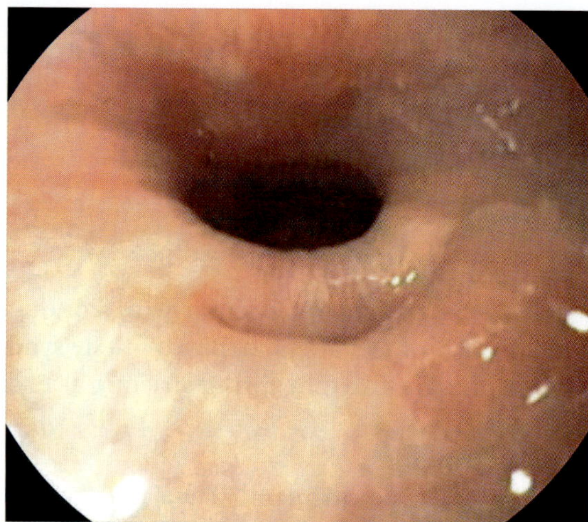

Fig. 33: Zenker's diverticulum.

- But in a typical case, you will notice (if you are careful) the presence of twin channel with you entering a blunt-ending pouch every time.
- The esophageal lumen is pushed anteriorly, and the diverticular opening is located posteriorly and often in line with the usual axis of the esophagus.
- Residual food material may be present in the bottom of a large pouch.
- Consider barium swallow or CT neck to evaluate further
- Elective endoscopic excision of Zenker's diverticulum is feasible in the hands of experts.
- Rarely, you may notice midthoracic traction type of diverticulum due to previous mediastinal nodal TB with scarring. Lower esophageal or epiphrenic diverticulum may be present in case of achalasia cardia.

Corrosive stricture ***(Fig. 34)****:*

- History of corrosive poisoning and long history of dysphagia, vomiting, and weight loss will be present.
- We should get either barium swallow or CT chest and abdomen.
- Endoscopy would reveal single or multiple areas of stricture in esophagus and stomach.
    - *Stricture in esophagus:*
        - Commonly found at 15, 25, and 40 cm level
        - Could be short web-like or long tortuous and could be multiple.
        - Associated mucosal changes like hyperemia or ulceration may be present.
    - *Antrum of stomach:* Usually present as a small contracted and deformed stomach with antral wall thickening and stricture making it difficult to find and pass through the pylorus

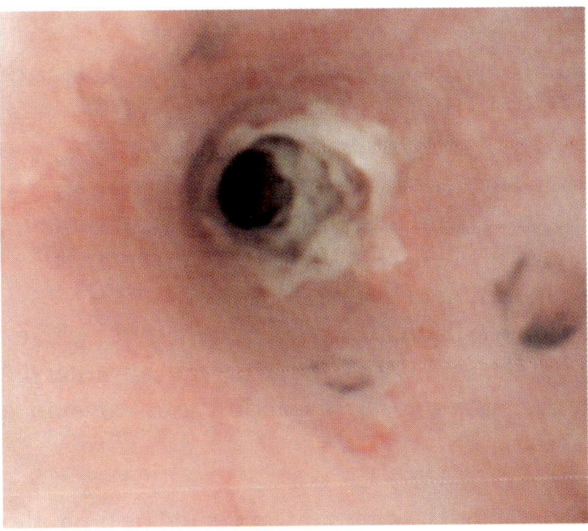

Fig. 34: Corrosive stricture.

Peptic stricture ***(Fig. 35)****:*

- Long-term complication of various grades of esophagitis due to GERD
- It is usually present in the lower esophagus just above the Z-line.
- It often appears as a short irregular stricture with associated ulceration
- We need to look for its relationship with Z-line and the level of opening of hiatus
- We should consider biopsy to rule out malignancy.
- Dilatation with a CRE balloon or Savary dilator may be needed to enter the stomach.
- We have to thoroughly examine the stomach including cardia during J-maneuver.

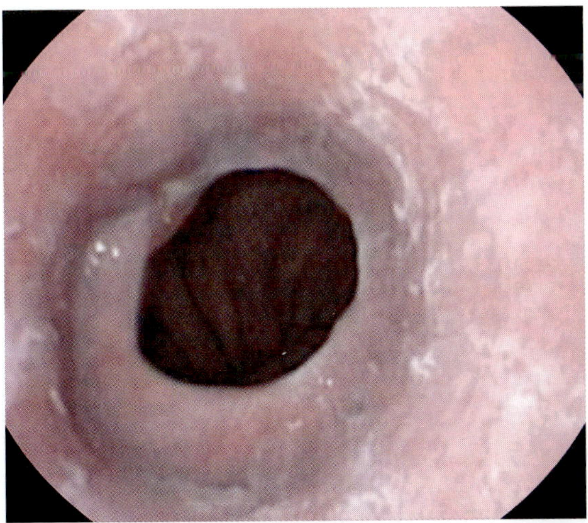

Fig. 35: Peptic stricture.

Benign Tumors of Esophagus

- *Fibroepithelial polyp*: Pedunculated lesion of variable size from a few mm to a few cm
- *Submucosal esophageal lesions:*
  - Leiomyoma and lipoma are common pathology.
  - Appear as an ill-defined submucosal lesion of variable size
  - Normal but stretched-out mucosa over the lump
  - Mucosa can be tented by biopsy forceps.
  - Routine biopsy will not be useful and interferes with excision later.
  - Endoscopic US or MRI is essential prior to any intervention
  - Endoscopic submucosal dissection and excision are feasible in selected cases.
- *Esophageal hemangioma:*
  - It appears as a bluish soft lesion and could be multiple.
  - We should avoid biopsy in such a situation and consider EUS.

Achalasia Cardia (Fig. 36)

- Present with a long history of intermittent dysphagia both for solids and liquids, history of recurrent aspiration pneumonia and vomiting
- *Classical endoscopy findings:*
  - The presence of frothy fluid and food debris in the esophagus is very typical.
  - Esophagus appears very dilated and capacious and lacks propulsive peristaltic contractions
  - Spastic ectopically located esophagus-gastric (OG) junction
  - Difficulty in entering the stomach

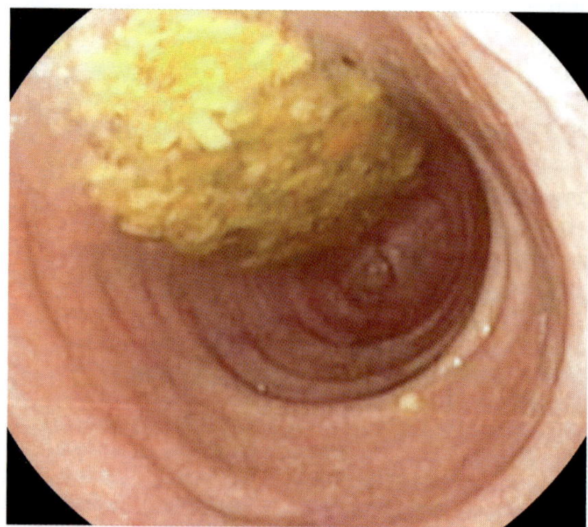

Fig. 36: Achalasia cardia.

- Perform J-maneuver to assess the cardia carefully to exclude any small scirrhous tumor (pseudoachalasia). Take multiple biopsies if needed.
- Barium swallow shows typical short smooth narrowing at the EG junction with the dilated esophagus (bird beak sign and sigmoid esophagus)
- Manometry is required before any therapy to confirm the diagnosis. It will show elevated pressure and failure of relaxation at lower esophageal sphincter (LES) level on wet swallow and absence of propulsive peristalsis.
- Endoscopic US would reveal muscular hypertrophy and exclude any small cancer at cardia.
- *Treatment options are as follows:*
  - Endoscopic pneumatic dilatation under image intensifier
  - Laparoscopic Heller's myotomy
  - Peroral endoscopic myotomy (POEM)

Malignant Tumor Esophagus (Fig. 37)

- Mostly squamous cell carcinoma (adenocarcinoma is common in the lower esophagus)
- Look for the level, length, size, and nature of the tumor
- Note the upper and lower limit of the tumor. The upper esophagus extends from 15 to 20 cm from the incisor teeth, the midesophagus from 20 to 30 cm, and the lower esophagus is beyond 30 cm. But the levels are just arbitrary.
- See the extent of involvement of esophageal circumference and degree of stenosis of the esophageal lumen
- For the carcinoma lower esophagus, look at the lower limit of the tumor with the Z-line, examine the cardia during the J-maneuver, and look for any tumor encroachment.

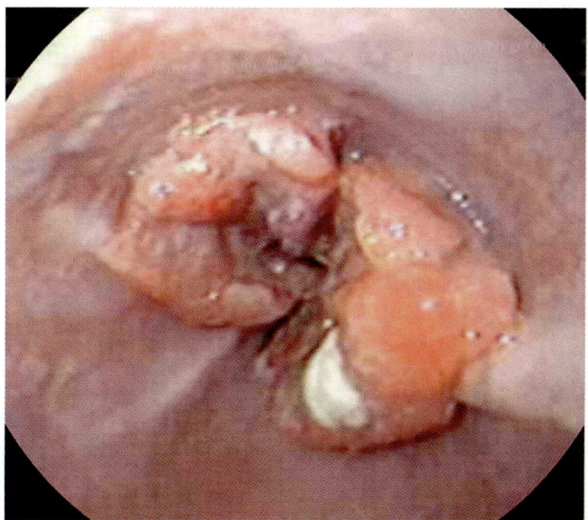

Fig. 37: Carcinoma esophagus.

- *Present as polypoidal, ulcerative, or infiltrative types:*
  - *Polypoidal tumor:* Often appears as a very vascular and soft and friable mass occluding the esophageal lumen
  - *Ulcerative/infiltrative type:* It appears as an indurated lesion with raised margins and necrotic base. Look for any fistula to airway in case of upper and midesophageal lesions. Perforation and false passage are likely if we use undue force during endoscopy and biopsy.
- Take multiple bits of tumor tissue for histological examination
- Consider CRE balloon or Savary dilatation if needed to cross the stricture area. But prior imaging with barium swallow and CT chest and upper abdomen would be preferable in difficult cases.
- NBI and endoscopic US could yield additional useful findings.
- Palliative treatment may entail the deployment of self-expanding metal (SEM) stent.

Case of Upper Gastrointestinal Bleeding

It is defined as bleeding from the esophagus, stomach, or duodenum and is usually present as hematemesis, melena, or anemia.

We should take a good history with regard to the duration and severity of symptoms, history of intake of drugs such as NSAIDs, aspirin, and steroids, and history of alcohol dependence and chronic liver disease.

One should look for the following findings during the clinical examination:

- Vital signs (if in shock, first resuscitate then investigate)
- Anemia, jaundice, and signs of liver failure
- Examination of the abdomen for hepatosplenomegaly
  Splenomegaly indicates portal HT
- PR to look for any melena

The following are the common causes for upper GI bleeding:

- *Esophagus:*
  - Esophagitis
  - Esophageal varices
  - Mallory–Weiss tear
- *Stomach:*
  - Erosive gastritis (drug-induced/alcohol)
  - Fundal varices
  - Gastric ulcer
- *Duodenum:* Duodenal ulcer

Esophagitis with Bleeding

Appears as linear erosions in the lower esophagus with oozing.

Esophageal Varices

- They are the endoscopic signs of portal hypertension
- Present as dilated submucosal esophageal veins (portosystemic collaterals between portal system) (left gastric and short gastric veins) and systemic veins (azygos and hemiazygos veins)
- Appear as dilated long, tortuous, submucosal venous columns from Z-line upward for variable distance
- 1–4 columns may be present.
- Note the size and length of the each variceal column and grade them (grades 1–4).

Grade of varices **(Figs. 38 to 40)**:

- *Grade 1:* It appears as small varices disappearing on insufflation of esophagus (missing varices)

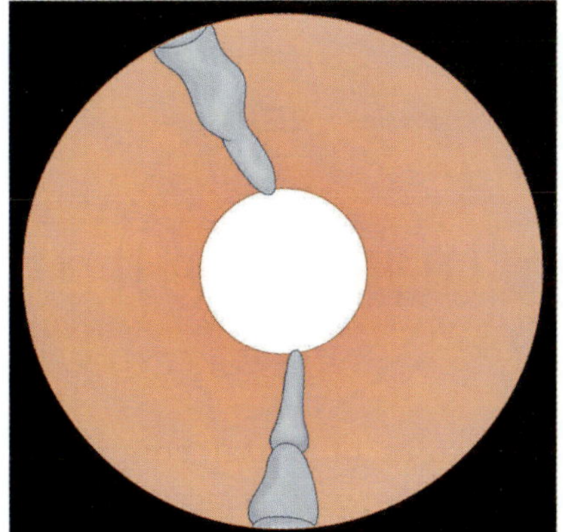

Fig. 38: Grade 1 varices.

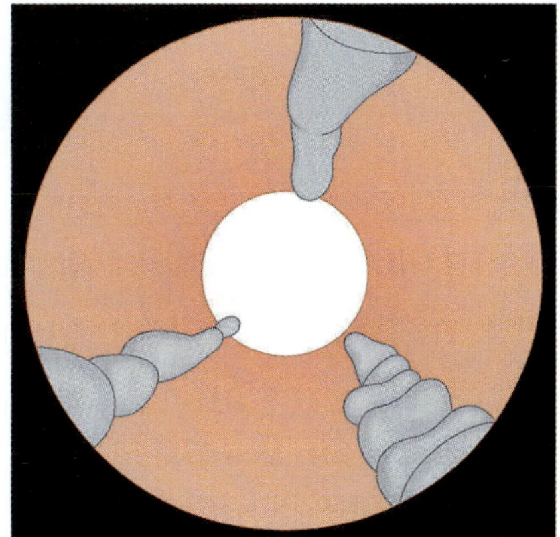

Fig. 39: Grade 2 varices.

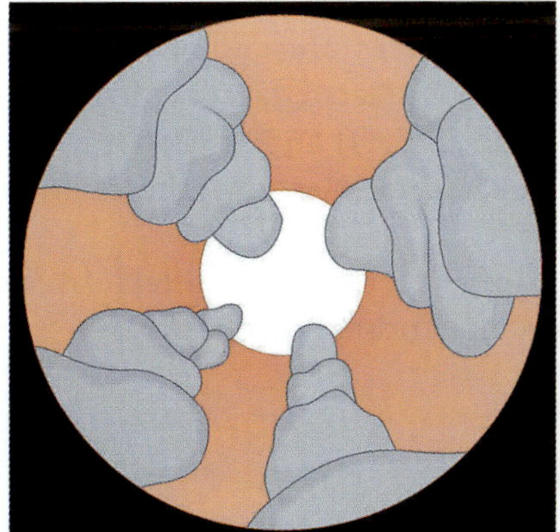

Fig. 40A: Grade 3 varices.

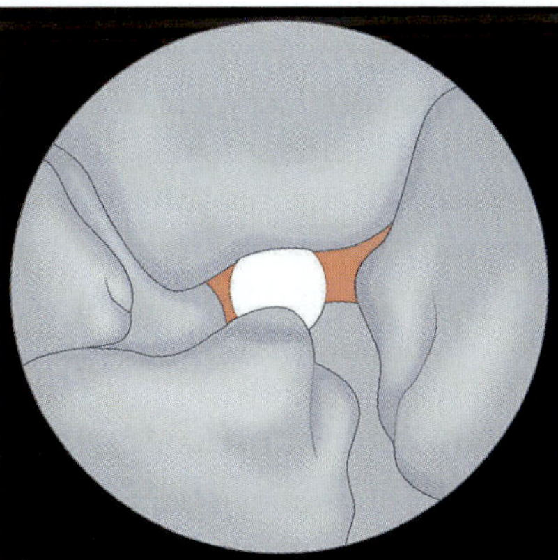

Fig. 40B: Grade 4 varices.

- *Grade 2:* It appears as varices <5 mm in width
- *Grade 3:* It appears as varices >5 mm in width
- *Grade 4:* Large varices almost filling the esophageal lumen (kissing varices)
    - Look for any cherry-red spot **(Fig. 41)** or red whale sign on the surface of the big varices. If present, they usually indicate the presence of intramucosal varices and denote an increased risk of bleeding

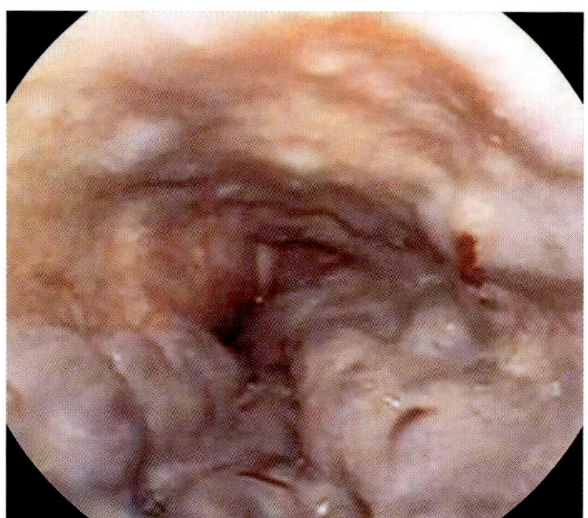

Fig. 41: Cherry red spot.

    - Look for associated severity and extent of portal congestive gastropathy, any fundal varix, varix in any other ectopic locations such as antrum or even duodenum
    - Risk of bleeding is high in grade 3 or 4 varices, fundal varices, and also in the presence of cherry-red spots and red whale streaks on the surface of varices.

Consider endotherapy for all cases of varices presenting with active bleeding or with a history of GI bleeding recently (secondary prophylaxis).

Consider banding for big varices (grade 3 or 4) and sclerotherapy for small varices or residual varices (grade 1 or 2). Glue injection is the treatment of choice for fundal varix.

Prophylactic endoscopic banding can be considered in select cases of grade 3 or 4 varices to prevent any GI bleeding (primary prophylaxis)

Mallory–Weiss Tear (Fig. 42)

- It often occurs after a bout of alcohol intake
- Typically, the patient complains of retching and vomiting a few times before any episode of hematemesis

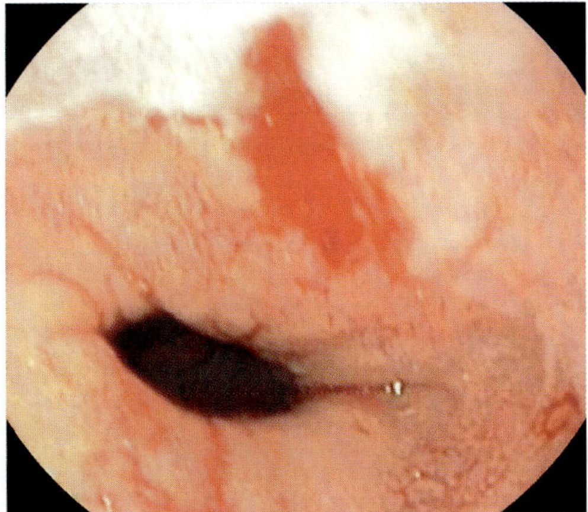

Fig. 42: Mallory–Weis ulcer.

- Diagnostic endoscopy shows linear mucosal tear of a few mm in length with oozing. It is commonly noted in the lower esophagus just above the Z-line or seen at the cardia during the J-maneuver.
- Boerhaave syndrome is a spontaneous rupture of the esophagus and presents with severe chest pain and dyspnea. Look for pneumomediastinum and pleural effusion. Gastrografin swallows or CT chest could be diagnostic.

Gastritis (Fig. 43)

- Note the type, extent, and severity of gastritis
- Multiple areas of erosions, hemorrhagic areas, or oozing are commonly noted.

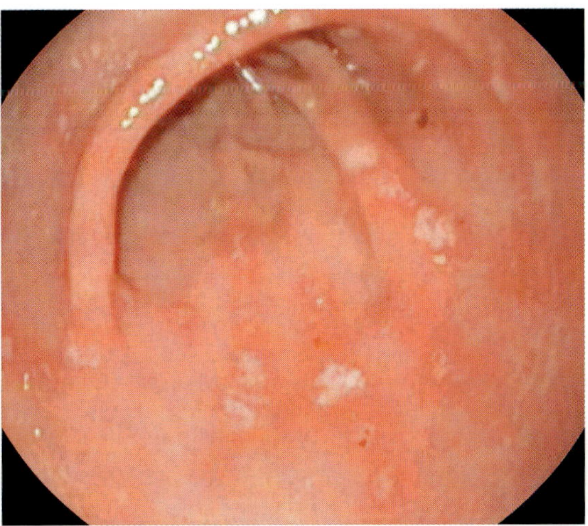

Fig. 43: Prepyloric erosions.

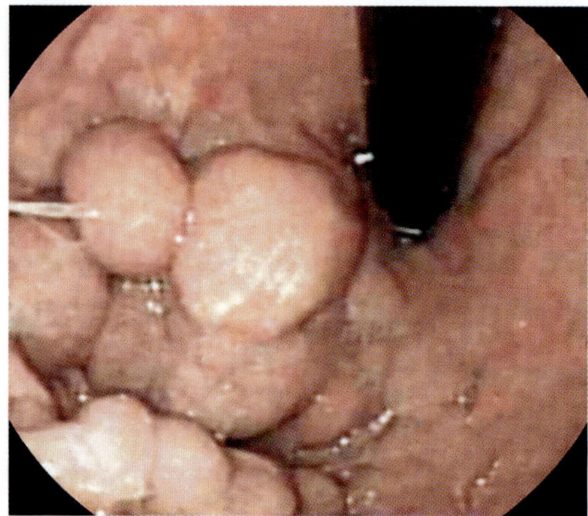

Fig. 44: Fundal varices.

Fundal Varices (Figs. 44 to 48)

- It is located in the fundal region and seen during the J-maneuver.
- It can be easily missed in an actively bleeding patient due to collected blood clots in the fundus masking the view. Adequate irrigation and suction are needed. Also, try changing the patient to a supine or sitting position to look at the cardia.
- Note the size and extent of fundal varices and evidence of any recent bleeding
- It usually appears as a bunch of grapes hanging from the roof. Differential diagnosis (DD): Leiomyoma of the stomach
- It can be seen either as an extension of esophageal varices to the stomach [gastroesophageal varices (GEV) 1 and 2] or as isolated gastric varices (IGV 1 and 2)

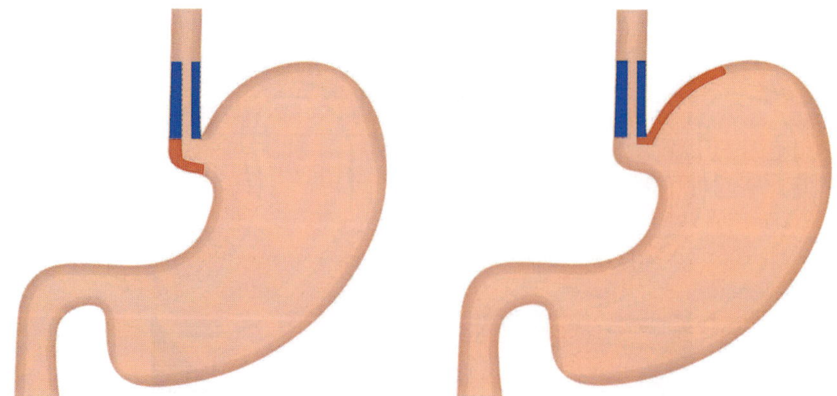

Fig. 45: Gastroesophageal varices (GEV) 1. **Fig. 46:** Gastroesophageal varices (GEV) 2.

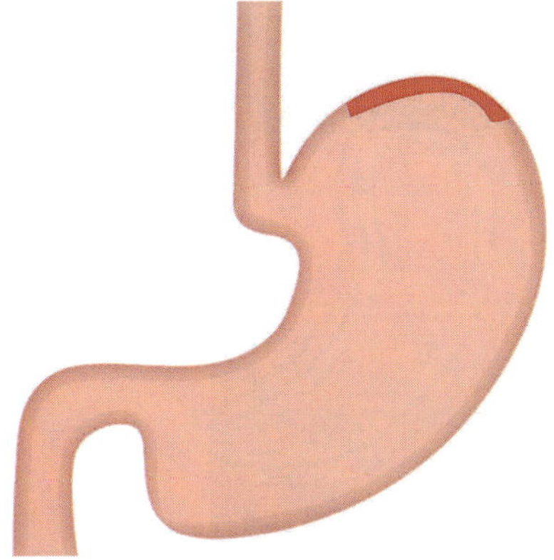

Fig. 47: Isolated gastric varices (IGV) 1.

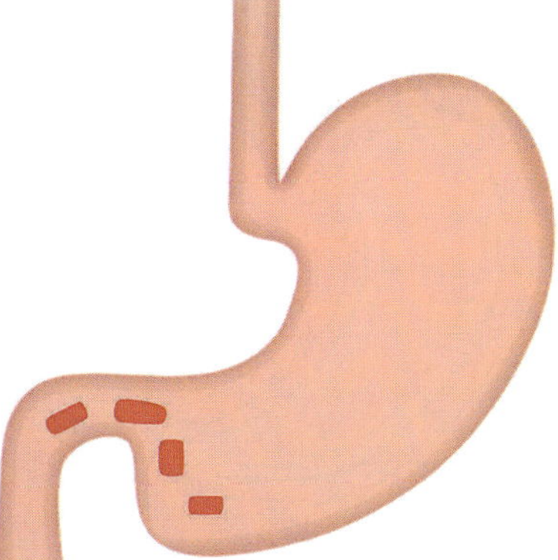

Fig. 48: Isolated gastric varices (IGV) 2.

Gastric and Duodenal Ulcers

- Note the site, size, and number of ulcers, margins, and surface
- Large posterior duodenal ulcer could bleed torrentially from gastroduodenal vessel
- High lesser curve or posterior gastric ulcer could also bleed heavily from left gastric or splenic artery.
- Classify them as per the Forrest grading to understand the risk of any further bleeding
  - *Forrest grading:*
    - *Grade 1:* Actively bleeding lesions
      - *Grade 1A:* With arterial spurting
      - *Grade 1B:* With constant or intermittent oozing
    - *Grade 2:* With stigmata of recent bleeding and risk for further future bleeding (potential bleeder)
      - *Grade 2A:* Nonbleeding visible vessel
      - *Grade 2B:* Surface covered by a blood clot and difficult to dislodge on irrigation
      - *Grade 2C:* Covered by black spot due to hematin pigment
    - *Grade 3:* Clean-based ulcers are unlikely to bleed.

Rare causes of Upper Gastrointestinal Bleeding

- *Angiodysplasia of esophagus, stomach, or duodenum* ***(Fig. 49)****:* Appears as a bright red flat or slightly elevated vascular lesion (as in Osler–Rendu–Weber syndrome, connective tissue disorders, irradiation, cirrhosis of the liver, and chronic renal failure)
- *Dieulafoy lesion:* Small, 1 mm papular lesion hidden in the rugal folds usually in the proximal stomach with intermittent bleeding due to arteriolar spurt. One may notice it on a lucky day.

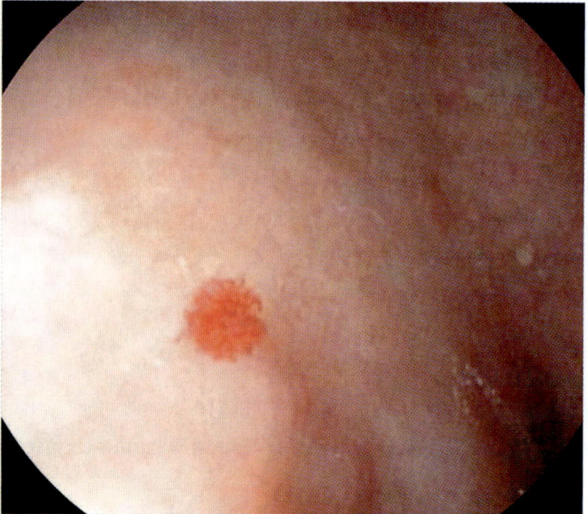

Fig. 49: Angiodysplasia.

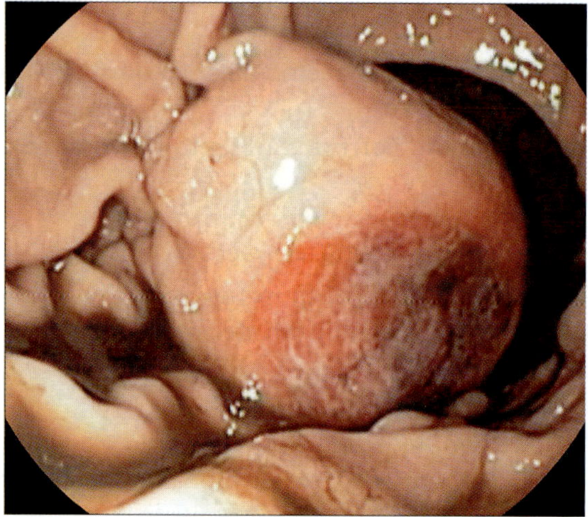

Fig. 50: Leiomyoma stomach.

- Watermelon stomach (GAVE syndrome)
- Leiomyoma or cancer stomach presenting as a bleeding source **(Fig. 50)**

A Case of Atypical Chest Pain

We need to consider the following causes namely:

- Various types of esophagitis and associated hiatus hernia
- Motility disorders, e.g., diffuse esophageal spasm

Hiatus Hernia

- *Types:* Sliding hiatus hernia, paraesophageal, and mixed type
    - *Sliding hiatus hernia (>80%)* ***(Figs. 51A and B)****:*
        - EG junction appears patulous with prolapsing gastric mucosa on retching
        - Note the double-ring configuration with intervening bell-shaped dilatation. The proximal ring is formed by LES and the distal ring by the esophageal hiatus

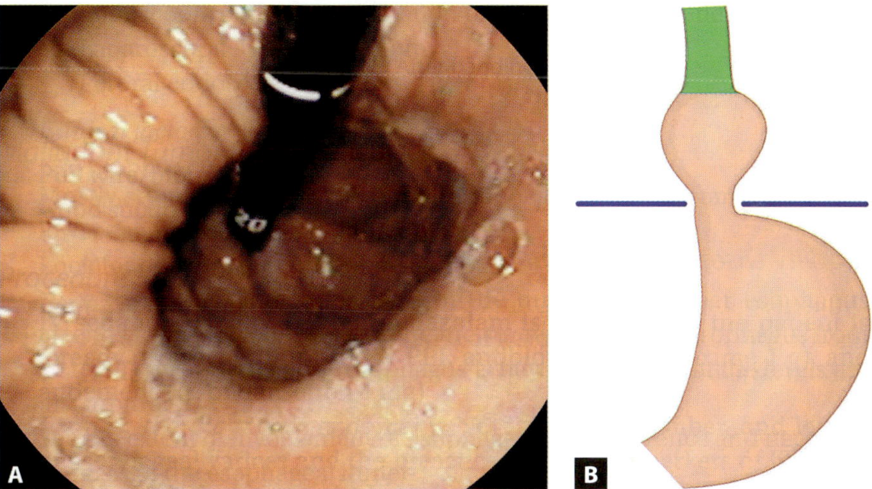

Figs. 51A and B: Sliding hiatus hernia.

        - Note the level of Z-line and hiatus from the incisor teeth
        - Note the shortened distance between the Z-line and incisor teeth
        - Note any associated reflux esophagitis
        - Sliding hiatus hernia is best appreciated on J-maneuver where you notice the endoscope passing through the cardia. The endoscope is not firmly clasped or gripped by the hiatus. There is significant space between the scope and hiatal opening depending on the size of the hernia. Hill's classification describes four grades of hiatus and grade 4 is usually considered as sliding hiatus hernia.
    - *Paraesophageal hernia* ***(Figs. 52A and B)****:*
        - It is seldom seen. EG junction appears normal.
        - On J-maneuver, one may notice an endoscope which is firmly gripped by the hiatus. But, one would also notice a separate defect in the diaphragm next to the hiatus through which stomach is seen herniating.
    - *Mixed type (very rare):* Both sliding and paraesophageal hernia coexist.

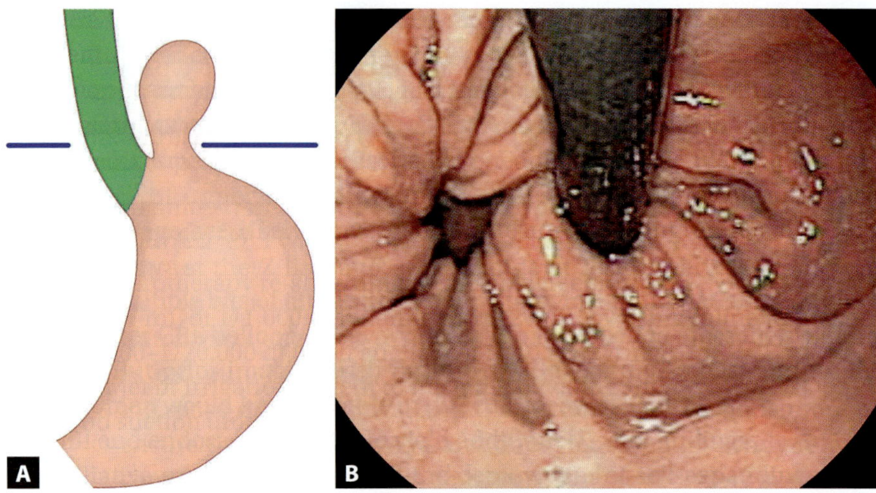

Figs. 52A and B: Paraesophageal hernia.

Motility Disorders

Diffuse esophageal spasm or nutcracker esophagus may not show any typical endoscopic abnormality but is recognized by high-resolution manometry. Barium swallow may show a corkscrew appearance of esophagus.

SURVEILLANCE ENDOSCOPY

- Barrett's esophagus
- Varices
- Postoperative cases

Barrett's Esophagus (Fig. 53)

- It is the complication of GERD due to metaplasia of squamous epithelium to columnar epithelium.
- It appears as salmon-pink gastric mucosa extending on to esophageal lumen
- It may appear as a circumferential sheet, as tongue-like projections creeping up from the EG junction or as isolated islands of columnar mucosa interspersed with squamous mucosa.
- Note the level of Z-line and level of hiatus from incisor teeth and also look for any hiatus hernia.
- The Z-line is at least 3 cm or more proximal to esophageal hiatus.
- Look for any associated ulceration, nodularity, polypoidal area, or stricture
- Apply NBI to find early lesions and also to assess the extent and severity of BE

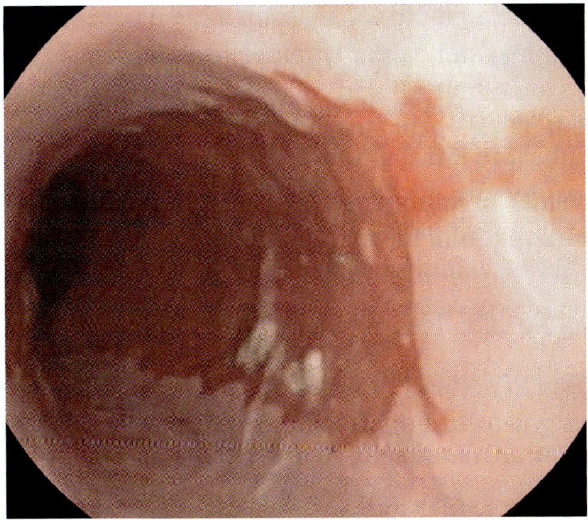

Fig. 53: Barrett's esophagus.

- Chromoendoscopy by spraying the esophagus with either methylene blue or iodine contrast also helps to delineate Barrett's mucosal patches.
- Brush cytology or four quadrant biopsy is needed to look for any dysplasia.
- Dysplasia is divided into four categories: (1) Negative for dysplasia, (2) indefinite for dysplasia (ID), (3) low-grade dysplasia (LGD), and (4) high-grade dysplasia (HGD).

LGD needs regular 3–6 months endoscopic surveillance while HGD merits endoscopic or surgical intervention as the risk of adenocarcinoma is high in such individuals.

Esophageal Varices

- All cases of esophageal varices need monthly endoscopy until all the varices are eradicated and then do surveillance endoscopy once in 6–12 months to look for any residual varix or development of fundal or ectopic varices.
- You may recognize the previous banding sites as whitish fibrotic areas.
- Small residual varix may benefit from injection of sclerosants to facilitate eradication.

Postoperative Conditions

- We should note detailed history regarding indication for surgery and timing and type of operation. We should study the patient record and the previous operative notes and radiological images carefully. Perform systematic endoscopic examination of esophagus, stomach, and duodenum and recognize the postoperative changes like stoma and also look for any associated pathology such as alkaline reflux gastritis, suture granuloma, stomal stenosis, any recurrent tumor, any bleeding lesion or ulcer at the stoma, nature and amount of gastric residue, bezoars, and so on.

- *Antireflux surgery:*
  - Check the EG junction and resistance to pass the hiatus
  - In J-maneuver, look for the tight cardia wrapped by fundal mucosal ring (Nissen's fundoplication) **(Figs. 54A and B)**

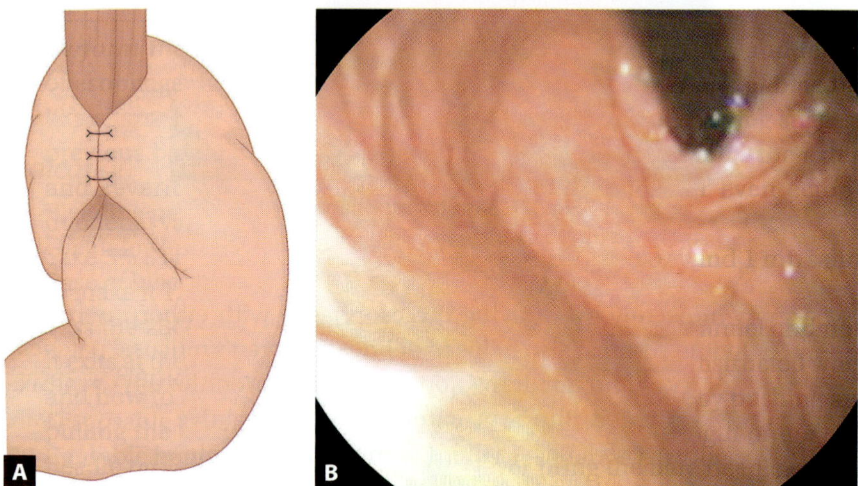

Figs. 54A and B: Post-Nissen's fundoplication.

- *After distal gastrectomy:*
  - Look at the size and nature of gastric remnant
  - *Billroth I type:* With gastroduodenal anastomosis **(Figs. 55A and B)**
    - Look for the size of the stoma and any stomal ulceration, granuloma, or stenosis
    - Any residual food or fluid
    - Extent and severity of bile reflux gastritis
    - Look for evidence of any recurrent tumor (luminal or extrinsic) in case of previous malignancy
  - *Billroth II type:* With gastrojejunostomy (GJ) **(Figs. 56A and B)**
    - Look for the size and nature of gastric remnant
    - Look at the GJ stoma and recognize efferent and afferent loops
- *Efferent loop:* Usually easy to locate and easy to enter. Usually, it is noted along the greater curve and appears at the bottom of the monitor. It usually appears empty and leads directly to distal jejunal loops. One may recognize the side-to-side (Braun) anastomosis in some cases. Look for any stenosis, ulcer, or tumor recurrence at the stoma.

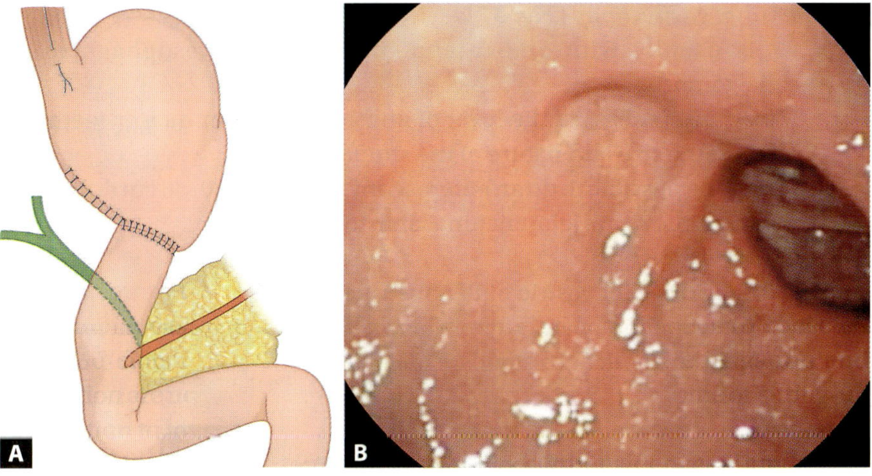

Figs. 55A and B: Billroth I gastrectomy.

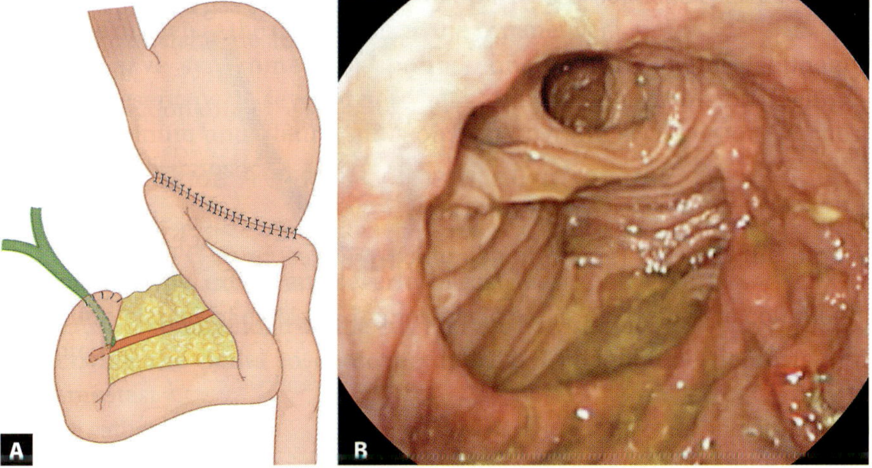

Figs. 56A and B: Billroth II gastrectomy.

- *Afferent loop:* Usually difficult to see and enter. It appears on the top part of the monitor often at 12–3 o'clock position. Often filled with frothy bile. Further distally you may be able to locate the ampulla of Vater sitting upside down at the bottom of the vertical duodenal mucosal fold. You will finally reach the blind-ending duodenal stump.
  - Side-to-side anastomosis can also be recognized in some cases
  - In cases of Roux-en-Y anastomosis, you will notice only one loop exiting gastric remnant which is further distally joined by the afferent limb. Bile reflux gastritis is absent in such cases.

- *After total gastrectomy* ***(Fig. 57)****:*
    - It is usually with end-to-end or end-to-side esophagojejunal anastomosis.
    - We should measure the level of anastomosis from incisor teeth and look at the size and nature of the stoma.
    - It may be possible to do an enteroscopy for further 20–30 cm downward as far as the distal jejunojejunal anastomosis.
- *After GJ* ***(Fig. 58)****:*
    - Usually done for gastric outlet obstruction
    - Locate the efferent and afferent loops and their adequacy and evidence of any stomal ulcer or stenosis

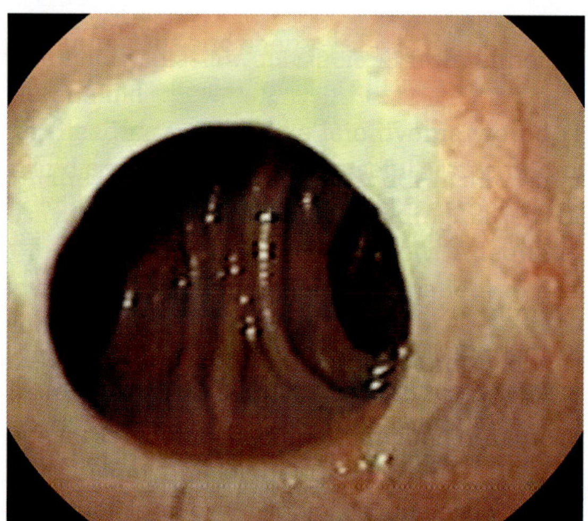

Fig. 57: Total gastrectomy.

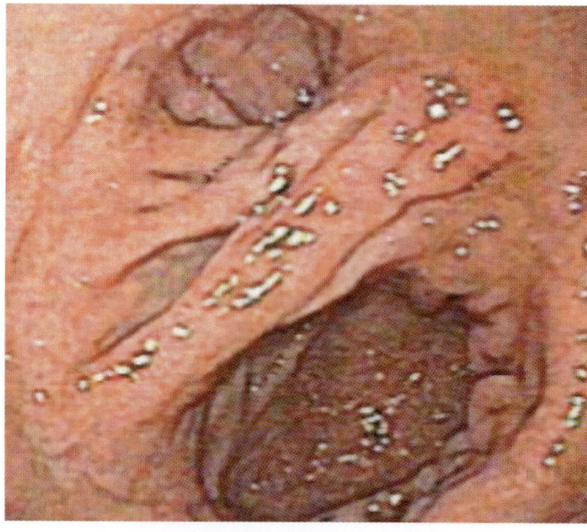

Fig. 58: Gastrojejunostomy.

- Look for the extent and severity of any gastritis and the presence of any bezoar or food residue

- *After esophagectomy with esophagogastric anastomosis:*
  - Note the level and nature of anastomosis
  - Look for any stomal stenosis or tumor recurrence and do biopsy in suspected cases
  - Look for any gastric residue and adequacy of pyloroplasty
- *After bariatric surgery:*
  - *Sleeve gastrectomy* (***Figs. 59A and B***): The sleeve gastrectomy produces a long tubular stomach limited in expansion by a staple line that parallels the lesser curvature. The staple line should be examined for defects and ulcerations. Endoscopy will then reach a normal-looking antrum and pylorus.
  - *Roux-en-Y gastric bypass* (***Figs. 60A and B***)*:* Very small capacity gastric remnant with scope entering the jejunum. The width of the anastomosis

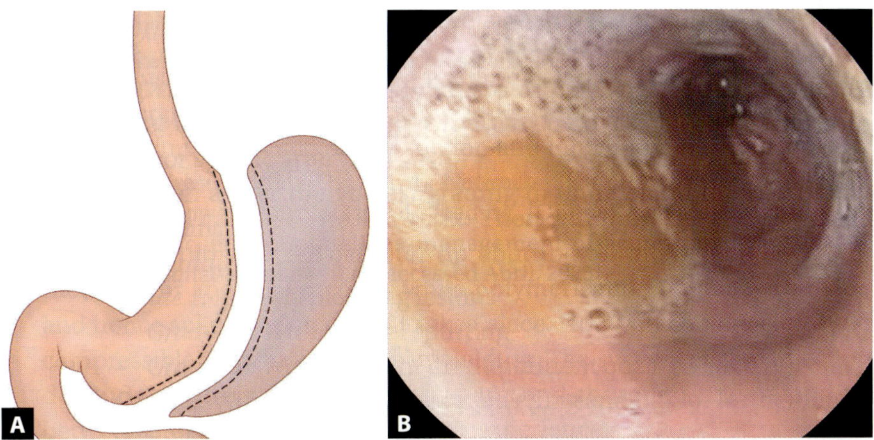

Figs. 59A and B: Sleeve gastrectomy.

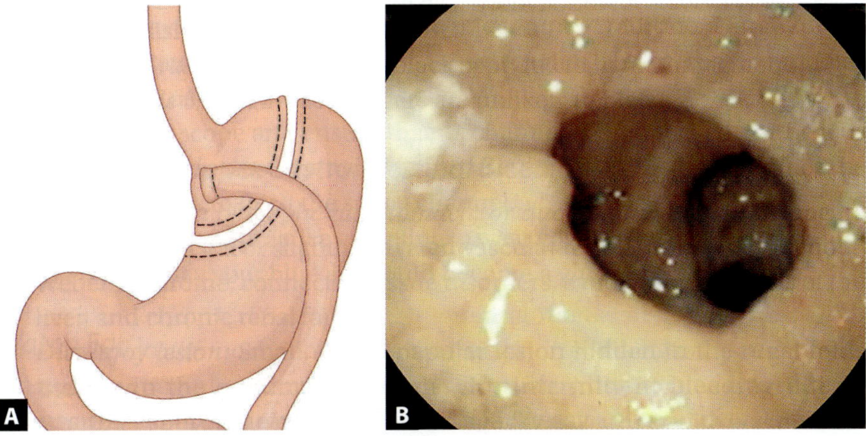

Figs. 60A and B: Post-Roux-en-Y bypass.

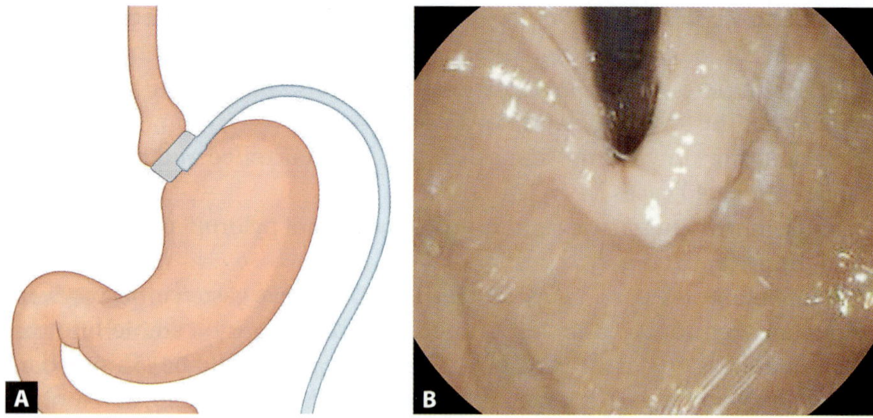

Figs. 61A and B: Post-gastric band.

is generally 10–12 mm in diameter. Beyond the anastomosis, a short, blind limb is often visible alongside the efferent jejunal limb. The jejunojejunal anastomosis can sometimes be reached with an upper endoscope, depending on the length of the Roux limb.

- *Gastric band* ***(Figs. 61A and B)****:* Laparoscopic adjustable gastric bands produce a variable amount of extrinsic circumferential compression on the proximal stomach that is evident on upper endoscopy.

Polyps in the Upper Gastrointestinal Tract

Classification

- Polypoidal lesions in esophagus
- *Polypoidal lesions in the stomach:*
  - Elster glandular cysts
  - Hyperplastic polyps
  - Focal inflammatory hyperplasia or chronic erosions
  - Adenomatous polyps
  - Peutz-Jeghers syndrome
- *Polypoidal lesions in duodenum:*
  - Inflammatory hyperplastic polyps
  - Heterotrophic gastric mucosa
  - Brunner gland hyperplasia
  - Pedunculated adenomatous polyps
  - Flat villous adenoma

Note the size, site, and number of polyps **(Fig. 62)**. Hyperplastic gastric polyps and Elster glandular cysts are common and with normal color of gastric mucosa and hence often overlooked. NBI and chromoendoscopy are helpful. Biopsy is done to confirm the diagnosis. There is no risk of malignancy.

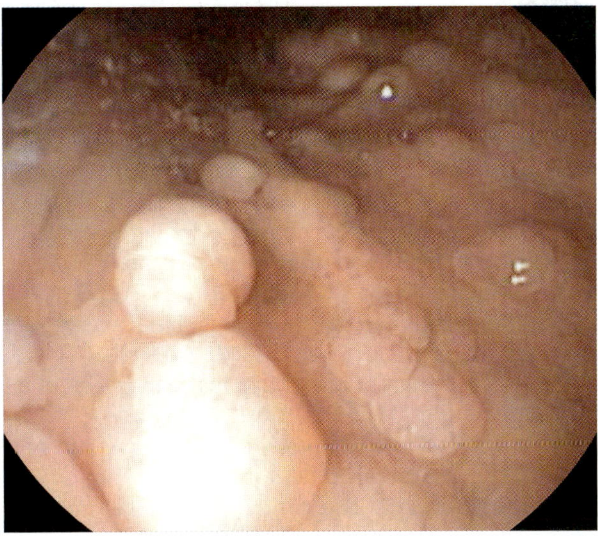

Fig. 62: Gastric polyps.

Elster glandular cysts are small glassy glistening polypoidal lesions in the fundus and body of the stomach and usually are multiple with size <5 mm. They can be easily plucked completely with the help of biopsy forceps.

Hyperplastic polyps are common in the body and antrum of the stomach and appear sessile, often multiple, and size usually <5 mm.

Adenomatous gastric polyps are rare and can be single or multiple and size varies from a few mm to even 1–2 cm and appear erythematous often with long pedicles.

Peutz–Jeghers syndrome can present with hamartomatous polyps in the stomach and duodenum.

CONCLUSION

A good history and examination are essential before endoscopy. We have to perform a thorough endoscopy and describe the findings accurately. Record and document the endoscopic findings using standard medical terminology and correlate with clinical diagnosis.

SUGGESTED READING

1. Calabrese C, Di Febo G, Brandi G, Morselli-Labate AM, Areni A, Scialpi C, et al. Correlation between endoscopic features of gastric antrum, histology and Helicobacter Pylori Infection in adults. Ital J Gastro Hepato. 1999;31(5):359-65.
2. Cotton PB, Price AB, Tighe JR, Beales JS. Preliminary evaluation of "duodenitis" by endoscopy and biopsy. Br Med J. 1973;3(5877):430-3.
3. Dacosta RS, Wilson BC, Marcon NE. New optical technologies for earlier endoscopic diagnosis of premalignant gastrointestinal lesions. J Gastroenterol Hepatol. 2002;17:S86-S105.

4. Dooley CP. Background and historical considerations of *Helicobacter pylori.* Gastroenterol Clin North Am. 1993;22(1):1-4.
5. Elta GH, Appelman HD, Behler EM, Wilson JA, Nostrant TJ. A study of the correlation between endoscopic and histological diagnoses in gastroduodenitis. Am J Gastroenterol. 1987;82(8):749-53.
6. Hecker R, Fitch R. The value of endoscopy and biopsy in the diagnosis of gastric carcinoma. Med J Aust. 1975;2(12):472-4.
7. Hopkins HH. Optical principles of endoscope. In: Berci G (Ed). Endoscopy, 2nd edition. New York: Appleton-Century-Crofts; 1976. pp. 3-26.
8. Joo YE, Park HK, Myung DS, Baik GH, Shin JE, Seo GS, et al. Prevalence and risk factors of atrophic gastritis and intestinal metaplasia: a nationwide multicenter prospective study in Korea. Gut Liver. 2013;7(3):303-10.
9. Levy N, Stermer E. Accuracy of endoscopy in the diagnosis of inflamed gastric and duodenal mucosa. Sr J Med Sci. 1985;21(7):564-8.
10. Marson BC, Dawon IMP. Gastrointestinal Pathology, 2nd edition. London: Blackwell Scientific Publications; 1998. pp. 148-51.
11. McBroom HM, Ramsay AD. The clinicopathological meeting: A means of auditing diagnostic performance. Am J Surg Pathol. 1993;17:75-80.
12. Ofman JJ, Shaheen NJ, Desai AA, Moody B, Bozymski EM, Weinstein WM. The quality of care in Barrett's esophagus: endoscopist and pathologist practices. Am J Gastroenterol. 2001;96(3):876-81.
13. Pailoor K, Sarpangala MK. Histopathological diagnosis of gastric biopsies in correlation with endoscopy- A study in a tertiary care center. Adv Lab Med Int. 2012;3(2):22-31.
14. Paymaster JC, Sanghvi LD, Gangadharan P. Cancer in the gastrointestinal tract in western India. Epidemiologic study. Cancer. 1968;21(2):279-88.
15. Qizibash AH, Stevenson GW. Early gastric cancer. In: Sommers SC, Rosen PP (Eds). Pathology Annals. New York: Appleton-Century-Crofts; 1979. pp. 14-24.
16. Rao DN, Desai PB, Ganesh B. Epidemiological observations on cancer of the oesophagus--a review of Indian studies. Indian J Cancer. 1996;33(2):55-75.
17. Shennak MM, Tarawneh MS, Al-Sheikh TM. Upper gastrointestinal diseases in symptomatic Jordanians: A prospective endoscopic study. Ann Saudi Med. 1997;17(4):471-4.
18. Vartanian RK, Leung JK, Davis JE, Kim YB, Owen DA. A novel Alcian yellow-toluidine blue (Leung) stain for Helicobacter species: comparison with standard stains, a cost-effectiveness analysis, and supplemental utilities. Mod Pathol. 1998;11(1):72-8.
19. Versalovic J. *Helicobacter pylori*: Pathology and Diagnostic Strategies. Am J Clin Pathol. 2003;119:403-12.

Expert's Comment

In this unique book, the approach to examining different lesions of the upper gastrointestinal tract is absolutely original. The primary criterion for exploring this subject is the classical scenario of a patient visiting the outpatient department (OPD) or emergency department to consult with the doctor. Presentations are approached one by one, ranging from common to rare, and all relevant theoretical and practical tips are discussed. This has never been done in any book so far. All possible scenarios, from esophagitis to postbariatric cases, are lucidly examined in detail. Learners and skilled surgeons performing for decades alike will benefit from the expansive information provided in this book. Every classification is analyzed to help the reader make the best of reports of international standards.

One should go through this book repeatedly on the path to becoming a perfect performer with excellent reporting skills. This book has created history by becoming the best textbook and atlas ever written.

Dr Satyapriya De Sarkar
Kolkata

6 CHAPTER

Foreign Body Upper Gastrointestinal Tract

Chapter Outline

Keywords: Coin esophagus, FB esophagus, button battery esophagus, food bolus obstruction, fishbone esophagus

INTRODUCTION

Foreign body ingestion and food bolus impaction occur commonly. Though the majority of ingested foreign bodies will pass spontaneously, at times it could be presented as a surgical emergency with acute dysphagia and odynophagia. Impaction, obstruction with risk of aspiration and rarely even perforation could occur due to ingested foreign body (FB). Hence swift and expert management is paramount in these challenging situations.

COMMON TYPES OF INGESTED FOREIGN BODIES

Accidental Ingestion

Children, mentally challenged adults:

- Coins, pins, and small toys
- Button batteries
- Food bolus
- Denture

Intentional Ingestion

- Razor blades and nails (prisoners)
- Heroin packs (smugglers)

APPROACH TO A CASE OF SUSPECTED FOREIGN BODY INGESTION

- *Take a good history:* Dysphagia, odynophagia, drooling of saliva, and pain in the neck or chest.
- *Clinical examination:*
  - Vital signs
  - Oral cavity, airway, and examination of chest and abdomen
  - Look for crepitus over the neck and chest.
- Do X-rays of the neck and chest and upper abdomen [anteroposterior (AP)/lateral] **(Fig. 1)**

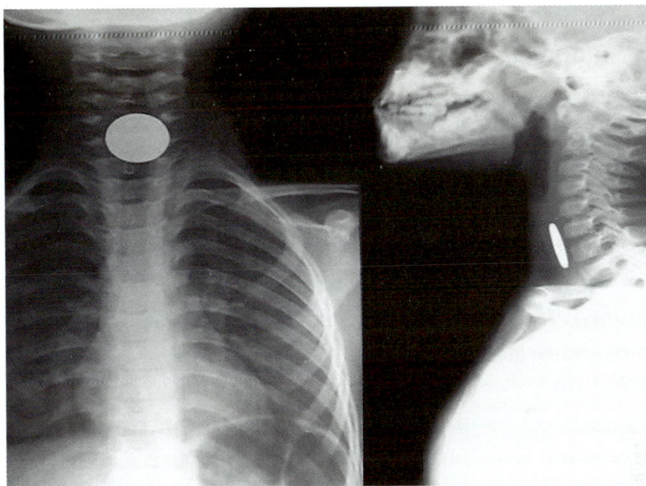

Fig. 1: Foreign body coin in X-ray anteroposterior (AP) and lateral view images.

  - Beware of radiolucent FB
    - *Examples:* Fish and chicken bone, wooden, glass and plastic objects
  - Coin will be seen as a round shadow in the AP view if it is in the esophagus.
  - *Look for signs of perforation:* Mediastinal and free peritoneal air.
  - CT abdomen may be useful if sharp FB with esophageal impaction or penetration is suspected.
  - Barium swallow is not indicated in cases of FB ingestion.
- *Diagnostic endoscopy:*
  - Locate the nature of FB and note its level in the esophagus.
  - Look for any local mucosal impaction and ulceration or even penetration.
  - FB with sharp edges or metal projection needs careful assessment and removal.

- You may notice severe chemical esophagitis in case button batteries that are left out for a long duration. Hence this situation warrants urgent endoscopy under short general anesthesia (GA).
- *Timing of endoscopy:*
    - Immediate endoscopy
        - Button battery in the esophagus
        - Sharp object in the esophagus
    - Urgent endoscopy (within 6 hours)
        - All FB in the esophagus
        - Long FB (>6 cm) or sharp FB in the stomach
        - Magnets within endoscopic reach
    - Non-urgent endoscopy (within 24 hours)
        - Objects in the stomach >2.5 cm diameter
        - Button batteries in the stomach for >2 days.

ENDOSCOPIC REMOVAL OF FOREIGN BODY

Foreign Body Accessories (Figs. 2A to E)

- *Rat-toothed forceps:* Universal use
- *Dormia basket:* Food bolus
- *2 and 3 prong forceps:* Coins and pins
- *Roth net basket:* Rounded objects such as ear studs, diamond rings, and even coins in the stomach.
- *Snare:* Denture
- *Magnet forceps:* For some metallic objects in a difficult location
- *Over tube/hood:* For sharp objects

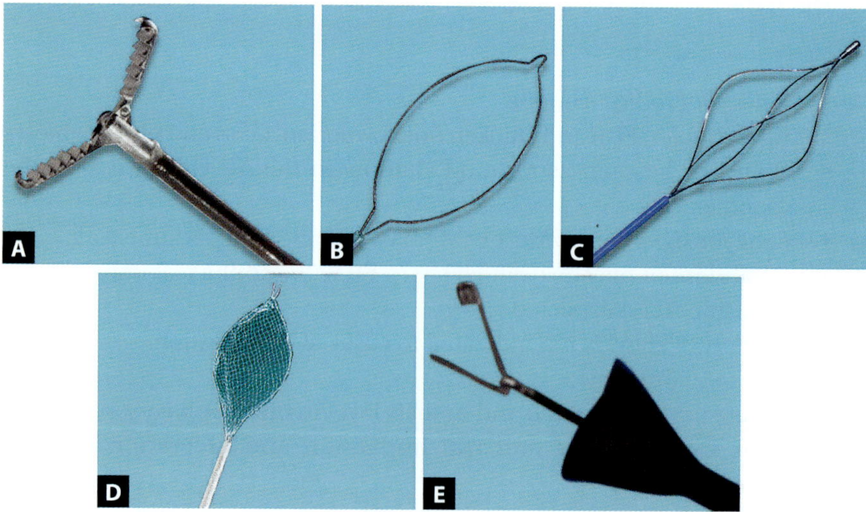

Figs. 2A to E: Foreign body removal accessories. (A) Rat-toothed forceps; (B) Snare; (C) Dormia; (D) Rothnet; and (E) Hood.

Practice Guidelines

- FB esophagus needs immediate attention and removal within 24 hours to avoid the risk of perforation and aspiration. If the FB is already in the stomach and beyond one may choose to observe for spontaneous expulsion in the next 2–5 days.
- Button batteries, dentures with sharp wire, and impacted fish or chicken bones are problem cases and need immediate attention from experts.
- Long or large FB stuck in the stomach or duodenum for >1 week may warrant intervention occasionally.
- Perform an X-ray neck, chest, and abdomen to look for the site and nature of FB. "Coin seen as coin" in the X-ray neck AP view and as a small ridge in the lateral view behind the tracheal air shadow confirms its position in the esophagus, usually either at or just below the cricopharynx.
- In adults, removal can be accomplished under xylocaine spray or conscious sedation but in children, it invariably requires the presence of an anesthetist and GA, as airway control is vital.
- Keep all different FB removal gadgets ready and if possible, do a "Dry run". Practice with similar types of FB such as coins, batteries, and pins kept outside and try to catch them with various types of accessories to decide which one is most suitable for the given occasion. "Dry run" gives us confidence and ensures success.
- Instruct the assistant exactly how to use appropriate accessories.
- Do diagnostic endoscopy and note the following:
  - The site and nature of FB
  - Any impaction or penetration
  - Any injurious sharp ends trailing or pointing up
  - Presence of food debris
  - Any associated distal stricture
- Use the appropriate FB forceps to catch hold of the FB. Gently remove the scope with the accessory as one unit keeping the FB under vision during the whole process of extraction. Take a pause at the cricopharynx to ensure it relaxes to let the FB out!
- In the case of a sharp FB, take care to keep the sharp end trailing, or else you may have to use a hood at the distal end of the scope or even an over tube **(Figs. 3A and B)**.

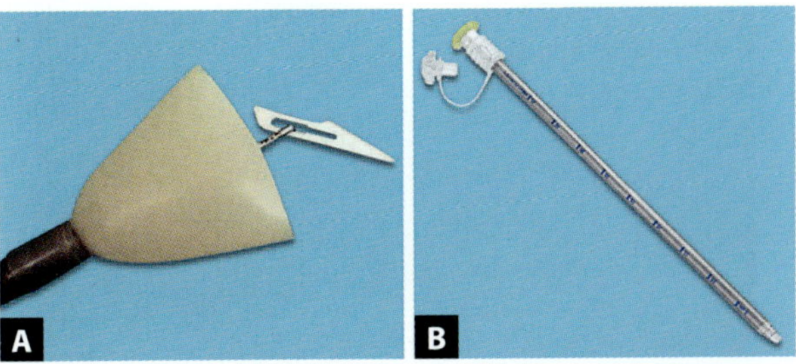

Figs. 3A and B: Sharp objects removal with hood and over the tube.

- FB in the stomach may be lying in the puddle of fluid in the fundus and difficult to see or grasp. You may choose a magnet forceps to grasp the coin and dock it again in the antral region before grasping with a two-prong coin forceps. Or else shift the patient to a semirecumbent position and try.
- Like the surgery for cases of the appendix, it may be the easiest FB to remove and some other day it could turn out to be the most challenging frustrating task.
- Be innovative and use all your knowledge, experience, and common sense!
- Check endoscopy after the removal of FB may be preferable to look for any damage at the site of FB or the presence of any distal stricture.

Watch For

Any bleeding, mucosal damage, or even perforation.

PRACTICE TIPS FOR CHALLENGING FOREIGN BODIES

- *Food bolus obstruction* ***(Fig. 4)****:*
    - It is common in elderly and edentulous patients.
    - Chunks of meat, vegetable parts, chicken bone, and fish bone are often the culprit.
    - Look for any local impaction or penetration of the esophagus by sharp objects.
    - Eosinophilic esophagitis and underlying malignancy have to be considered.
    - Radiological imaging may be needed including computed tomography (CT) neck and chest in selected cases if impaction or perforation is suspected.

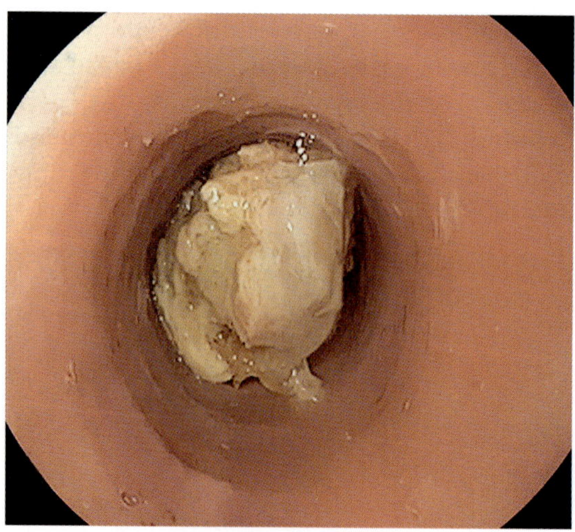

Fig. 4: Food bolus obstruction.

  - Injection glucagon is seldom used and is rather expensive.
  - Keep all different FB removal accessories ready during the procedure.
  - Often the food bolus can be gently pushed into the stomach
  - Associated peptic stricture or Schatzki's ring would warrant dilatation
  - Your experience, expertise, common sense, and luck would determine the outcome.
- *Disk/button batteries* ***(Figs. 5A and B)****:*
  - Button batteries are usually from toys, watches, calculators, and hearing aids.

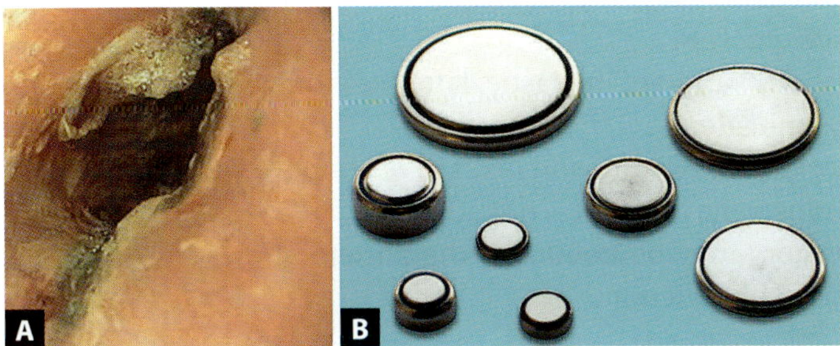

Figs. 5A and B: (A) Foreign body esophagus; and (B) Button battery.

  - Common in children <6 years.
  - Disk battery in esophagus needs urgent removal to prevent severe chemical esophagitis with risk of perforation
  - Use of Roth net or Dormia basket is recommended.
  - Consider endotracheal intubation and overtube for safe retrieval of FB.
- *Sharp objects* ***(Figs. 6A and B)****:*
  - Fishbone, a denture with metal hooks, toothpicks, sharp pins, and razor blades.
  - Risk of impaction and perforation arc real.
  - CT neck and chest would assist in a detailed evaluation.
  - Rat-toothed forceps, Polypectomy snare, or Roth net can be used.

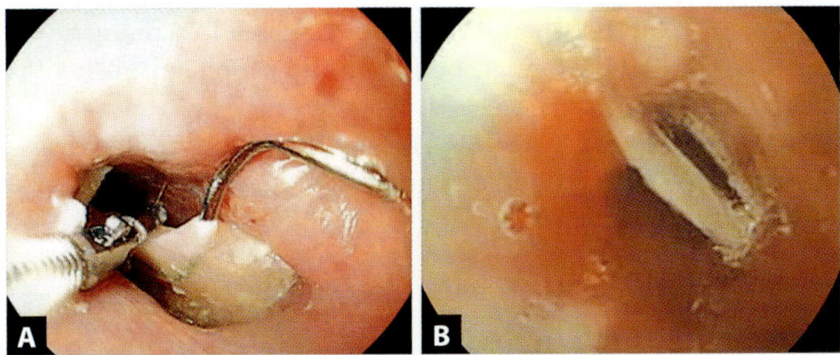

Figs. 6A and B: Denture and fishbone.

    - Ensure the sharp end is trailing during removal to avoid esophageal injury.
    - Consider overtube or placing a rubber hood at the endoscope tip for safe removal of FB.
    - Check endoscopy is usually recommended immediately after FB removal to assess any mucosal damage or perforation.
    - In case of suspected perforation consider CT, neck, and chest and keep the patient nil oral.
- *Magnets:* Multiple magnets or magnets with metal object ingestion could risk necrosis and perforation of the trapped bowel wall. Hence early removal of the magnet is advisable.
- *Narcotic packets:*
    - Usually wrapped in plastic, latex condom, or balloon and taken orally by smugglers.
    - Accidental rupture and leakage of content could be lethal, and hence endoscopic removal is not advisable.
    - Surgery may be needed if the patient shows signs of impaction or bowel obstruction.

CONCLUSION

An FB upper GI tract can be safely and efficiently managed by following the above guidelines. >80% of FB passes out spontaneously and endoscopic removal is indicated only in 10–20% of cases. Surgery is rarely indicated. Our experience, expertise, common sense, and luck would determine the nature of the outcome!

SUGGESTED READING

1. Athanassiadi K, Gerazounis M, Metaxas E, Kalantzi N. Management of esophageal foreign bodies: a retrospective review of 400 cases. Eur J Cardiothorac Surg. 2002;21(4):653-56.
2. Ciriza C, García L, Suárez P, Jiménez C, Romero MJ, Urquiza O, et al. What predictive parameters best indicate the need for emergent gastrointestinal endoscopy after foreign body ingestion? J Clin Gastroenterol. 2000;31(1):23-8.
3. Dahshan A. Management of ingested foreign bodies in children. J Okla State Med Assoc 2001;94(6):183-6.
4. Lin HH, Lee SC, Chu HC, Chang WK, Chao YC, Hsieh TY. Emergency endoscopic management of dietary foreign bodies in the esophagus. Am J Emerg Med. 2007;25(6):662-5.
5. Yong PT, Teh CH, Look M, Wee SB, Tan JC, Chew SP, et al. Removal of a dinner fork from the stomach by double-snare endoscopic extraction. Hong Kong Med J. 2006;6(3):319-21.

Expert's Comment

Foreign body (FB) ingestion of the upper gastrointestinal tract is a frequent clinical challenge, most often accidental in children or intentional in adults, such as prisoners and smugglers. While over 80% pass spontaneously, a subset presents as emergencies with dysphagia, odynophagia, obstruction, aspiration, or even perforation, demanding swift evaluation.

The approach begins with a detailed history and examination, supported by X-rays of the neck, chest, and abdomen. CT scans are valuable for radiolucent or sharp FBs, while barium swallow has no role. Endoscopy remains the gold standard for both diagnosis and treatment. Urgency of intervention depends on object type: Button batteries and sharp FBs in the esophagus need immediate removal; large objects, long FBs, or magnets require urgent endoscopy; and selected gastric FBs may allow short observation.

A wide range of retrieval devices—Rat-toothed forceps, Dormia baskets, Roth nets, snares, magnets, and protective hoods—enhance safety and success. Practical guidelines emphasize preparation, airway safety in children, and careful extraction techniques. Difficult scenarios such as food bolus impaction, button batteries, sharp dentures, fish bones, magnets, and narcotic packets require innovation, experience, and sound judgment.

Ultimately, successful outcomes rely on timely diagnosis, appropriate tools, and clinical expertise.

Dr S Easwaramoorthy, the author, is deeply passionate about writing on endoscopy. Having authored the acclaimed Art and Science of Endoscopy and now preparing its revised edition, he continues to inspire the field through his academic dedication and mastery.

Dr T Sivakumar
Eathamozhi

CHAPTER 7

Role of Endoscopy in Upper Gastrointestinal Bleeding

Chapter Outline

- Causes of Upper Gastrointestinal Bleeding
- Approach to Cases of Upper Gastrointestinal Bleeding
- Management of Esophageal Varices
- Management of Fundal Varices
- Management of Nonvariceal Bleeding
  - Diagnostic Endoscopy in Nonvariceal Bleeding
- Risk Factors for Recurrent Bleeding in Case of Nonvariceal Causes
- Guidelines for Initial Management of Nonvariceal Upper Gastrointestinal Bleeding
- Endotherapy for Nonvariceal Causes of Upper Gastrointestinal Bleeding
  - Injection with Dilute Adrenaline
  - Thermal Method
  - Hemoclip Application
  - Argon Plasma Coagulation
- Guidelines for Endotherapy in Cases of Nonvariceal Bleeding

Keywords: Hematemesis, malena, upper GI bleeding, variceal bleeding, bleeding peptic ulcer, endoscopic hemostasis

INTRODUCTION

Upper gastrointestinal (GI) bleeding is defined as bleeding from the lesion in the esophagus, stomach, or duodenum above the ligament of Treitz. It usually presents with hematemesis, malena, or anemia. It is broadly classified as due to variceal and nonvariceal causes. Immediate resuscitation, early diagnosis, and effective therapy would help to minimize the morbidity and mortality due to upper GI bleeding.

CAUSES OF UPPER GASTROINTESTINAL BLEEDING

Esophagus

- Esophagitis
- Esophageal varices
- Mallory-Weiss tear

Stomach

- Erosive gastritis (drug-induced/alcohol)
- Fundal varices
- Gastric ulcer

Duodenum

Duodenal ulcer.

APPROACH TO CASES OF UPPER GASTROINTESTINAL BLEEDING

Take a Good History

- Assess the duration and severity of symptoms.
- History of (H/O) Alcoholism, drug intake, such as steroids, nonsteroidal anti-inflammatory drugs (NSAIDs), or aspirin
- Known cases of chronic liver disease?

Clinical Examination

- Vital signs (if in shock, first resuscitate then investigate)
- Anemia, jaundice, signs of liver failure
- *Examination of the abdomen*: Splenomegaly indicates portal HT.
- PR to look for any malena.

MANAGEMENT OF ESOPHAGEAL VARICES

- *Diagnostic endoscopy in cases of esophageal varices*:
  - Esophageal varices are the endoscopic signs of portal hypertension.
  - Appear as dilated long, tortuous, submucosal venous columns from Z line upward for variable distance.
  - They are due to portosystemic collaterals between the portal system (left gastric and short gastric veins) and systemic veins (Azygos and hemi azygos veins).
  - One to four columns may be present.
  - Note the size and length of each variceal column and grade them (grades 1–4)
- *Grades of varices and treatment options:*
  - Grades **(Figs. 1 to 4)**
  - *Grade:* Small varices disappearing on insufflation (missing varices).
  - *Grade II:* Varices <5 mm width.
  - *Grade III:* Large prominent varices >5 mm width.
  - *Grade IV:* Varices occluding the lumen (kissing varices).
  - Look for any cherry red spot or red whale sign on the surface of the big varices. If present, they indicate the presence of intramucosal varices and denote an increased risk of bleeding.

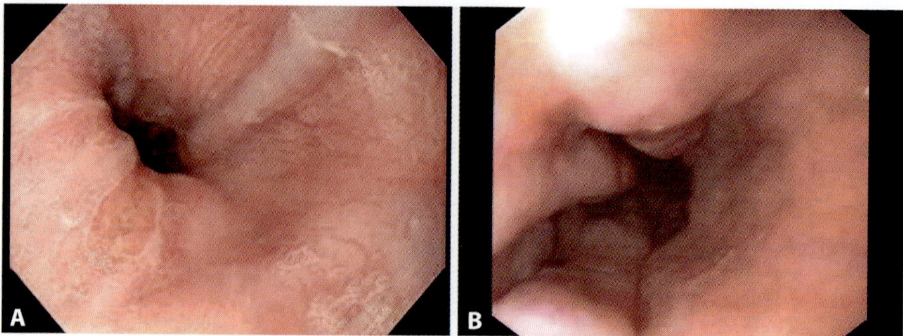

Figs. 1A and B: Grade 1 and 2 varices.

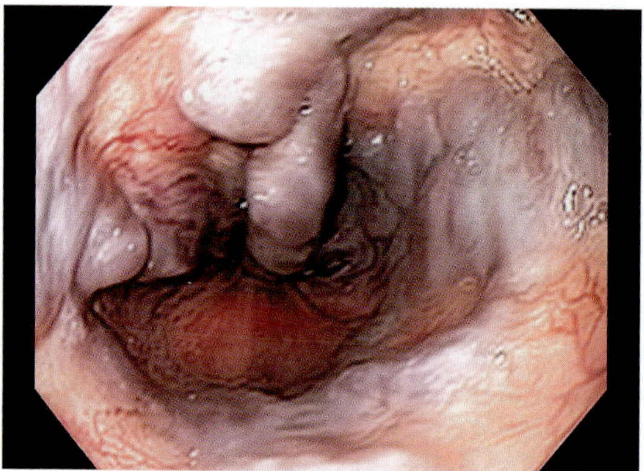

Fig. 2: Grade 3 varices.

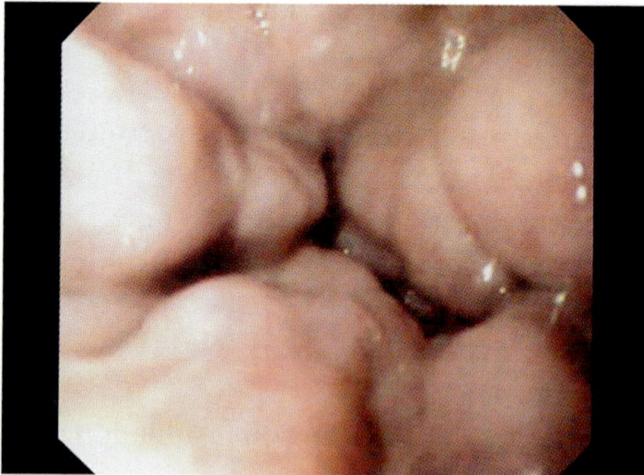

Fig. 3: Grade 4 varices.

- Look for associated severity and extent of portal congestive gastropathy, any fundal varix, varix in any other ectopic locations like antrum or even duodenum.

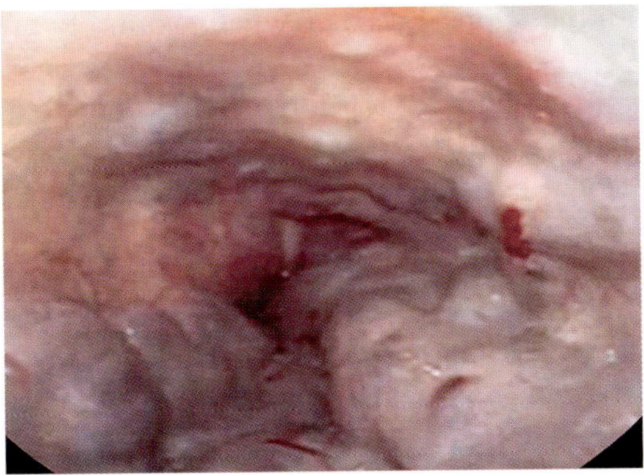

Fig. 4: Cherry red spots.

- *Risk of bleeding* is high in grade 3 or 4 varices, fundal varices, and also in the presence of cherry red spots and red whale streaks on the surface of varices.
- Consider endotherapy for all cases of varices presenting with active bleeding or with a history of GI bleeding recently (Secondary prophylaxis).
- Consider banding for big varices (Grade 3 or 4) and sclerotherapy for small varices or residual varices (Grade 1 or 2). Glue injection is the treatment of choice for fundal varix.
- Prophylactic endoscopic banding can be considered in select cases of Grade 3 or 4 varices to prevent any GI bleeding (Primary prophylaxis)

INITIAL MANAGEMENT OF BLEEDING ESOPHAGEAL VARICES

- Immediate assessment of vital signs and initiate resuscitation
- Avoid infusion of large volumes of saline
- Consider infusion of frozen plasma, 20% human albumin, and blood transfusion
- Admit to high dependency unit and do baseline blood investigation, clotting screen and liver profile, and serum ammonia level
- *Pharmacotherapy for esophageal varices*:
  - *In case of acute bleeding*: Intravenous (IV) terlipressin, somatostatin, or octreotide
  - *For prevention of bleeding:*
    - Nonselective beta blocker: Propranolol, nadolol, and carvedilol.
- Use of Sengstaken tube is rare nowadays
- No need for nasogastric tube insertion (retching might worsen blood vomiting).

- Initiate IV antibiotic prophylaxis (IV cefotaxime) to prevent bacterial peritonitis.
- IV proton pump inhibitor (PPI) is not indicated if there is no evidence of peptic ulcer disease.
- Plan for immediate endotherapy (banding/sclerotherapy).
- *Commence hepatic encephalopathy prophylaxis*:
  - Oral rifaximin and oral lactulose and rectal lactulose enema
- *Correct coagulopathy*:
  - IV vitamin K 10 mg/day for 3 days.
  - If the international normalized ratio (INR) >1.5, consider transfusion of fresh frozen plasma (FFP).
  - Consider platelet transfusion only in case of active bleeding with a platelet level <50,000.
- Consider preemptive intubation before endotherapy if the patient is restless and the risk of aspiration or airway compromise is high.

ENDOTHERAPY FOR ESOPHAGEAL VARICES

- Endoscopic band ligation
- Endoscopic sclerotherapy

Endoscopic Band Ligation (Figs. 5 and 6)

Indication

Grade III and IV esophageal varices:

- With a history of previous upper GI bleeding (secondary prophylaxis).
- Without any previous upper GI bleeding (primary prophylaxis).

Things required:

- 6 band barrel
- Release handle

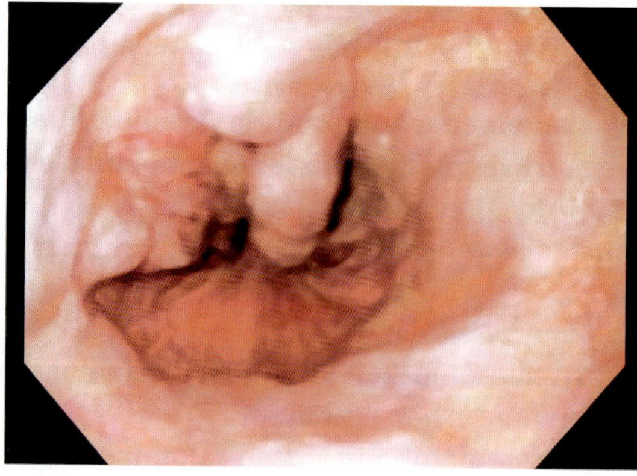

Fig. 5: Before banding.

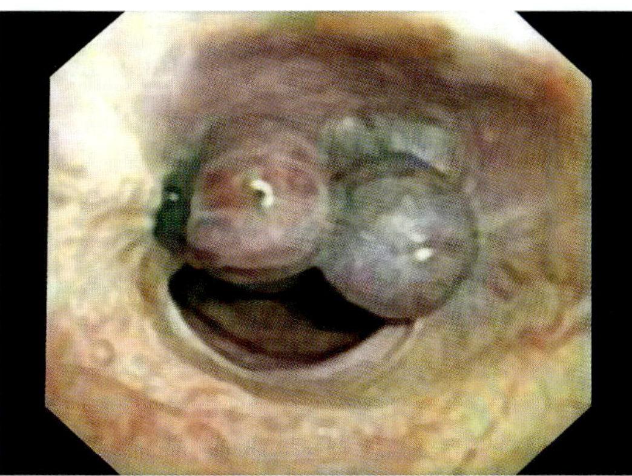

Fig. 6: After banding.

- Pull wire/biopsy forceps
- Good suction unit

Procedure

- IV sedation usually 1–2 mg midazolam is given unless the patient is already drowsy. Administer IV PPI, antibiotic (IV cefotaxime 1 g), and antiemetic (IV ondansetron 4 mg)
- *Perform the diagnostic endoscopy*: Note the size, number, and length of esophageal varices and the presence of any risk markers of bleeding like cherry red spot or red whale sign. The presence of scarring denotes the previous banding site. Examine the stomach and duodenum for the extent and severity of gastropathy, fundal varices, and any ectopic antral or duodenal varices.
- Large fundal varices need attention before esophageal varices.
- *Loading of bands*: (Read the manufacturer's instructions carefully).
  - Fix the "band release handle" in the biopsy channel.
  - Pass the pull catheter or biopsy forceps through the hole in the release handle and see it coming out at the distal end of the scope.
  - Fix the thread of the 6-band barrel to the hook-like end of the pull catheter and start pulling the catheter with the thread through the biopsy channel until the barrel comes close to the tip of the scope (Railroad technique).
  - Fix the band barrel snugly to the end of the scope. Align the thread in line with the biopsy channel, e.g., 5'o clock position in Pentax scope and 7'o clock position in monitor for Olympus scope.
  - Dock the end of the thread to a groove in the release handle and rotate the handle clockwise till the assembly is snugly fit and ready to deploy the bands.

- *Check the power of suction*: Suction determines the success of band deployment. Hence place your gloved finger at the barrel end and apply suction and see. If the finger stalls balloons inside the barrel as soon as suction is applied, then it means suction is sufficient. Each varix is going to be similarly suctioned inside the barrel and engaged well prior to band deployment.
- *Deployment of bands:*
  - Start at the Z line and apply bands at 1 cm intervals in a spiral fashion to avoid luminal narrowing. Once the suction is applied, watch varix engaging inside the barrel and creating what we see as red out. Then gently turn the release handle clockwise till the sense of giving way. Keep the suction a few seconds more to ensure that the deployed band does not slip out! Gently release your finger from the suction to see the banded varix appearing like a bluish grape and slipping out of the barrel. One may notice the collapsing of the proximal column of the varix after banding. So now proceed to the next varix 1 cm higher in different quadrants and apply the band. Twisting or torque of the scope and turning of the body brings each varix to the desirable banding position.
  - Ensure the patient is not retched during the procedure.

Watch For

- Risk of procedure-related bleeding (usually minimal).
- Risk of aspiration (in actively bleeding patients or if the stomach is full of blood). Consider intubation in selected cases.

Follow-up

- Following endoscopic banding starts the patient on a liquid diet after 4 hours and maintained in a liquid diet for 24–48 hours. Continue with IV terlipressin infusion until endoscopic hemostasis is ensured (up to 3–5 days).
- Repeat endoscopy and banding after 3–4 weeks.
- Perform further endoscopy at monthly intervals until all the varices are eradicated and the risk of bleeding is eliminated.
- Surveillance endoscopy at 3–6 monthly intervals to look for any residual varices. If present, consider endoscopic sclerotherapy.
- Failure of endoscopic banding to control bleeding from varices would warrant a transjugular intrahepatic portosystemic shunt (TIPS) procedure or endoscopic deployment of a removable covered metal stent in the lower esophagus (Ella Danis stent).

ENDOSCOPIC SCLEROTHERAPY OF VARICES (FIGS. 7 AND 8)

Indication

- *Grade I and II esophageal varices*: Banding is the procedure of choice for esophageal varices because of the ease of the procedure and very little procedure-related complications. However subsequent residual varices may not be suitable for banding because of smaller size and surrounding fibrosis. In that situation, consider endoscopic sclerotherapy for eradication of the varices.
- Remember that Small varices need sclerotherapy and big varices require banding! (S for S and B for B).

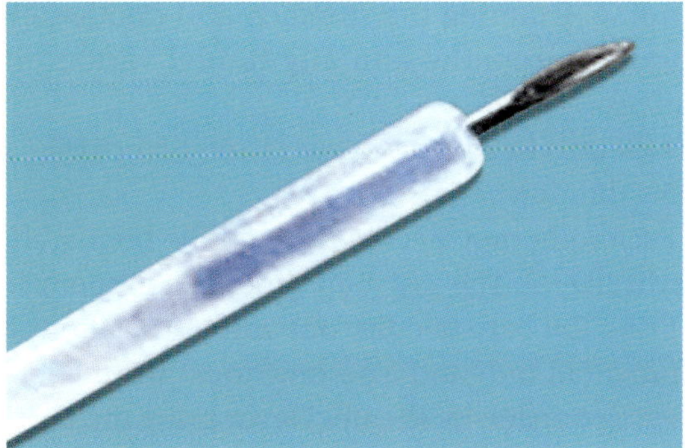

Fig. 7: 23G sclerotherapy needle.

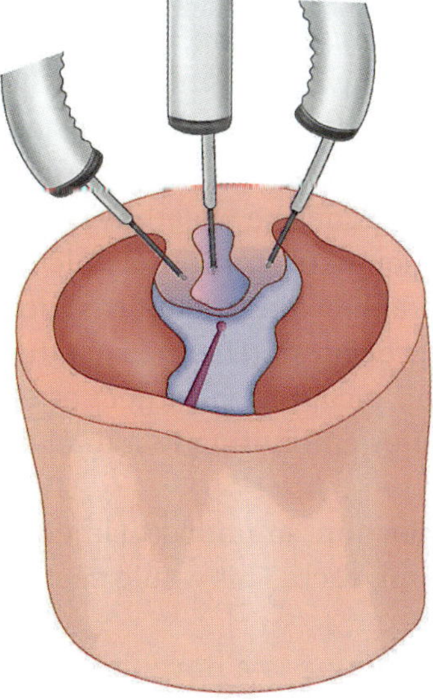

Fig. 8: Technique of sclerotherapy.

Things Needed

- 23G and 160 cm sclerotherapy resheathing retractable needle.
- *Sclerosing agent*: 3% sodium tetradecyl sulfate (STD)/ethanolamine/polidocanol

Procedure

- IV sedation usually 1–2 mg midazolam is given unless the patient is already drowsy. Administer IV PPI, antibiotic IV cefotaxime 1 g) and antiemetic (IV ondansetron 4 mg).
- *Perform the diagnostic endoscopy*: Note the size, number, and length of esophageal varices and the presence of any risk markers of bleeding like cherry red spot or red whale sign. The presence of scarring suggests previous banding. Examine the stomach and duodenum for the extent and severity of gastropathy and any fundal varices or even ectopic duodenal varices.
- Take 3% STD (Setrol) in 2 mL syringes (1 mL of the drug and 1 mL saline to make it 1.5% dilution).
- Pass the 23G sclerotherapy needle through the biopsy channel and note it exits at the distal end. The assistant should be properly instructed when and how to bring the bare needle "out and in" positions by pushing and pulling the proximal hub and also how to adjust the length of the bare needle projecting outside its sheath. Never bring the bare needle outside its sheath, when it is still inside the biopsy channel of the scope to avoid any damage to the channel.
- Start the injection just above the Z-line.
- *Intravariceal/paravariceal injection*: There are many different methods of sclerotherapy. In intravariceal injection, the needle is brought out tangentially in line with the varix to be injected. Now gently pierce the varix for about 1–2 mm, inject 1 cc of the drug, and ask the assistant to take the needle back inside the sheath while you maintain the sheath over the site of injection like a plug on a hole for a minute to ensure no undue post-procedural bleeding. Patients should also cooperate by not retching during the procedure. Then torque the scope to bring the next varix in the preferred location and inject at the level of Z line. Inject up to three to four sites amounting to a total of 5–6 mL of drug during each sitting.
    - In paravariceal injection, submucosal injection is given on either side of varix about 0.5 mL each. This would cause peri variceal fibrosis and chemical phlebitis.
    - The sandwich technique is a novel technique where you start with paravariceal injection for each varix and then inject intravariceally to obtain satisfactory results with minimal bleeding.

Watch For

- Procedure-related bleeding.
- Mediastinitis with retrosternal pain.
- Dysphagia and fever that require IV antibiotics and analgesics.

MANAGEMENT OF FUNDAL VARICES (FIGS. 9 AND 10)

Diagnostic Endoscopy

- Located in the fundal region and seen during the J maneuver.
- It can be easily missed in an actively bleeding patient due to collected blood clots in the fundus masking the view. Adequate irrigation and suction are needed. Also, try to change the patient to a supine or sitting-up position to look at the cardia.
- Note the size and extent of fundal varices and evidence of any recent bleeding.

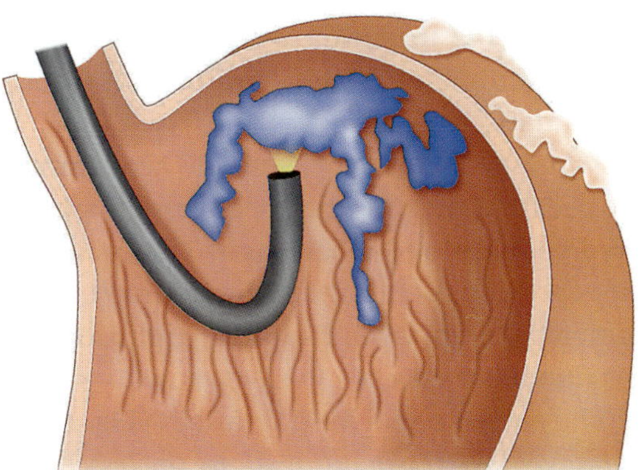

Fig. 9: Technique of glue injection.

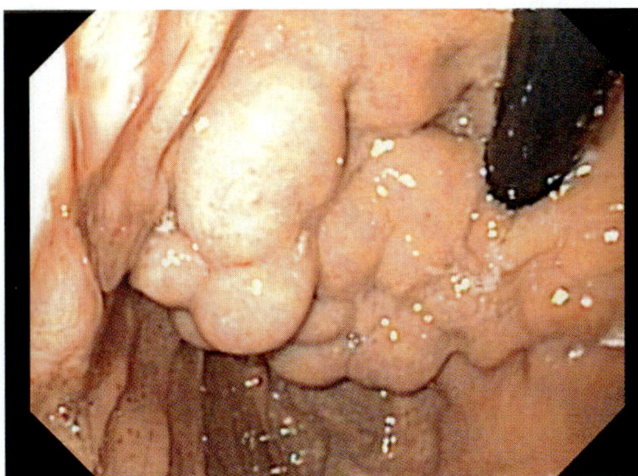

Fig. 10: Huge fundal varix.

- Appear as a bunch of grapes hanging on the roof!
  - *DD:* Leiomyoma of the stomach.
- Can be seen as an extension of esophageal varices to the stomach [gastroesophageal varices (GOV) 1 and 2] or found as isolated gastric varices [isolated gastric varices (IGV) 1 and 2]

Glue Injection of Fundal Varices

Things Needed

- 21G and 160 cm sclerotherapy resheathing retractable needle.
- N butyl cyanoacrylate 1 mL ampoules/ensure at least three more spare ampoules are available.
- 2 mL syringes with distilled water for flushing.
- Acetone for cleaning lens and channels.
- Goggles

Procedure

- IV sedation usually 1–2 mg midazolam is given unless the patient is already drowsy. Administer IV PPI, antibiotic (IV cefotaxime 1 g) and antiemetic (IV ondansetron 4 mg).
- *Perform the diagnostic endoscopy*: Note the size, number, and length of esophageal varices and the presence of any risk markers of bleeding such as a cherry red spot and red whale sign. The presence of any scarring usually suggests previous banding or sclerotherapy. Examine the stomach and duodenum for the extent and severity of gastropathy, fundal varices, or any ectopic duodenal varices.
- Note the size, site and extent of fundal varices **(Fig. 11)**.
  - *Gastroesophageal varix extending along the lesser curve (GOV 1)*: 75%.
  - *Gastroesophageal varix extending onto the fundus (GOV 2)*: 20%

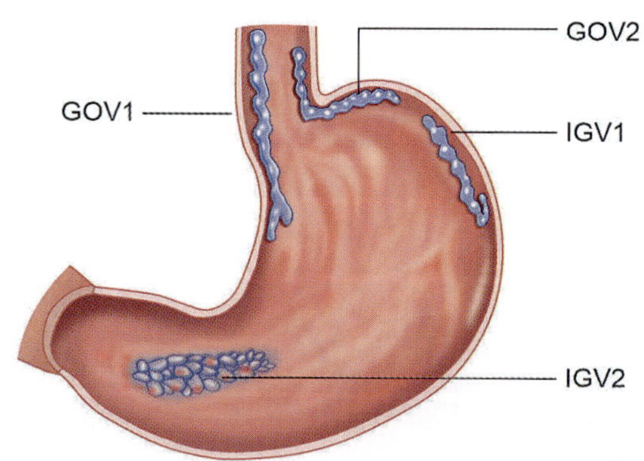

Fig. 11: Types of fundal varices.
(GOV: gastroesophageal varices; IGV: isolated gastric varices)

- *Isolated gastric varix confined to fundus (IGV1)*: 4%
- *Isolated gastric varix in an ectopic place like antrum (IGV2)*: 1%

- Ensure you have an agile and competent assistant who is ready with all the required things on a trolley.
- The assistant should be properly instructed when and how to keep the "needle out and needle in" positions by pushing and pulling the proximal hub and how to adjust the length of the bare needle projecting outside its sheath. Never bring the needle sharpened out when it is still inside the biopsy channel of the scope to avoid any damage to the channel.
- Pass the 21G glue injection needle catheter through the biopsy channel while the scope is straight and note that it reaches just near the endoscope tip but not projecting outside.
- Now do the J maneuver to see the fundus. By shortening the scope and torque, the scope should reach the fundal varix at firing distance!
- Perform a "Dry run" of rehearing by bringing the needle out of its sheath and seeing its trajectory!
- Once you are satisfied and the patient is comfortable and not retching. Gently push the bare needle into the fundal varix at the selected site and give the command for the injection sequence.
- The assistant will switch off the suction and then immediately inject 0.5–1 mL of the glue followed by 1.5 mL of distilled water to flush the glue from the injection catheter into the varix. Then withdraw the needle inside while you still keep the catheter tip abutting on the needle hole over the varix for about 30 seconds while polymerization of glue with blood and hence solidification of varix takes place. Now you could feel the soft compressible varix had become unyielding. The success of glue injection depends on the agility of the assistant and thorough understanding between the team members and their experience.
- Avoid the tip of the scope in contact with blood or glue.
- Ensure there is no undue postprocedural bleeding.
- Patient may require more than one injection to eradicate a large fundal varix and total volume may reach 4–5 mL of glue. Hence, spare ampoules of glue and needles are a must.
- Remove the scope and ensure that its channel is not blocked, or the lens is covered with glue. Acetone can be used to clean the distal end of the scope and also to flush the scope channel.
- It is always a good practice guideline to wear goggles during the procedure or else one day your blue eye could become a glued eye. So, beware.

Watch For

- Bleeding
- *Blockage of suction channel or hazy view*: Clean or flush with acetone.

- Rarely patient could develop glue embolism to pulmonary or cerebral vessels risking stroke or other serious consequences!

MANAGEMENT OF NONVARICEAL BLEEDING

Diagnostic Endoscopy in Nonvariceal Bleeding

Mallory Weiss Tear

- Often after a bout of alcohol intake.
- Typically, the patient complains of retching and vomiting a few times before any hematemesis!
- Appear as small linear mucosal tears with oozing.
- Commonly noted in the lower esophagus just above the Z line or seen at the cardia during the J maneuver.
- Boerhaave syndrome is a spontaneous rupture of the esophagus and presents with severe chest pain and dyspnea. Look for pneumomediastinum and pleural effusion. Gastrografin swallows or computed tomography (CT) chests could be diagnostic.

Gastritis

- Note the type, extent, and severity of gastritis.
- Multiple areas of erosions, hemorrhagic areas, or oozing are commonly noted.

Gastric and Duodenal Ulcers

- Note the site, size, and number of ulcers, margins, and surface.
- Large posterior duodenal ulcers could bleed torrentially from the gastroduodenal vessel.
- High lesser curve or posterior gastric ulcer could also bleed heavily from the left gastric or splenic artery. So, beware.
- Classify them as per the Forrest grading to understand the risk of any further bleeding.

Forrest grading:

- *Grade 1*: Actively bleeding lesions.
  - *Grade 1A*: With arterial spurting.
  - *Grade 1B*: With constant or intermittent oozing.
- *Grade 2*: With stigmata of recent bleeding and risk for further future bleeding.
  - *Grade 2A*: Nonbleeding visible vessel.
  - *Grade 2B:* Surface covered by a blood clot and difficult to dislodge on irrigation.
  - *Grade 2C:* Covered by black spot due to hematin pigment.
- *Grade 3:* Clean-based ulcer and unlikely to bleed.

- *Rare causes of upper GI bleeding:*
    - *Angiodysplasia of esophagus, stomach, or duodenum:* Appears as a bright red flat or slightly elevated vascular lesion (as in Osler–Rendu–Weber syndrome, connective tissue disorders, irradiation, cirrhosis of the liver, and chronic renal failure).
    - *Dieulafoy lesion:* Small 1 mm papular lesion hidden in the rugal folds usually in the proximal stomach with intermittent bleeding due to arteriolar spurt. You may notice it on a lucky day!
    - Watermelon stomach [gastric antral vascular ectasia (GAVE) syndrome].
    - Leiomyoma or cancer stomach presenting as a bleeding source.

RISK FACTORS FOR RECURRENT BLEEDING IN CASE OF NONVARICEAL CAUSES

- *Clinical factors:*
    - Age >60 years
    - Shock on admission
    - Hemoglobin (Hb) on admission <8 g
    - Blood transfusion >5 units
- *Endoscopic factors:*
    - Forrest Grade 1A, 1B, and 2A type of lesions
    - Doppler positive lesion

GUIDELINES FOR INITIAL MANAGEMENT OF NONVARICEAL UPPER GASTROINTESTINAL BLEEDING

- Immediate assessment of hemodynamic status in patients who present with acute upper GI bleeding with prompt intravascular volume replacement initially using crystalloids if hemodynamic instability exists.
- Consider packed cell transfusion if Hb is below 8 g.
- Give high dose IV PPI (injection pantoprazole 80 mg IV bolus followed by 8 mg/h infusion).
- No need for routine nasogastric tube insertion and or aspiration.
- No role of IV tranexamic acid or somatostatin/octreotide infusion in nonvariceal causes.
- Consider early endoscopy (<24 hours) to establish the cause and plan therapy accordingly.
- Give *Helicobacter pylori* eradication therapy in case of proven infection (rapid urease test).

ENDOTHERAPY FOR NONVARICEAL CAUSES OF UPPER GASTROINTESTINAL BLEEDING

- Injection with diluted adrenaline.
- *Thermal methods:* Monopolar and bipolar diathermy and heater probe

- *Laser:* Neodymium-doped yttrium aluminum garnet (Nd:YAG) laser
- Hemoclips
- Argon plasma coagulation
- *Topical hemostatic sprays*: Hemospray and EndoClot

Injection with Dilute Adrenaline (Fig. 12)

Things Required

- 23G sclerotherapy re-sheathing retractable needle.
- Dilute 1 mL of 1/1,000 adrenaline to 10–20 mL by using saline to make it 1/10,000–1/20,000 dilution and take it in 10 mL syringes.
- Water jet or irrigation system to flush the bleeding site.
- Good suction unit.

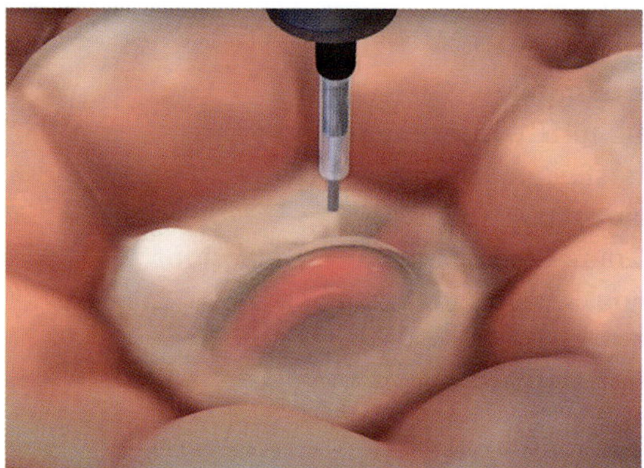

Fig. 12: Injection of dilute adrenaline.

Indication for using Dilute Adrenaline Injection

- Bleeding benign gastric ulcer or erosions
- Bleeding duodenal ulcers
- Mallory Weiss tear
- Dieulafoy lesion
- Base/stalk of a polyp

Tricks of the Trade: Bleeding Peptic Ulcer

- Check endoscopy under local anesthesia (LA)/conscious sedation. Consider IV buscopan 20 mg IV. Give one dose of IV antibiotic (cefotaxime 1 g).
- Locate the site and nature of the bleeding ulcer and its grade as per Forrest classification
- Forrest type 1a, 1b, and 2a require therapy to prevent any re-bleeding.
- Reach and dock the endoscope at a satisfactory position.

- Pass the sclerotherapy needle through the biopsy channel and once seen at the distal end, instruct the assistant to push the bare "needle out" from the sheath for about 5 mm.
- Pass it perpendicularly on four quadrants just outside the margin of the bleeding lesion.
- Inject 1 cc of diluted adrenaline in each quadrant to achieve blanching by tamponade effect which initiates vasospasm and inflammatory reaction and thrombosis.
- Subsequently one may choose to inject the base of the ulcer also with one to two injections of 1 mL at each site.
- If bleeding persists, one may choose a combination of modalities such as adding a thermal method (e.g., bipolar diathermy using a Gold probe) or even hemoclip application.
- Keep the patient under close observation in the high-dependency unit.
- Give high-dose IV pantoprazole (for adults: 8 mg/h infusion or 80 mg/ 8 hourly).
- Consider second look endoscopy after 48 hours to ensure satisfactory hemostasis.
- Injection of adrenaline is an easy, cheap, and effective modality to consider as the first line of endoscopic hemostasis.

Thermal Method

- Heater probe or bipolar diathermy using the "Gold Probe **(Fig. 13)**."
- Usually as a combined method following the injection with dilute adrenaline
- Apply the gold probe over the bleeding ulcer to achieve a pressure effect and then activate the diathermy to achieve superficial coagulative thrombosis.
- Simultaneous application of pressure and heat causes coaptive coagulation.

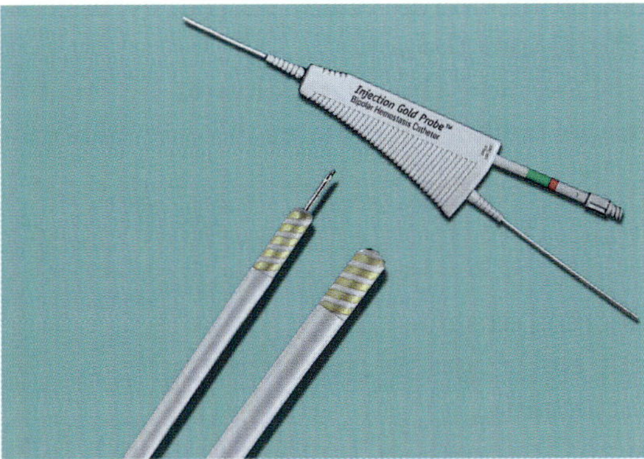

Fig. 13: Gold Probe.

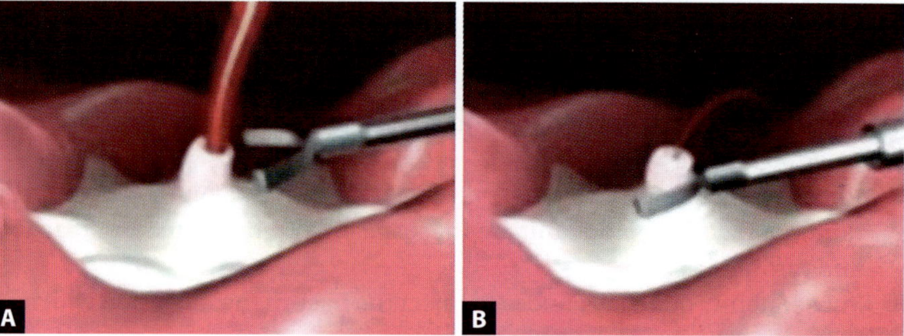

Figs. 14A and B: Hemoclip for bleeding.

Hemoclip Application (Figs. 14A and B)

Indication

- Bleeding peptic ulcer
- Dieulafoy lesion
- Base of bleeding polyps
- To close any defect following ESD/NOTES/POEM procedures

Types of Hemoclip

- Disposable preloaded hemoclips.
- Reusable hemoclip applicator with clips in separate cartridges.
- Choose the one that can be rotatable and with adjustable width.

Tricks of the Trade

- Dock the endoscopy at the satisfactory position.
- Load the clip from the cartridge onto the applicator.
- Pass the hemoclip applicator with the clip hidden in the retractable sheath through the biopsy channel.
- Bring out the clip and adjust the trajectory angle and its width.
- Release the clip by pushing the thumb grip handle once you have grabbed the tissue at the desired position.
- You may need a few more clips depending on the situation.
- Avoid any thermal methods at the site following hemoclip.

Argon Plasma Coagulation (Figs. 15A and B)

Indication

- Superficial bleeding erosions
- Gave syndrome and congestive gastropathy
- Radiation proctocolitis
- To ablate tumor ingrowth or tumor overgrowth following previous stenting for ca esophagus

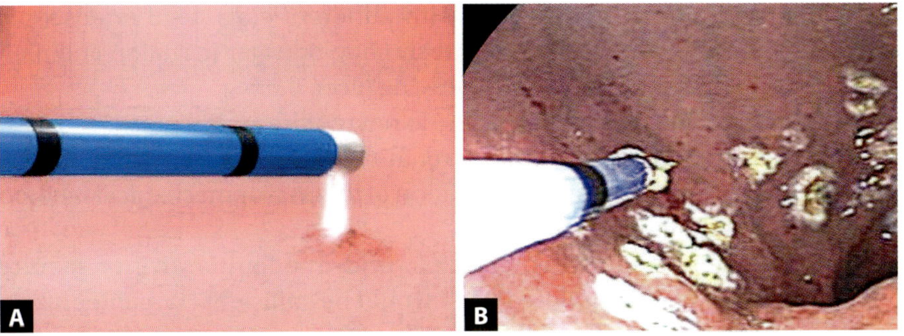

Figs. 15A and B: APC for GAVE syndrome. (APC: argon plasma coagulation; GAVE: gastric antral vascular ectasia)

Things Required

- Diathermy with argon plasma coagulation (APC) provisions (ERBE or Valley laboratory)
- Argon plasma gas cylinder
- *Spray catheter*: Side and end firing types
- Water jet
- Good suction unit

Tricks of the Trade: A Case of Congestive Gastropathy

- Check endoscopy.
- Take the APC spray catheter (side or end firing) through the biopsy channel.
- Ensure recommended diathermy and gas flow setting.
- Activate the pedal to achieve superficial coagulative necrosis and hemostasis.
- The catheter is close to but not touching the mucosa ("noncontact" mode).
- Either adjust the catheter to direct it toward the lesion each time or keep the spray catheter still projecting 1 cm from the distal end and manipulate the endoscopy and catheter as one unit to spray the area with APC (called "paintbrush technique").

Watch For

Any bleeding, mucosal damage, or even perforation.

GUIDELINES FOR ENDOTHERAPY IN CASES OF NONVARICEAL BLEEDING

- Consider Forrest classification in all patients with peptic ulcer bleeding to identify patients with a high risk of recurrent bleeding.
- Forrest 1A and 1B and 2A need endoscopic therapy.

- Patients with Forrest 2B (Ulcer with adherent clot) need endoscopic clot removal using a cold snaring technique or water irrigation and plan according to the status of the underlying ulcer
- Forrest 2C and 3-type peptic ulcers do not require endotherapy.
- Injection therapy with dilute adrenaline as sole therapy may not be effective in most cases and the addition of thermal or mechanical method is strongly recommended
- Patients with esophagitis, gastritis, and duodenitis do not require endotherapy, and high dose IV PPI would be sufficient (IV pantoprazole 8 mg/h or 80 mg IV 8 hourly).
- Patients with Mallory–Weiss tear or Dieulafoy lesion with persisting bleeding would benefit from endotherapy like an injection with dilute adrenaline or hemoclip.
- Patients with angiodysplasia would benefit from either APC or injection with dilute adrenaline
- Patients with bleeding tumors like leiomyoma would require surgical intervention and endotherapy may be useful as a temporary measure.
- Second-look endoscopy is indicated only if there is clinical evidence of recurrent bleeding.

SUGGESTED READING

1. Blatchford O, Murray W, Blatchford M. A risk score to predict need for treatment for upper-gastrointestinal haemorrhage. Lancet. 2000;356(9238):1318-21.
2. Button L, Roberts S, Evans PA, Goldacre MJ, Akbari A, Dsilva R, et al. Hospitalized incidence and case fatality for upper gastrointestinal bleeding from 1999 to 2007: a record linkage study. Aliment Pharmacol Ther. 2011;33(1):64-76.
3. Cook D, Guyatt G, Salena B, Laine LA. Endoscopic therapy for acute nonvariceal upper gastrointestinal hemorrhage: a meta-analysis. Gastroenterology. 1992; 102(1):139-48.
4. Fiaccadori F, Pedretti G, Biraghi M, Arcidiacono R. Terlypressin and endoscopic sclerotherapy control variceal bleeding and prevent early rebleeding in cirrhotic patients. Current Therapeutic Research. 1993;54(5):519-28.
5. Fried M, Krabshuis J. Can 'Cascades' make guidelines global? J Eval Clin Pract. 2008;14(5):874-9.
6. Gralnek IM, Dumonceau JM, Kuipers EJ, Lanas A, Sanders DS, Kurien M, et al. Diagnosis and management of nonvariceal upper gastrointestinal hemorrhage: European Society of Gastrointestinal Endoscopy (ESGE) Guideline. Endoscopy. 2015;47(10):a1-46.
7. In: Block B, Schachschal G, Schmidt H. Endoscopy of Upper GI tract: Training Manual. Germany: George Thieme Verlag; 2004.
8. In: Easwaramoorthy S (Ed). Art and Science of Endoscopy, 1st edition. Tamil Nadu: Lotus Laparoscopic and Endoscopic Training Center; 2016.
9. In: Walsh CM, Ahmad A, Saunders BP, Chonen J, Cotton BP, William CB (Eds). Cotton and Williams' Practical Gastrointestinal Endoscopy: The Fundamentals. New Jersey: Wiley-Blackwel; 2023.

10. Ishaq S, Nunn L. Optimal interval times for rescoping after an acute variceal haemorrhage. Frontline Gastroenterol. 2016;7(4):332-3.
11. Kahi C, Jensen D, Sung J, Bleau BL, Jung HK, Eckert G, et al. Endoscopic therapy versus medical therapy for bleeding peptic ulcer with adherent clot: a meta-analysis. Gastroenterology. 2005;129(3):855-62.
12. Laine L, Cooke D. Endoscopic ligation compared with sclerotherapy for treatment of esophageal variceal bleeding. A meta-analysis. Ann Intern Med. 1995;123(4):280-7.
13. Lau J, Sung JJ, Lee KK, Yung MY, Wong SK, Wu JC, et al. Effect of intravenous omeprazole on recurrent bleeding after endoscopic treatment of bleeding peptic ulcers. N Engl J Med. 2000;343(5):310-6.
14. Malagelada JR, Bazzoli F, Boeckxstaens G, De Looze D, Fried M, Kahrilas P, et al. World Gastroenterology Organisation Global Guidelines: Dysphagia—global guidelines and cascades update September 2014. J Clin Gastroenterol. 2015;49(5):370-8.
15. National Confidential Enquiry into Patient Outcome and Death (NCEPOD). Gastrointestinal Haemorrhage: Time to get control? [Online] Available from https://www.ncepod.org.uk/2015gih.html [Last accessed April, 2025].
16. Rockall T, Logan R, Devlin H, Northfield TC. Risk assessment after acute upper gastrointestinal haemorrhage. Gut. 1996;38(3):316-21.
17. SAGES. Handbooks for Endoscopic and Laparoscopic Surgery. [Online] Available from https://www.sages.org/publications/sages-manuals/ [Last accessed April, 2025].
18. Scottish Intercollegiate Guidelines Network (SIGN). Management of acute upper and lower gastrointestinal bleeding. [Online] Available from https://www.sign.ac.uk/our-guidelines/management-of-acute-upper-and-lower-gastrointestinal-bleeding/ [Last accessed April, 2025].

Expert's Comment

Upper gastrointestinal (UGI) bleeding remains a major clinical emergency worldwide, demanding timely intervention and multidisciplinary care. Endoscopy has transformed this field by offering both diagnostic precision and therapeutic efficacy. Today, practicing surgeons can draw from a wide armamentarium of modalities, each with defined strengths and indications.

Injection therapy with dilute epinephrine provides rapid but temporary hemostasis and often serves as the first step before definitive measures. Thermal methods such as heater probe and bipolar coagulation ensure deep tissue coagulation with durable results. Mechanical approaches, including endoscopic clips and variceal band ligation, are frequently definitive and are considered the standard of care for peptic ulcer bleeding and variceal hemorrhage. Argon plasma coagulation (APC) has become indispensable for managing diffuse or flat lesions such as gastric antral vascular ectasia (GAVE) or radiation-induced mucosal bleeding, with its noncontact application and controlled depth of injury. Newer techniques—such as over-the-scope clips and topical hemostatic powders—are expanding our therapeutic reach.

For variceal bleeding, endoscopy remains the first-line therapy, yet in refractory or recurrent cases, transjugular intrahepatic portosystemic shunt (TIPS) plays a vital salvage role by decompressing the portal system. Its timely consideration, in close collaboration with interventional radiology, can be life-saving in patients who fail endoscopic and pharmacologic therapy.

Ultimately, the success of managing UGI bleeding does not rest in any single technique but in the skillful, patient-specific combination of modalities, guided by clinical judgment and supported by pharmacological and critical care measures.

Five key principles for clinical practice:

1. Early endoscopy within 24 hours is essential for diagnosis, risk stratification, and therapy.
2. Injection, thermal, mechanical, and APC modalities all have distinct and complementary roles—no single method is universally sufficient.
3. Combination therapy offers superior hemostasis in high-risk nonvariceal bleeding.
4. TIPS must be considered in refractory variceal hemorrhage where endoscopic and pharmacologic therapies fail.
5. Multidisciplinary care—integrating resuscitation, proton-pump inhibitors, interventional radiology, and surgical backup—is the foundation of optimal outcomes.

Professor Dr Sunil D Popat
Ahmedabad

8

CHAPTER

Role of Endoscopy in Gastroesophageal Reflux Disease and Achalasia

Chapter Outline

Role of Endoscopy in Gastroesophageal Reflux Disease

- Endoscopic Assessment of Gastroesophageal Disease
  - Endoscopic Evaluation of Sliding Hiatus Hernia
  - Hill Classification of Laxity of Lower Esophageal Sphincter
  - Endoscopic Evaluation of Barrett's Esophagus
  - Prague Classification of the Extent of Barrett's Esophagus
  - Seattle Protocol
  - Types of Hiatus Hernia
- Functional Assessment of Gastroesophageal Reflux Disease
  - 24-Hour pH Study
  - High-resolution Manometry
  - Impedance PH Study
- Role of Endotherapy for Gastroesophageal Reflux Disease
  - Stretta Procedure
  - EsophyX (Transoral Incisionless Fundoplication)
  - Antireflux Mucosal Resection Procedure
- Rationale and Ways of Endotherapy for Barrett's Esophagus
- Role of Endoscopy in Evaluation for the Complications after Fundoplication
  - Endoscopic Findings of Complications after Fundoplication

Role of Endoscopy in Achalasia

- Presentation Symptoms
- Investigation Tools
- Endoscopic Findings in Achalasia
  - Treatment

Keywords: Barrett's esophagus, Savary–Miller classification, Hill's classification, Stretta procedure, high resolution manometry, impedance study, endoFLIP

ROLE OF ENDOSCOPY IN GASTROESOPHAGEAL REFLUX DISEASE

INTRODUCTION

Gastroesophageal reflux disease is a very common clinical situation we encounter on a daily basis. Normal antireflux mechanism **(Fig. 1)** depends on the pinch-cock effect of the crus of the diaphragm, competence of the lower esophageal sphincter (LES), flap valve effect of the angle of His, and due to the flutter effect of intra-abdominal pressure on the abdominal part of the esophagus. These defense mechanisms often fail in case of a hiatus hernia **(Fig. 2)**.

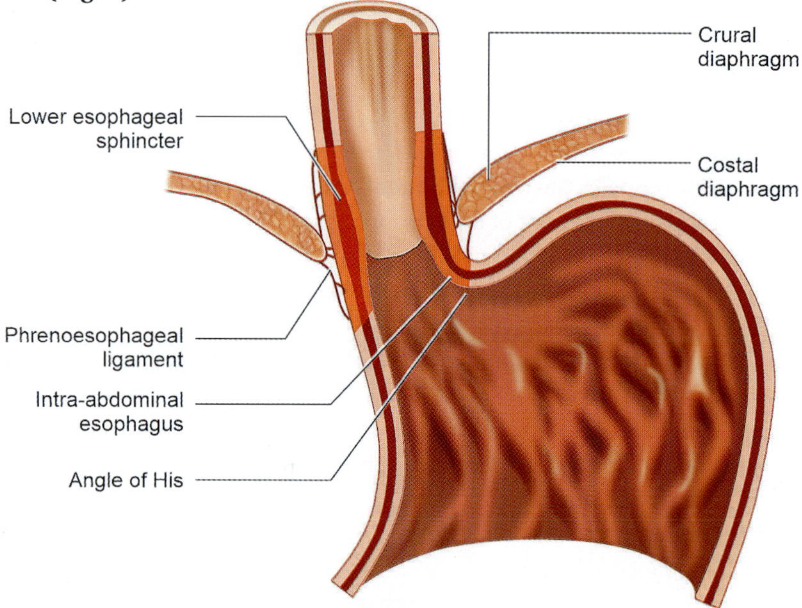

Fig. 1: Normal antireflux defense mechanism.

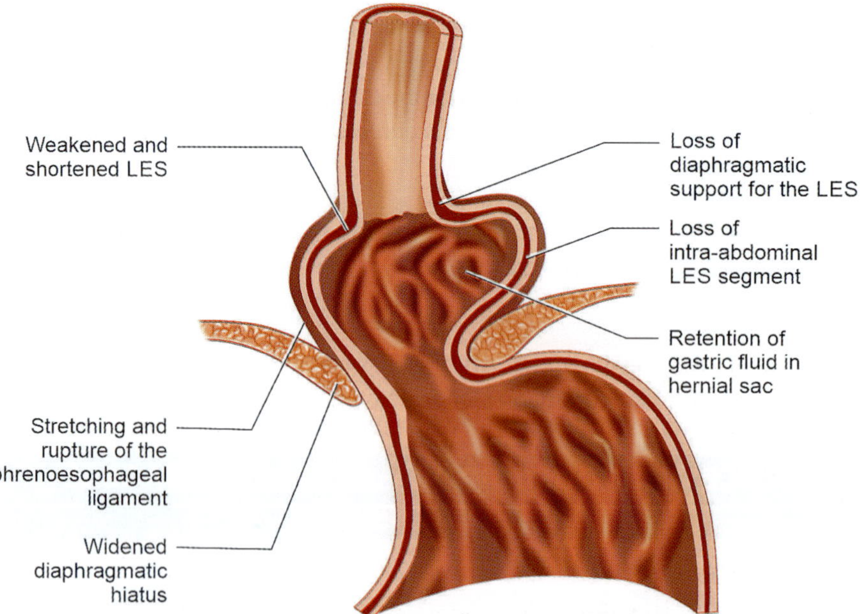

Fig. 2: Sliding hiatus hernia. (LES: lower esophageal sphincter)

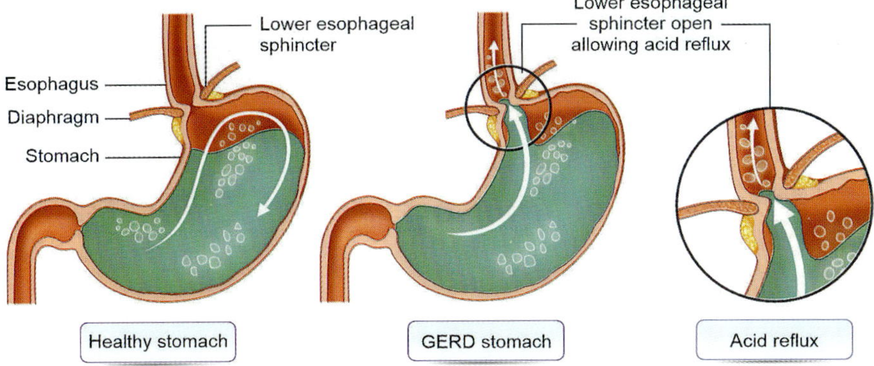

Fig. 3: Acid reflux in gastroesophageal reflux disease (GERD).

But more commonly it is the increase in the transient relaxation of the LES that results in reflux episodes **(Fig. 3)**, especially in the subset of patients with obesity, faulty food habits, stressful life, smoking habits, and alcoholism.

Retrosternal discomfort, belching, and acid reflux are the common symptoms but could present to various specialists with a vast array of symptoms **(Box 1)**.

BOX 1: Clinical presentation of GERD.

- *Typical symptoms:*
  - Heartburn
  - Water brash
- *Atypical symptoms:*
  - Atypical chest pain
  - Asthma, cough, and LRI
  - Laryngitis, URI
  - Dental plaque, oral ulcers
- *Alarm symptoms:*
  - Dysphagia
  - GI bleeding

(GERD: gastroesophageal reflux disease; GI: gastrointestinal; URI: upper respiratory infection)

ENDOSCOPIC ASSESSMENT OF GASTROESOPHAGEAL DISEASE

Endoscopic Evaluation of Sliding Hiatus Hernia (Figs. 4A to D)

Endoscopy is one of the common investigations **(Box 2)** considered in the evaluation of patients with symptoms due to GERD.

In patients with reflux symptoms, endoscopy is an essential investigational tool in addition to the PH study and Impedance study. Unless a proton pump inhibitor (PPI) is withheld for a week, endoscopy could miss inflammatory signs of GERD. So, beware.

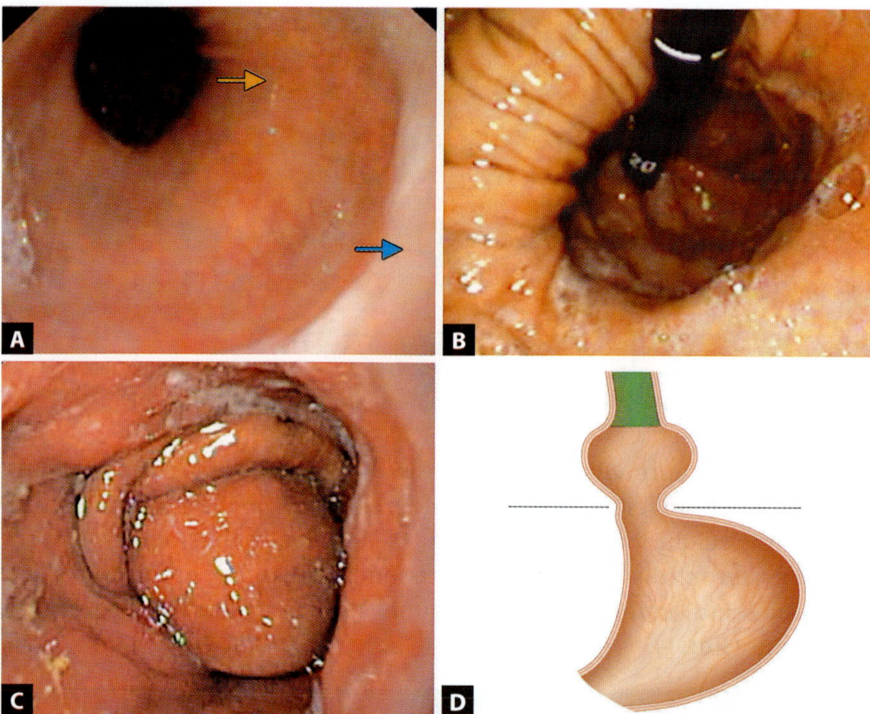

Figs. 4A to D: (A) Z line (blue arrow) and hiatus (orange arrow); (B) Large hiatal hernia on retroflexion; (C) Gastric mucosal prolapse; and (D) Schematic diagram of sliding hiatus hernia.

BOX 2: Investigations of GERD.

- Barium swallow study
- HD image enhancement endoscopy
- 24-hour pH monitoring
- High-resolution manometry
- Impedance study
- CT imaging with oral contrast in selected cases

(CT: computed tomography; GERD: gastroesophageal reflux disease; HD: high-definition)

High-definition (HD) endoscopy with image enhancement technology is essential for proper evaluation and grading of severity of esophagitis. The surgeon should look for the level of the Z line, the level of hiatus, and whether the hiatus is very patulous with mucosal prolapse and degree of esophagitis.

Z line is the transition line between pale esophageal squamous epithelium and pinkish gastric columnar epithelium. It is better appreciated in image enhancement endoscopic images than white light images. Usually, it is at the level of 38–40 cm from incisor teeth in an adult.

Then locate the level of hiatus by asking the patient to sneeze and thereby, we will be able to appreciate the pinchcock mechanism of LES.

It would be normally at the level of 40 cm from the incisor teeth. If the distance between the Z line and the hiatus is >2 cm, we can assume there is some proximal migration of the stomach leading to a sliding type of hiatus hernia. In addition, we will be able to observe the prolapse of fundic mucosal folds across the hiatal opening when the patient retches during the endoscopic procedure. In addition, we also need to look for the horizontal width of the hiatus hernia on retroflexion of the endoscope.

The less common paraesophageal hiatus hernia will look like a diverticular opening in the J maneuver.

Paraesophageal hiatus hernia ***(Figs. 5A and B)****:* Also, one should carefully inspect the lower esophagus above the Z line for the presence and severity of esophagitis. Once again narrow-band imaging (NBI) or similar image enhancement modality would make the assessment more accurate. Los Angeles classification or Savary-Miller classification for the degree of esophagitis is recommended (Refer to Chapter 5). Even in the absence of a hiatus hernia, we should assess the laxity of LES on the J maneuver using Hill's classification.

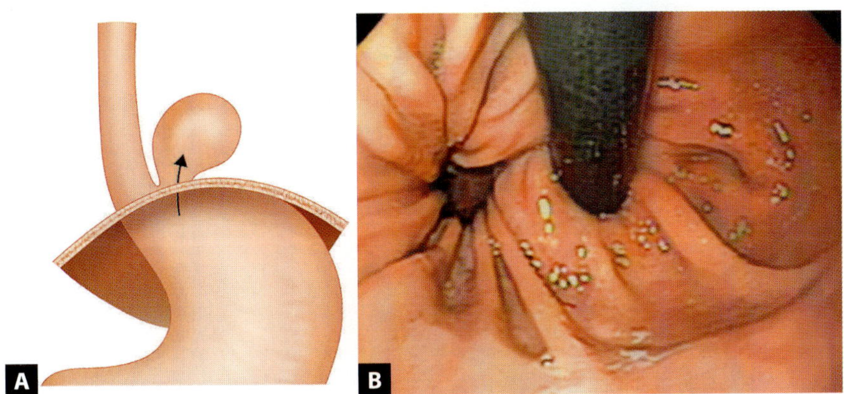

Figs. 5A and B: Paraesophageal hernia.

Hill Classification of Laxity of Lower Esophageal Sphincter (Fig. 6A to D)

To make a precise assessment of the competence of the esophagogastric (OG) sphincter mechanism, Hill et al. presented a practical classification in 1996. The gastroesophageal flap valve is inspected in the J maneuver and classified into one of four categories as given next.

There may be associated peptic stricture, Barrett's changes, or even early cancer. We should be very watchful and consider HD endoscopy with electronic chromoendoscopy and biopsy where it is indicated.

Peptic stricture is shown in **Figure 7**.

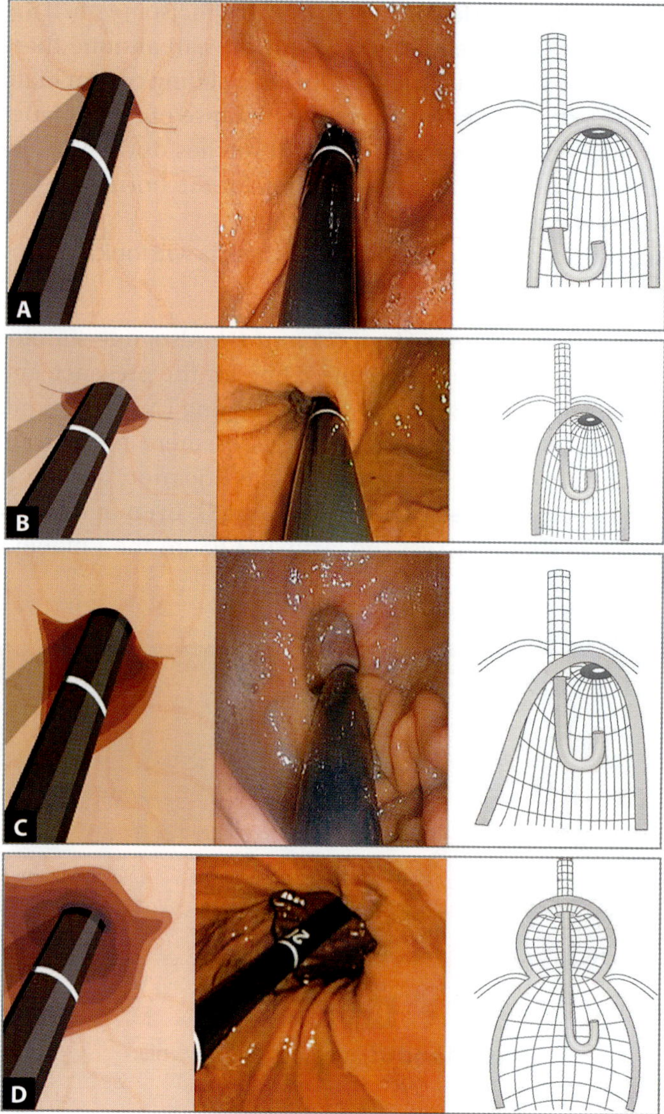

Figs. 6A to D: (A) Grade 1: Gastroesophageal flap valve tightly closed around the shaft of endoscopy at all times; (B) Grade II: Gastroesophageal flap valve becomes lax during inspiration; (C) Grade III: Gastroesophageal flap valve is absent with a constant gap between the shaft of the endoscopy and LES; and (D) Grade IV: Absent gastroesophageal flap valve and proximal migration of stomach with large hiatus opening around the shaft of endoscopy.

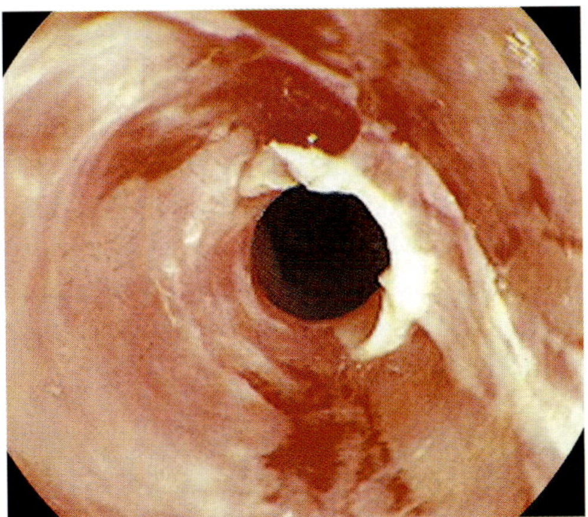

Fig. 7: Peptic stricture.

Endoscopic Evaluation of Barrett's Esophagus (Figs. 8A and B)

Barrett's esophagus is the metaplastic changes of the esophageal squamous epithelium to specialized intestinal columnar epithelium. It appears as salmon-pink mucosa, creeping into the esophageal lumen. It may appear as a circumferential sheet, as tongue-like projections creeping up from the esophagogastric junction (EGJ), or as isolated islands of columnar mucosa interspersed with squamous mucosa. We should note the level of the Z line and level of hiatus from incisor teeth and also look for any hiatus hernia. Then turn on the electronic chromoendoscopy (NBI or similar) to find early lesions and also to assess the extent and severity of Barrett's esophagus.

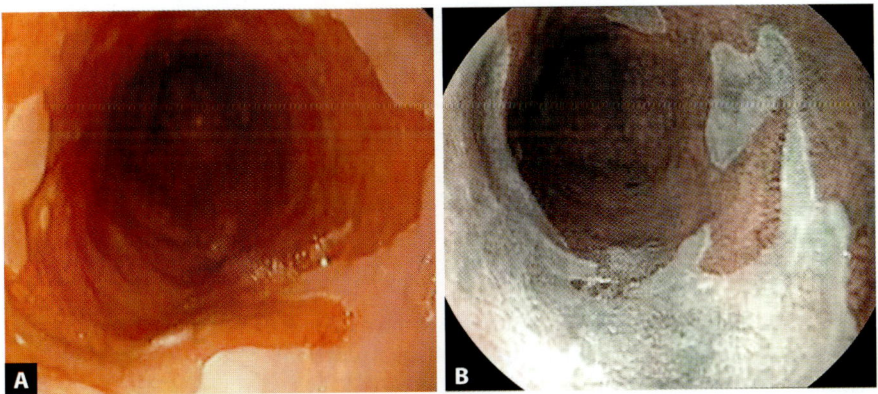

Figs. 8A and B: While light endoscopy and narrow-band imaging (NBI) of Barrett's esophagus.

Prague Classification of the Extent of Barrett's Esophagus (Figs. 9A and B)

Prague classification is commonly used to measure the extent of Barrett's changes. First, locate the top of the gastric rugal folds. Measure the circumferential extent of Barrett's mucosa in cm (C) and maximum height of tongues of Barrett's mucosa (M) and mention in the endoscopy report. If the maximum length of Barrett's is >3 cm, then it is called a *long segment,* and if it is <3 cm, then it is classified as a short segment of Barrett's esophagus which has less propensity for dysplasia.

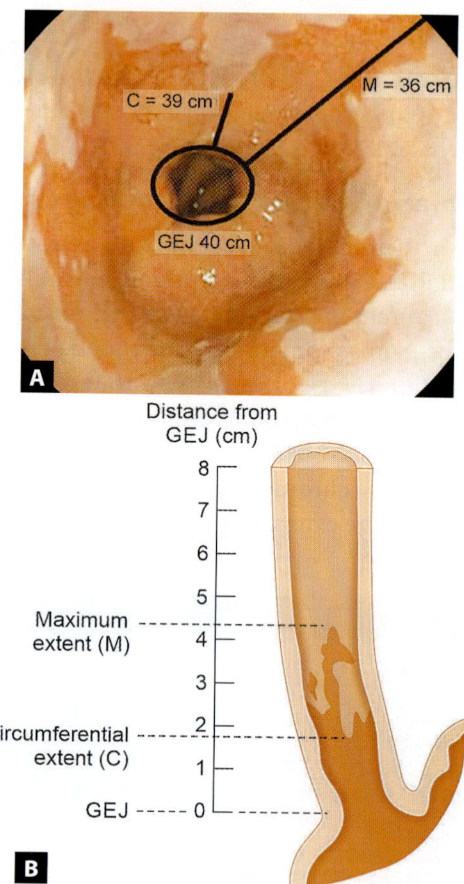

Figs. 9A and B: Prague classification of the extent of Barrett's esophagus. (GEJ: gastroesophageal junction)

Seattle Protocol (Fig. 10)

Biopsy is a must in all cases of Barrett's esophagus. Seattle protocol advocates a four-quadrant biopsy of Barrett's segment at 2 cm intervals to look for any dysplasia. More recently, we have followed the policy of target biopsy of only

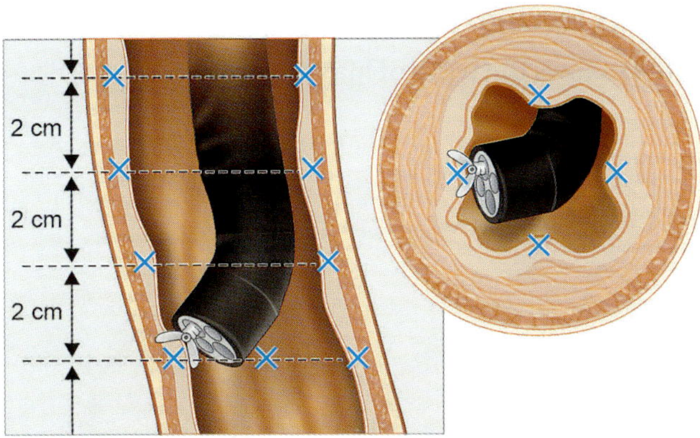

Fig. 10: Seattle protocol for biopsy.

areas showing mucosal or vascular irregularity in image enhancement mode to look for any dysplasia. We should look for dilatation, meandering, irregular caliber, and form variation in the intrapapillary capillary loops (IPCL).

Chromoendoscopy by spraying the esophagus with either methylene blue, Lugol's iodine, or acetic acid also helps to delineate Barrett's mucosal patches.

Dysplasia is divided into four categories: (1) Negative for dysplasia, (2) indefinite for dysplasia (ID), (3) low-grade dysplasia (LGD), and (4) high-grade dysplasia (HGD).

Low-grade dysplasia needs regular 3–6 months of endoscopic surveillance while high-grade dysplasia merits endoscopic or surgical intervention as the risk of adenocarcinoma is high in such individuals.

Young patients with classical reflux symptoms which are easily controlled by a course of acid suppression therapy may not require endoscopic evaluation as the first line, but we need to keep the endoscopic evaluation in the investigation algorithm in all other cases of GERD as given in **Box 3**.

BOX 3: Indications for diagnostic upper GI endoscopy in a case of GERD.

- GERD symptoms that are persistent or progressive despite appropriate medical therapy
- Dysphagia or odynophagia
- Significant weight loss
- Evidence of GI bleeding or anemia
- Finding of a mass, stricture, or ulcer in imaging studies
- Screening for Barrett's esophagus in selected patients (as clinically indicated)
- Persistent vomiting (7–10 days)
- Evaluation of patients before or with recurrent symptoms after endoscopic or surgical anti-reflux procedures
- Placement of wireless pH monitoring

(GERD: gastroesophageal reflux disease; GI: gastrointestinal)

Types of Hiatus Hernia

Figures 11A to D shows the types of hiatus hernia.

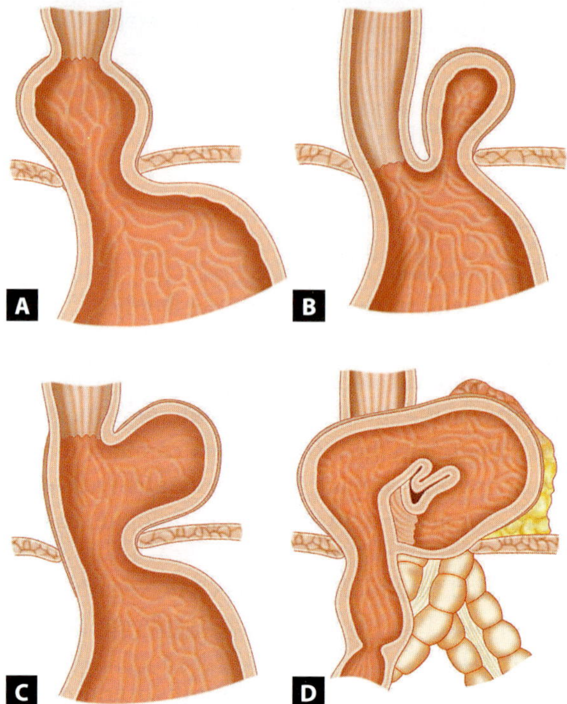

Figs. 11A to D: Types of hiatal hernia: (A) Type 1: Sliding hiatus hernia; (B) Type 2: Paraesophageal hiatus hernia; (C) Type 3: Mixed sliding and para esophageal type of hiatus hernia; and (D) Type 4: Mixed type of hiatus hernia along with other viscera namely colon and other solid viscera.

FUNCTIONAL ASSESSMENT OF GASTROESOPHAGEAL REFLUX DISEASE

Prior to any intervention, we ought to consider a 24-hour PH study along with high-resolution manometry (HRM) to precisely and accurately evaluate the present and severity of reflux disease.

24-Hour pH Study

We need to find the DeMeester score on evaluating the six components of 24-hour esophageal pH monitoring, namely:

1. Percent total time pH <4
2. Percent upright time pH <4
3. Percent supine time pH <4
4. Number of reflux episodes

5. Number of reflux episodes ≥5 minutes
6. Longest reflux episode (minutes)

The DeMeester score is a composite score used to diagnose gastroesophageal reflux disease (GERD). It measures the degree of esophageal reflux and how well the esophagus clears it. The composite score can be obtained by adding the scores calculated for each of the six components, called the DeMeester score [17], where >14.72 is considered abnormal, 14.72–50 is regarded as mild GERD, 51–100 is regarded as moderate GERD, and >100 is regarded as severe GERD.

High-resolution Manometry

High-resolution manometry may alter the surgical decision by assessment of esophageal peristaltic function and exclusion of esophageal outflow obstruction before antireflux surgery. In patients with poor peristaltic function, one may choose partial fundoplication over the classic Nissen's fundoplication.

Impedance PH Study

Esophageal impedance monitoring is considered the most sensitive tool for assessing all types of gastroesophageal reflux (acidic, weakly acidic, and weakly alkaline), their composition, proximal extent, duration, and clearing.

Impedance techniques are based on measurements of the electrical impedance between closely arranged electrodes mounted on a thin intraluminal probe. The impedance is inversely proportional to the electrical conductivity of the luminal contents and the cross-sectional area between the two electrodes. Air has low conductivity and causes an increase in impedance, whereas swallowed or refluxed material has high conductivity and causes a decrease in impedance.

The changes in the temporal-spatial patterns in impedance have been identified at various levels within the esophagus, allowing differentiation between antegrade (i.e., swallow) and retrograde (i.e., reflux) bolus movement. In this manner, the impedance can be used to evaluate the intraesophageal liquid movements (bolus transit tests and reflux monitoring) or gas movement (aerophagia and belching).

ROLE OF ENDOTHERAPY FOR GASTROESOPHAGEAL REFLUX DISEASE

Proton pump inhibitors are the cornerstone in the management of the majority of patients. However, 10–20% of the patients are refractory to PPI, and hence alternative treatment modalities should be considered in this subgroup. The treatment objectives of GERD are to relieve the reflux symptoms, improve quality of life, and to prevent the development of complications.

Surgery is associated with high morbidity, as well as a greater possibility of early therapeutic failure.

Moreover, many patients will not agree for the surgery due to its invasive nature and risk of complications, such as dysphagia, flatulence, and gas bloat. In such select subgroups of patients, endoscopic antireflux therapy can be considered.

Stretta procedure is radiofrequency ablation (RFA) of LES while EsophyX and GERDX are transoral endoscopic fundoplication procedures. In addition, antireflux mucosal resection (ARMS) and antireflux mucosal ablation (ARMA) using argon plasma coagulation (APC) are evolving novel therapies. Endoscopy will be also helpful in evaluating the patients after antireflux surgery if they present with any complications.

Stretta Procedure (Fig. 12)

The Stretta system (Mederi Therapeutics, Norwalk, CT, USA) involves the application of RF energy to the LES. The Stretta system delivers RF energy to the LES and gastric cardia leading to remodeling of the smooth muscle by potentially increasing the thickness of the musculature as well as the size and amount of smooth muscle fibers in the treatment zone. This leads to the strengthening of the OG barrier and possibly decreasing the rate of transient LES relaxation. It is an appropriate procedure for adult patients with GERD who wish to be off PPI and refuse laparoscopic fundoplication. Stretta is a viable low cost and safe procedure. Most importantly, Stretta does not preclude other therapies if needed and can be repeated when necessary.

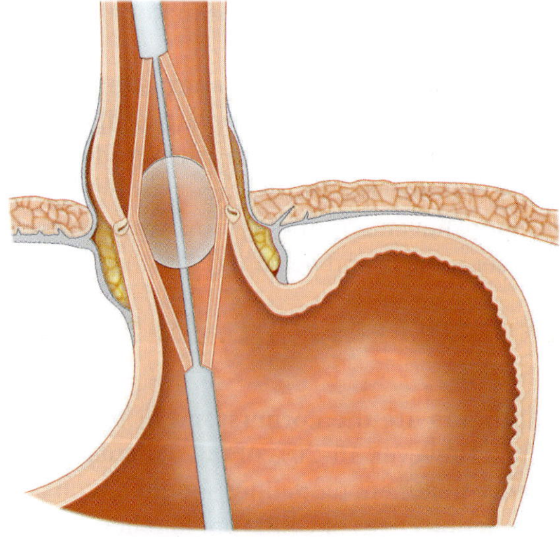

Fig. 12: Stretta procedure.

EsophyX (Transoral Incisionless Fundoplication) (Fig. 13A)

In this endoscopic procedure, check endoscopy and dilatation of the cricopharynx is done first to aid insertion of the EsophyX device along with the pediatric endoscope. The device is retroflexed in the stomach and an esophagogastric 270° wrap was done under endoscopic vision. GERDX is a similar procedure achieving tightening of the LES mechanism, especially in patients with Hill-type 2 or 3 types of LES **(Fig. 13B)**.

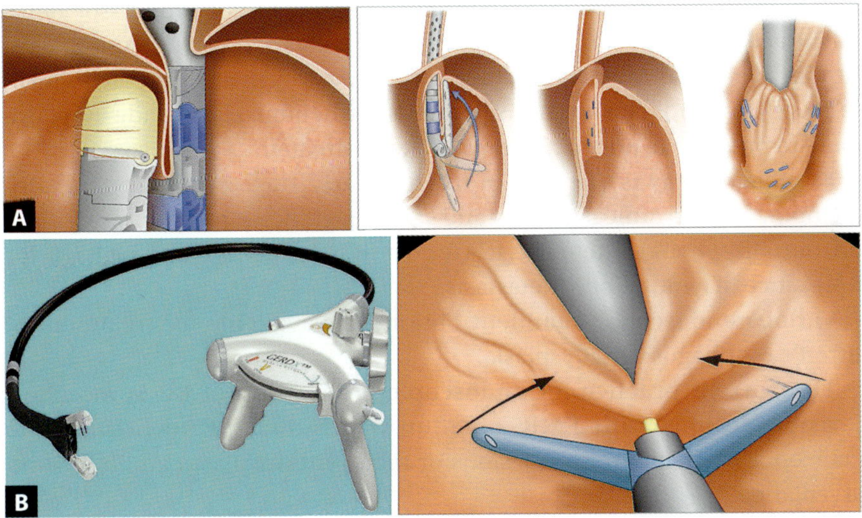

Figs. 13A and B: (A) EsophyX and (B) GERDX.

Antireflux Mucosal Resection Procedure (Figs. 14A and B)

The ARMS procedure is based on the principle that after mucosal resection, the mucosal healing results in scar formation. This in turn results in shrinkage and remodeling of the gastric cardia flap valve; thereby, reducing reflux events. About 270° circumferential endoscopic mucosal resection (EMR) is performed around the gastroesophageal junction (GEJ), which then contracts and tightens during healing.

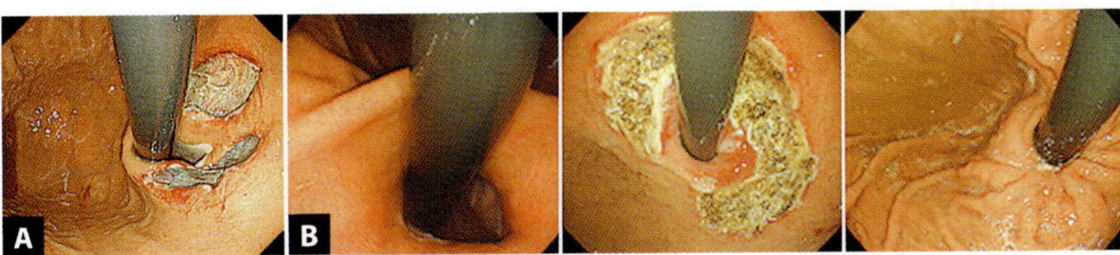

Figs. 14A and B: (A) Antireflux mucosal resection (ARMS) procedure; and (B) antireflux mucosal ablation procedure.

Antireflux mucosal ablation is a relatively easy procedure wherein a horseshoe-shaped area of mucosal ablation is achieved around cardia using APC.

RATIONALE AND WAYS OF ENDOTHERAPY FOR BARRETT'S ESOPHAGUS

Barrett's esophagus (BR) has the potential to progress to esophageal adenocarcinoma by genetic alteration of intestinal metaplasia, where there is unregulated cell growth due to the inactivation of tumor suppressor genes and the activation of oncogenes. This causes dysplasia in Barrett's esophagus. The aim of ablation/eradication therapy is to destroy this abnormal lining of the esophagus and reinstate nonsquamous epithelium. High-grade dysplasia is sure to progress to adenocarcinoma if left untreated.

Esophagectomy is effective in treating early-stage esophageal adenocarcinoma but is a radical therapy and carries significant morbidity (30–40%) and mortality (1–4%). Therefore, it is used only for patients with a high risk for or presence of lymph node metastasis.

Various endoscopic treatment options are available for treatment of Barrett's esophagus with dysplasia.

The current practice for endoscopic eradication of BE is resection of visible lesions with EMR, ablation of residual BE to prevent the occurrence of metachronous lesions or recurrent neoplasm and follow-up surveillance.

ENDOTHERAPY FOR BARRETT'S ESOPHAGUS

- *Thermal ablation therapy:*
  - Multipolar electrocoagulation
  - APC
  - Laser therapy
- *Nonthermal ablation therapy:*
  - Photodynamic therapy (PDT)
  - Radiofrequency ablation
  - Cryotherapy
- *Endoscopic resection:*
  - EMR
  - Endoscopic submucosal dissection (ESD)

Endoscopic mucosal resection and ESD are indicated for nodular areas while ablative therapy using PDT, RFA, cryotherapy or APC are applicable for flat dysplastic areas.

Endoscopic mucosal resection can be done by using a cap or band. In cap EMR, a special cap is applied to the endoscope tip. Submucosal injection of saline is given prior to applying suction of the affected mucosa into the cap. Subsequently, a diathermy snare is used to resect the lesion within the suction cap.

Suction EMR Band Mucosectomy device (Cook Medical, Limerick, and Ireland) is a modified version of the variceal band ligator that allows the passage of a snare into the working channel of the endoscope. Submucosal injections and lifting of the mucosa are not used in any such cases.

Radiofrequency ablation devices **(Figs. 15A and B)** are available in circumferential and focal configurations (which can be over the scope or through the scope). For longer and circumferential segments, the Barrx TM 360 (Medtronic, MN, USA) Express catheter can be used. It has a balloon 4 cm in length and is able to treat 4 cm with a single application. Following a spray of diluted N-acetyl cysteine (which acts as a mucolytic), facilitating optimal mucosal contact with the balloon, the treatment catheter is advanced over a wire into the esophagus. Under the vision, the proximal edge of the balloon catheter is placed 1 cm proximal to the BE segment and ablation is begun. The balloon is moved down sequentially to complete the ablation of the entire segment. The dose is 10 J per application and two applications are recommended at every site. Cleaning between applications is optional.

Shorter noncircumferential segments are treated with focal devices which are available in three configurations: two over the scope, the Barrx TM 90 and Barrx TM 60 (Medtronic, MN, USA), and one through the scope, the channel catheter. The device is placed in close contact with the BE mucosa and a preset energy dose (12 or 15 J) is delivered (three applications sequentially if no cleaning, or two-clean-two applications if cleaning between applications). The Barrx TM catheter is useful in those in whom intubation may be somewhat challenging or in those with minimal residual disease.

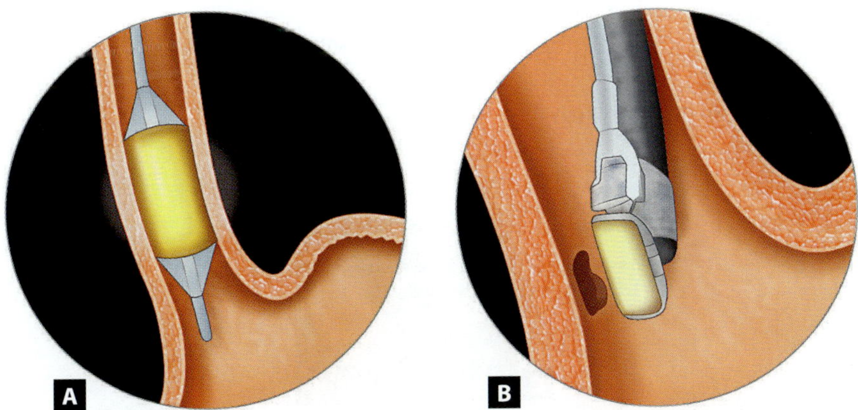

Figs. 15A and B: Radiofrequency ablation (RFA) devices.

Photodynamic therapy is a treatment with a photosensitizing drug administered in the circulation and activated with light of a specific wavelength that destroys the tumor cells. PDT for eradicating Barrett's esophagus has been abandoned because of ineffectiveness and practicality.

ROLE OF ENDOSCOPY IN EVALUATION FOR THE COMPLICATIONS AFTER FUNDOPLICATION

In patients with persisting or recurrent reflux symptoms or dysphagia would warrant endoscopic and radiological evaluation. Endoscopic evaluation by the operating surgeon would have more diagnostic yield. We need to get familiarized with endoscopic anatomy after various types of fundoplication **(Figs. 16A to C)**.

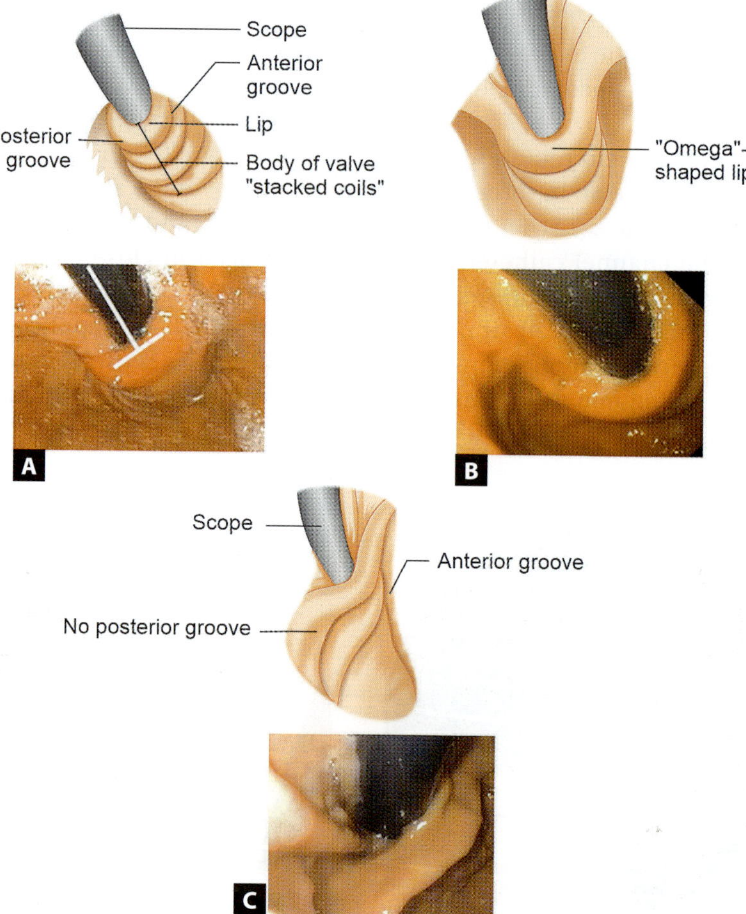

Figs. 16A to C: Endoscopy after various types of fundoplication. (A) Nissen's total fundoplication; (B) Toupet's partial fundoplication; and (C) Dor's anterior fundoplication.

Endoscopic Findings of Complications after Fundoplication

Figures 17A to G shows the endoscopic findings of complications after fundoplication.

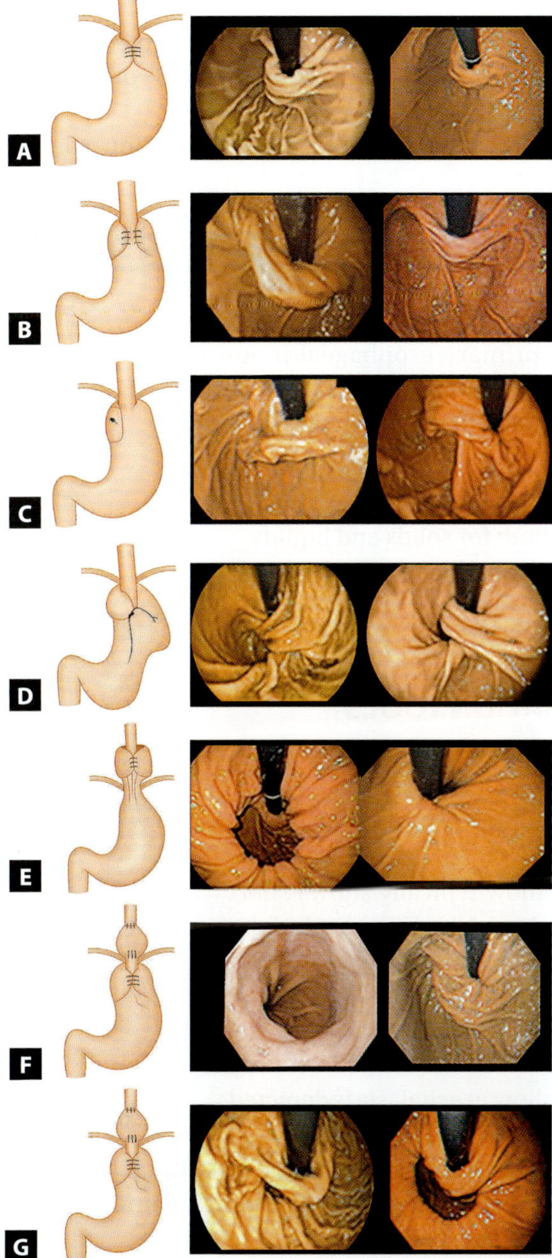

Figs. 17A to G: Various complications after fundoplication. (A) Normal aspect of Nissen fundoplication; (B) Partial fundoplication; (C) Disrupted fundoplication; (D) Twisted fundoplication; (E) Migrated fundoplication; (F) Slipped fundoplication; and (G) Paraesophageal hernia.

KEY MESSAGES

- HD endoscopy with NBI is essential in the evaluation of GERD.
- Impedance pH study with manometry is preferable prior to surgical intervention.
- Lap Nissen's fundoplication is the most preferred surgical options.
- Endotherapy for GERD is under evolution and could soon be the standard of care.
- Lifestyle modification and PPI are the cornerstones in the management of GERD.

ROLE OF ENDOSCOPY IN ACHALASIA

INTRODUCTION

Achalasia is a primary esophageal motor disorder of unknown etiology characterized by impaired relaxation of the EGJ, along with the loss of organized peristalsis in the esophageal body.

PRESENTATION SYMPTOMS

- Dysphagia both for solids and liquids
- Regurgitation and heartburn
- Chest pain
- Weight loss

INVESTIGATION TOOLS

- Barium swallow
- Flexible upper GI endoscopy
- HRM
- EndoFLIP

Barium swallow typically shows short smooth narrowing of the lower end of the esophagus like a "bird beak;" with a dilated sigmoid-like dilated esophageal body with poor emptying of contrast into the stomach.

Barium swallow in achalasia is depicted in **Figure 18**.

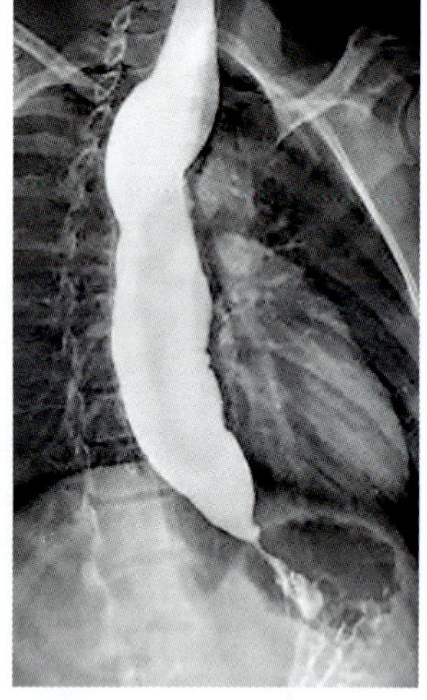

Fig. 18: Barium swallow in achalasia.

Though HRM is the test of choice, endoscopy is essential in all cases of achalasia which reveals the following findings, namely:

- Dilated sigmoid esophagus
- Fluid, and food residue in the esophagus
- Spastic lower esophageal Sphincter
- Absent peristalsis in the esophagus

ENDOSCOPIC FINDINGS IN ACHALASIA (FIGS. 19A TO C)

Endoscopy is also helpful to exclude the diagnosis of pseudo achalasia due to short scirrhous tumors at the cardia.

High-resolution manometry confirms and classifies the condition into three subtypes as per the Chicago classification. It shows typically incomplete relaxation of the EGJ coupled with the absence of organized peristalsis.

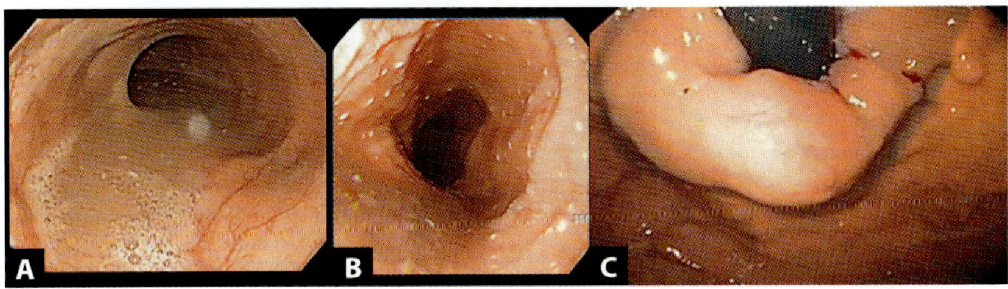

Figs. 19A to C: Endoscopic pictures of achalasia. (A) Fluid-filled esophagus; (B) Dilated esophagus with absent peristalsis; and (C) Spastic lower esophageal sphincter (LES).

Type I: Classic achalasia with low intraesophageal pressure.

Type II: Achalasia with panesophageal pressurization.

Type III: Achalasia with high-amplitude spastic contractions.

High-resolution manometry showing three types of achalasia **(Fig. 20)**.

The endoluminal functional lumen imaging probe (EndoFLIP, Crospon, Galway, Ireland) is a new technology that enables the assessment of the mechanical properties of the esophagus and EGJ. The EndoFLIP

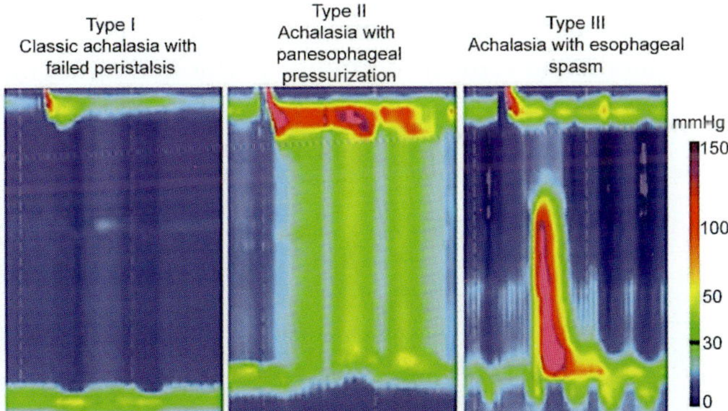

Fig. 20: High-resolution manometry images in achalasia.

(Figs. 21A and B) (EndoFLIP, Crospon, Galway, Ireland) is a new technology that enables assessment of the mechanical properties of the esophagus and EGJ and soon it will be considered in all cases of achalasia during surgery to monitor the adequacy of myotomy!

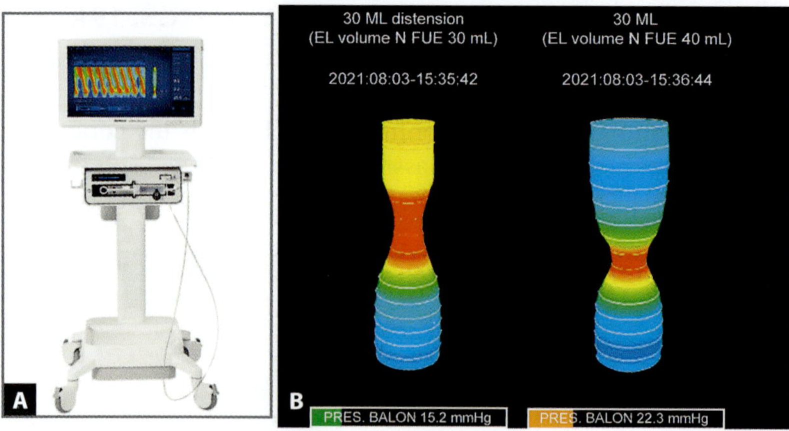

Figs. 21A and B: EndoFLIP.

Treatment

Based on available data, pneumatic dilation, laparoscopic Heller myotomy, and peroral endoscopic myotomy (POEM) are all believed to be efficacious for achalasia types I and II, whereas POEM has emerged as the preferred treatment for achalasia type III.

The Eckardt score is based on the summation of four symptoms (dysphagia, regurgitation, chest pain, and weight loss) that are graded according to severity, and treatment success. Eckardt score is used to measure the success of various therapeutic modalities for achalasia.

Pneumatic Balloon Dilation (Figs. 22A to C)

Pneumatic dilation disrupts the LES fibers through intraluminal dilation of a pressurized balloon and is most commonly performed under fluoroscopic

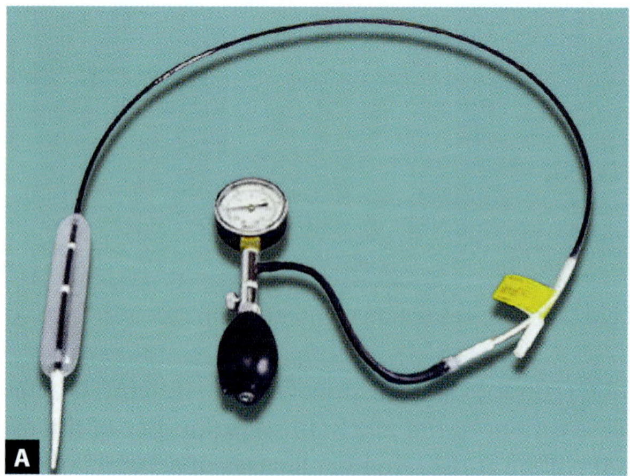

Fig. 22A

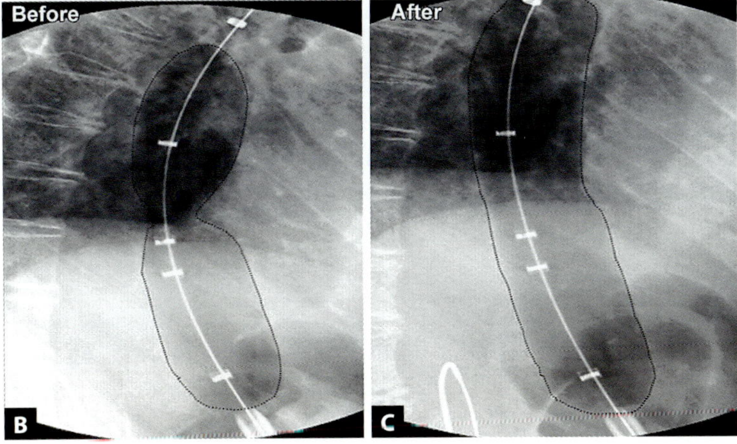

Figs. 22B and C

Figs. 22A to C: Pneumatic dilation.

guidance. Three balloon sizes (30, 35, and 40 mm diameter) are available for pneumatic dilation. The conventional approach is to start with the 30-mm balloon in most patients, progressing to bigger diameter balloons if a response is not achieved. Though this is very effective but not durable. It is typically indicated in patients not fit or unwilling for any surgical or endoscopic procedures. There is about a 3% risk of perforation and a 9% risk of reflux symptoms after dilatation.

Endoscopic Botox Injection (Fig. 23)

Endoscopy-based injection of botulinum toxin reduces LES pressure by inhibiting the release of acetylcholine from nerve endings. It is considered

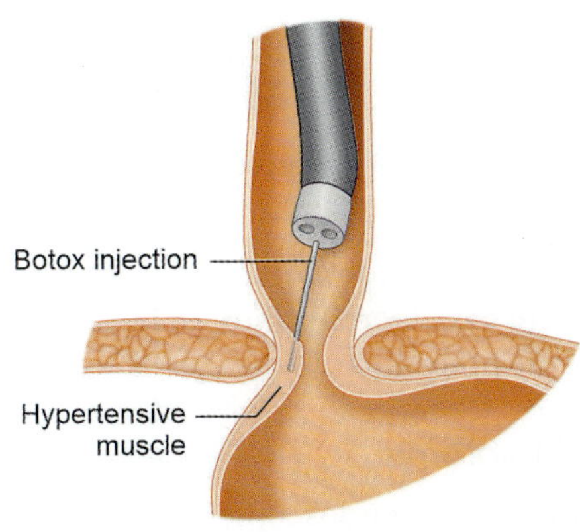

Fig. 23: Endoscopic botox.

to be generally very safe, and serious adverse events such as mediastinitis or allergic reactions are exceedingly rare.

Laparoscopic Heller's Myotomy (Figs. 24A and B)

Laparoscopic exposure and mobilization of lower 8–10 cm of esophagus. Anterior myotomy is done 5–6 cm on the esophagus and 2–3 cm in the stomach taking care to avoid any mucosal injury. This is accompanied by

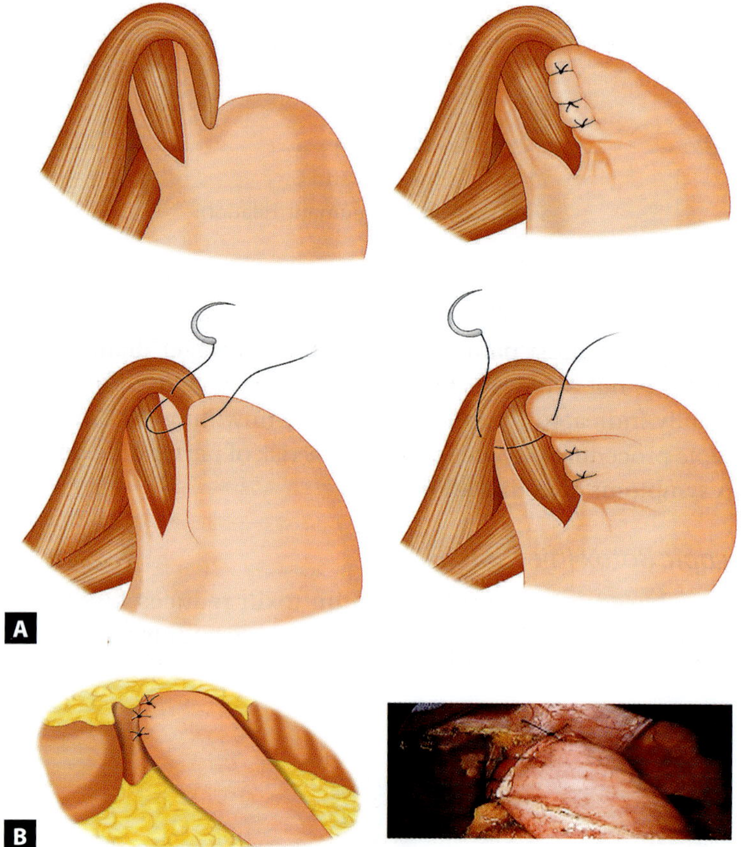

Figs. 24A and B: Laparoscopic myotomy.

anterior Dor fundoplication. Endoscopic assistance has been favored in recent times to facilitate easy identification of LEC and check for mucosal integrity at the end of the procedure.

Peroral Esophageal Myotomy

In POEM **(Figs. 25A to E)**, the endoscopic surgeon creates a submucosal tunnel from 25 cm downward to 3 cm beyond LES onto the gastric side.

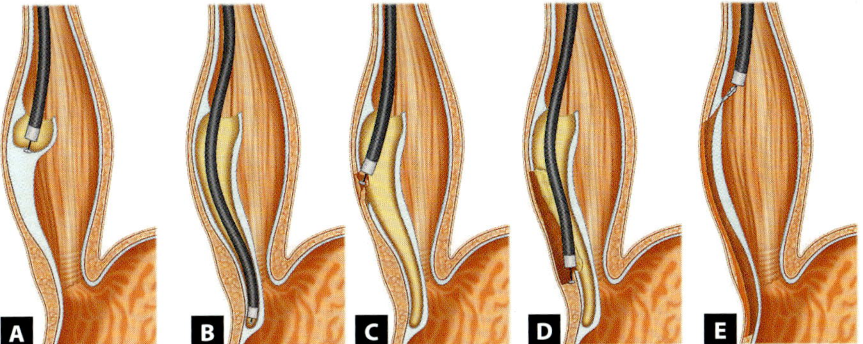

Figs. 25A to E: POEM images.

Thanks to the insulation-tipped (IT) knife and HD magnifying endoscope, we are able to perform precision myotomy with hemostasis.

KEY STEPS

- Mucosal incision.
- Creation of a submucous tunnel using an IT knife.
- Complete myotomy including 2–3 cm on the gastric side.
- Closure of mucosal incision with hemoclips.

In view of the preservation of sling fibers at LES and the nondisturbance of the phrenoesophageal ligament, POEM is expected to have less incidence of reflux compared to surgery. Nowadays, fundoplication can also be done endoscopically (POEM-F).

Peroral endoscopic myotomy can involve either anterior or posterior myotomy. POEM is ideally suited for type 3 achalasia cardia. POEM is also useful as a rescue procedure for failed laparoscopic Heller's myotomy.

KEY MESSAGES (TABLE 1)

- POEM and laparoscopic Heller myotomy are comparable treatment options for the management of patients with achalasia types I and II.

TABLE 1: Comparison of various treatment modalities of achalasia.

Comparison	*Balloon dilatation*	*Lap Heller's myotomy*	*Peroral endoscopic myotomy*
Type of procedure	Least invasive	Most invasive	Less invasive
Ease of procedure	Very easy	Easy to master	Steep learning curve
Effectiveness	Short term	Long term	Long-term results awaited
Incidence of reflux	Significant	Less with antireflux procedures	Matter of debate

- POEM is preferred for type III achalasia.
- Antireflux procedure is indicated along with laparoscopic Heller's myotomy.
- Botox injection and balloon dilatation are reserved for high-risk surgical patients.

SUGGESTED READING

1. ASGE Standards of Practice Committee; Evans JA, Early DS, Fukami N, Ben-Menachem T, Chandrasekhara V, et al. The role of endoscopy in Barrett's esophagus and other premalignant conditions of the esophagus. Gastrointest Endosc. 2012;76(6):1087-94.
2. ASGE Standards of Practice Committee; Pasha SF, Acosta RD, Chandrasekhara V, Chathadi KV, Decker GA, et al. The role of endoscopy in the evaluation and management of dysphagia. Gastrointest Endosc. 2014;79(2):191-201.
3. DeVault KR, Castell DO; American College of Gastroenterology. Updated guidelines for the diagnosis and treatment of gastroesophageal reflux disease. Am J Gastroenterol. 2005;100(1):190-200.
4. Dughera L, Rotondano G, De Cento M, Cassolino P, Cisarò F. Durability of Stretta radiofrequency treatment for GERD: results of an 8-year follow-up. Gastroenterol Res Pract. 2014;2014:531907.
5. Fock KM, Talley N, Hunt R, Fass R, Nandurkar S, Lam SK, et al. Report of the Asia-Pacific consensus on the management of gastroesophageal reflux disease. J Gastroenterol Hepatol. 2004;19(4):357-67.
6. Kahrilas PJ, Shaheen NJ, Vaezi MF, Hiltz SW, Black E, Modlin IM, et al. American Gastroenterological Association Medical Position Statement on the management of gastroesophageal reflux disease. Gastroenterology. 2008;35(4):1383-91; 1391.e1-5.
7. Lieberman DA, Oehlke M, Helfand M. Risk factors for Barrett's esophagus in community-based practice. GORGE consortium. Gastroenterology Outcomes Research Group in Endoscopy. Am J Gastroenterol. 1997;92(8):1293-7.
8. Moayyedi P, Talley NJ. Gastro-oesophageal reflux disease. Lancet. 2006; 367(9528):2086-100.
9. Modiano N, Gerson LB. Risk factors for the detection of Barrett's esophagus in patients with erosive esophagitis. Gastrointest Endosc. 2009;69(6):1014-20.
10. Noar M, Squires P, Noar E, Lee M. Long-term maintenance effect of radio-frequency energy delivery for refractory GERD: a decade later. Surg Endosc. 2014;28(8):2323-33.
11. Richter JE. Diagnostic tests for gastroesophageal reflux disease. Am J Med Sci. 2003;326(5):300-8.
12. Rodriguez S, Mattek N, Lieberman D, Fennerty B, Eisen G. Barrett's esophagus on repeat endoscopy: should we look more than once? Am J Gastroenterol. 2008; 103(8):1892-7.
13. Shaheen NJ, Weinberg DS, Denberg TD, Chou R, Qaseem A, Shekelle P, et al. Upper endoscopy for gastroesophageal reflux disease: best practice advice from the clinical guidelines committee of the American College of Physicians. Ann Intern Med. 2012;157(11):808-16.

14. Spechler SJ, Sharma P, Souza RF, Inadomi JM, Shaheen NJ. American Gastroenterological Association medical position statement on the management of Barrett's esophagus. Gastroenterology. 2011;140(3):1084-91.
15. Spechler SJ. Barrett esophagus and risk of esophageal cancer: a clinical review. JAMA. 2013;310(6):627-36.
16. Standards of Practice Committee; Lichtenstein DR, Cash BD, Davila R, Baron TH, Adler DG, et al. Role of endoscopy in the management of GERD. Gastrointest Endosc. 2007;66(2):219-24.
17. Wendling MR, Melvin WS, Perry KA. Impact of transoral incisionless fundoplication (TIF) on subjective and objective GERD indices: a systematic review of the published literature. Surg Endosc. 2013;27(10):3754-61.
18. Wo JM, Mendez C, Harrell S, Joubran R, Bressoud PF, McKinney WP. Clinical impact of upper endoscopy in the management of patients with gastroesophageal reflux disease. Am J Gastroenterol. 2004;99(12):2311-6.

Expert's Comment

Gastrointestinal reflux disease (GERD) is diagnosed mostly clinically. Esophageal reflux disease (EGD) is needed for grading in patients who develop symptoms due to complications such as dysphagia, odynophagia, significant weight loss, gastrointestinal (GI) bleeding, and anorexia. It is also done for the surveillance of Barrett's esophagus—a sequel of chronic reflux, patients not responding to proton-pump inhibitor (PPI), and for the follow-up after antireflux interventions. In addition to conventional white light endoscopy, high-resolution and high-magnification endoscopy and optical chromoendoscopy play a vital role in the diagnosis of GERD.

Therapeutic use of endoscopy in GERD, like the Sterra procedure, transoral fundoplication, mucosectomy, endoscopic submucosal dissection (ESD), and endoscopic mucosal resection (EMR), is limited to a few centers.

In achalasia cardia, endoscopy plays roles in both diagnostic and therapeutic purposes. Dilated esophagus and retained food and fluid with spastic lower esophageal sphincter (LES) is diagnostic of achalasia. It also helps to exclude pseudoachalasia. Therapeutic implication to relieve symptoms by disrupting LES through interventions like pneumatic balloon dilatation and peroral endoscopic myotomy (POEM) offers good results, which are comparable to surgery.

Endoscopy is a rapidly developing technology. Endoscopic surgery has undergone dramatic improvement since its introduction in India and in neighboring countries like Bangladesh. The proper, safe, and effective use of endoscopy is highly dependent on the user, which has a major impact on the patient's overall benefit. In fact, the skill and training of the user are often more important than the instrument used. For this reason, IAGES is conducting training programs on endoscopy regularly; moreover, they have taken the initiative to publish books on endoscopy, compiling the knowledge and experience of surgeons, which is something new and more informative, particularly in the interventional aspect. I am really grateful to IAGES on behalf of Bangladeshi surgeons for including me in this journey.

Professor Dr AHM Towhidul Alam
Bangladesh

CHAPTER 9

Role of Endoscopy in Upper Gastrointestinal Malignancy

Chapter Outline

- Endoscopy in Barrett's Esophagus
- Esophageal Leiomyoma
- Gastrointestinal Stromal Tumor Upper Gastrointestinal Tract
- Carcinoma Esophagus
- Gastric Polyps
  - Fundic Polyp
  - Hyperplastic Polyp
  - Adenomatous Polyp
  - Ectopic Pancreas
  - Peutz–Jeghers Polyps and Syndrome
- Neuroendocrine Tumors (Formerly Called Carcinoids)
- Carcinoma Stomach
  - Locally Advanced Gastric Cancers
  - Early Gastric Cancers
- Endotherapy for Barrett's Esophagus
  - Cap Endoscopic Mucosal Resection
  - Endoscopic Submucosal Dissection
- Endoscopic Management of Leiomyoma
- Endoscopy Laparoscopy Cooperative Surgery for Gastric Gastrointestinal Stromal Tumor
- Endoscopic Polypectomy for Gastric Polyps
  - Tools Required
  - Key Steps
  - Complications
- Role of Endoscopic Submucosal Dissection for Gastric Lesions
- Endoscopic Savary Dilatation
- Endoscopic Controlled Radial Expansion Balloon Dilatation
- Endoscopic Stent Deployment
- Endoscopic Rescue for Surgical Complications

Keywords: Barrett's esophagus, gastroinstestinal stromal tumor, neuroendocrine tumor, early gastric cancer, Savary dilatation, stent deployment

Thanks to HD endoscopy with image enhancement and a vast array of endoscopic accessories, early diagnosis and therapy are possible for upper GI tumors.

1. ROLE OF DIAGNOSTIC ENDOSCOPY IN UPPER GASTROINTESTINAL TUMORS

ENDOSCOPY IN BARRETT'S ESOPHAGUS (FIGS. 1A AND B)

- High-definition (HD) endoscopy with image enhancement modality [narrow-band imaging (NBI), i-scan, or flexible spectral imaging color enhancement (FICE)] would enable easy recognition of Barrett's esophagus (BE).
- Chromoendoscopy using methylene blue, Lugol's iodine, or acetic acid as a reactive dye will be also helpful.

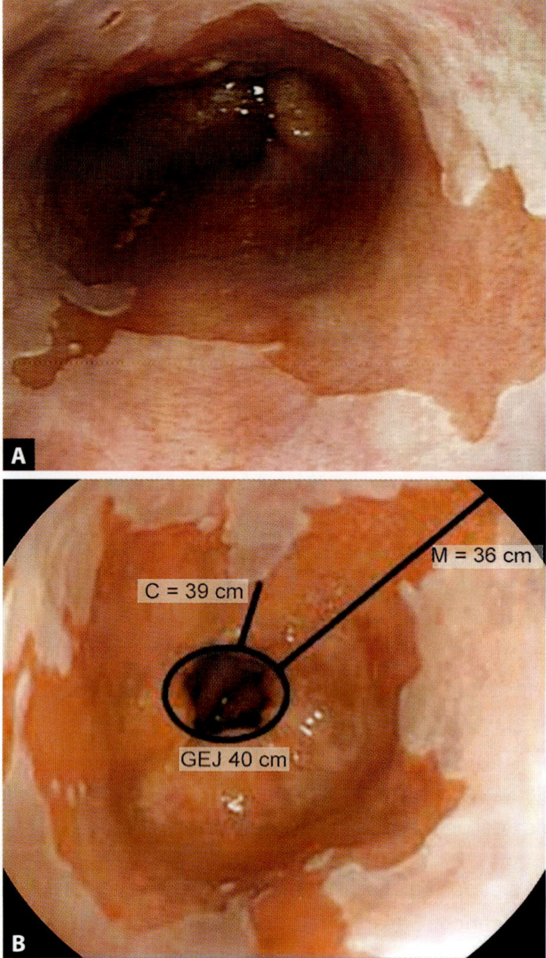

Figs. 1A and B: Barrett's esophagus. (GEJ: gastroesophageal junction)

- We need to assess the extent of BE by using the Prague classification. We need to consider either Seattle protocol of four quadrant biopsy or target biopsy of suspicious areas showing mucosal surface irregularity or vascular irregularity as per the Bing classification. (Barrett's international NBI group).
- Biopsy report showing dysplasia warrants careful follow-up and endotherapy.

ESOPHAGEAL LEIOMYOMA (FIGS. 2A AND B)

- Esophageal leiomyoma is a rare type of benign esophageal neoplasm found in cases presenting with chest pain and dysphagia.
- Endoscopy shows a submucosal firm mass in the lower two-thirds of the esophagus. An endoscopic biopsy is not advisable.
- Endoscopic ultrasound (US) or computed tomography (CT) scan chest or MRI imaging will delineate the exact size, nature, and location of the tumor and assist in the treatment plan.
- Either thoracoscopic or endoscopic excision is needed in large and symptomatic lesions.

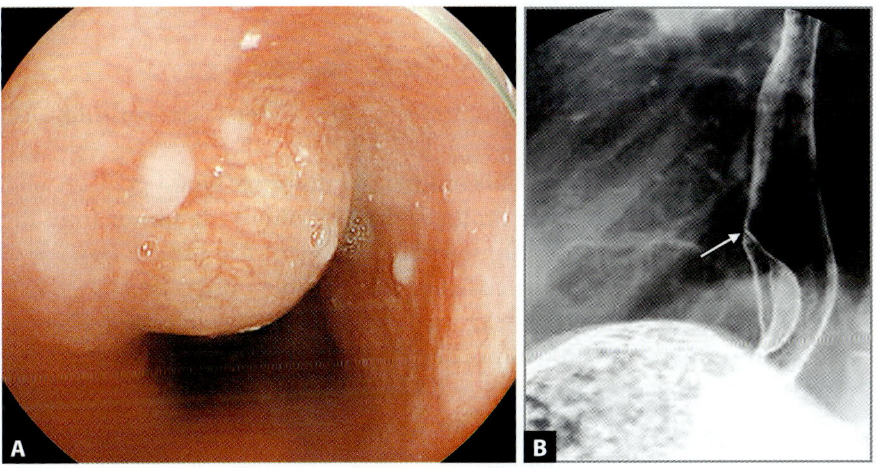

Figs. 2A and B: Esophageal leiomyoma.

GASTROINTESTINAL STROMAL TUMOR UPPER GASTROINTESTINAL TRACT (FIGS. 3A AND B)

- Gastrointestinal stromal tumors (GISTs) are rare mesenchymal tumors that originate from the interstitial cells of Cajal.
- They represent <1% of all neoplasms in the gastrointestinal tract. The stomach is the most common site of GIST (60%), followed by the small intestines (35%), and lastly by the colon and rectum (5%). <1% of tumors are found in the esophagus and gastroesophageal junction.

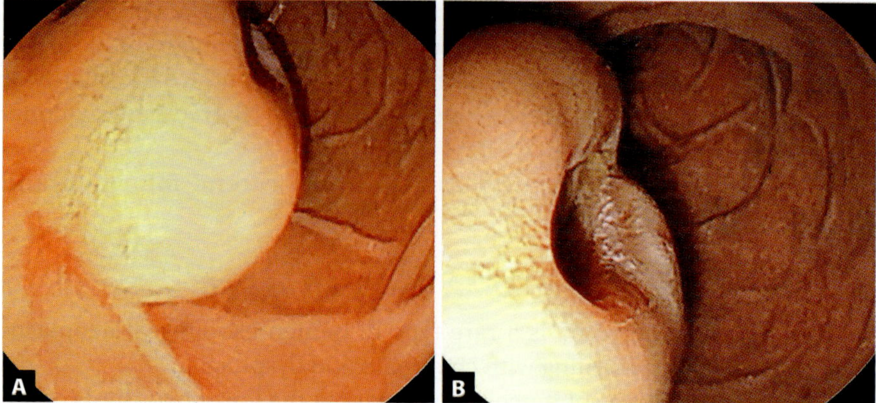

Figs. 3A and B: Gist upper gastrointestinal tract.

- They are presented as polypoidal masses with central umbilication.
- In suspected gastric GIST, a biopsy has to be sent for immunohistochemistry (IHC). The immunohistochemical markers CD117 (KIT) and DOG1 have become standard in routine diagnostics. GIST could present as acute upper GI bleeding.

CARCINOMA ESOPHAGUS (FIGS. 4A TO C)

- Esophageal carcinoma is common in the elderly, presenting with progressive dysphagia with weight loss.
- Can present as a polypoidal, ulcerative, or infiltrative type.
- We need to find the upper limit and lower limit of the tumor from the incisor teeth and the circumferential extent of the tumor. Beware of associated tracheo esophageal fistula in the upper third tumors.
- In case of tight malignant stricture, it might be better to take the biopsy from the upper part of the tumor and avoid any attempt at blind dilatation to evaluate the lesion completely. CT imaging and barium swallow would provide the road map, and dilatation should be done at the second sitting under C-arm image guidance.

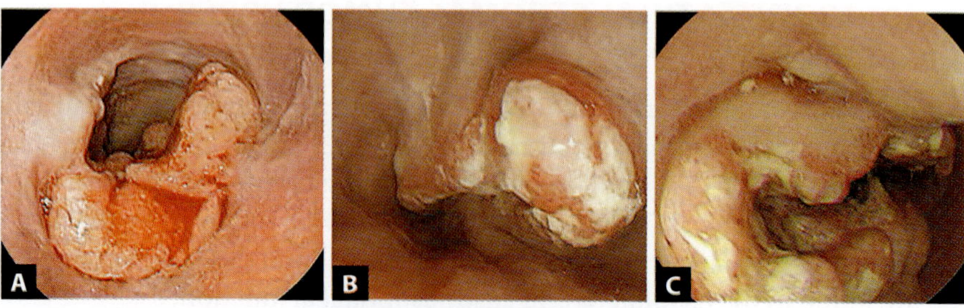

Figs. 4A to C: Carcinoma esophagus.

- Squamous cell carcinoma is common in the upper two-thirds and adenocarcinoma is prevalent in the lower third of the esophagus and esophagogastric (OG) junction.
- PET CT and endoscopic US are the common modalities to stage the tumor more accurately before any treatment plan.

GASTRIC POLYPS

Gastric polyps are a heterogeneous group of epithelial and subepithelial lesions that can vary in histology, neoplastic potential, and management.

Fundic Polyp (Figs. 5A and B)

They are normally present in the fundus and body in middle-aged women as hyperemic, glistening, smooth-surfaced sessile lesions of 1–8 mm in size. They blend with surrounding normal gastric mucosa and could be easily overlooked. They present themselves as sporadic lesions, in patients with long-term proton pump inhibitor (PPI) or patients with familial polyposis. The risk of malignancy is very low (<1%). Surveillance is not needed for sporadic fundic polyps. But in a suspected case of familial adenomatous polyposis (FAP), one has to proceed to a colonoscopy.

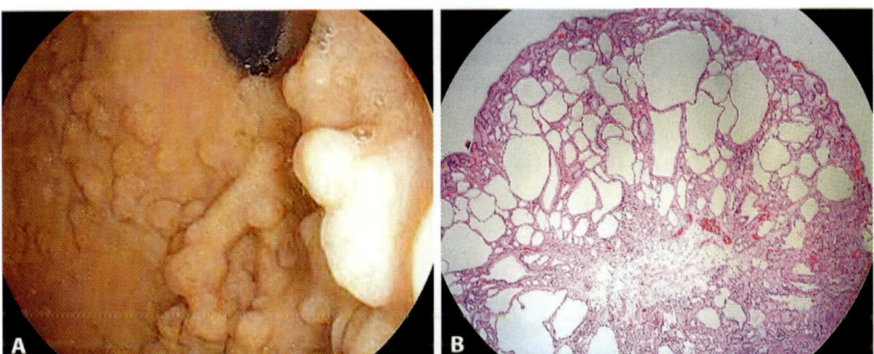

Figs. 5A and B: Fundic polyp.

Hyperplastic Polyp (Figs. 6A and B)

They normally present in the gastric antrum as sessile or pedunculated polyps of size up to 2 cm. There is often associated with *Helicobacter pylori* gastritis. Though they have low dysplastic potential, there is a high risk of synchronous cancer elsewhere in the stomach due to underlying chronic gastritis. Hence, surveillance endoscopy is recommended after the excision of a polyp.

Adenomatous Polyp (Figs. 7A and B)

They are rare and present in the gastric antrum as a solitary sessile or pedunculated polyp of size up to 2 cm. There is high dysplastic potential, and endoscopic submucosal resection is warranted.

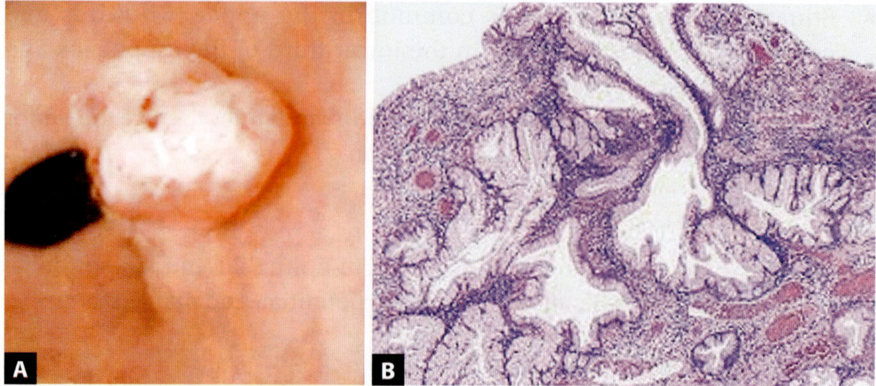

Figs. 6A and B: Hyperplastic polyp.

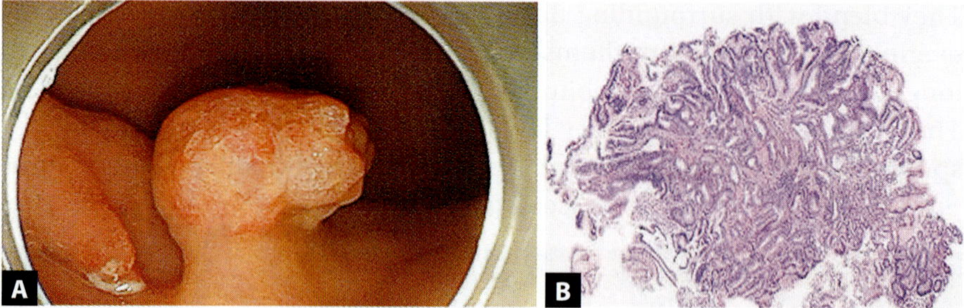

Figs. 7A and B: Adenomatous polyp.

Ectopic Pancreas (Figs. 8A and B)

Present as a submucosal lesion with umbilication in the antrum with the least malignant potential.

Peutz–Jeghers Polyps and Syndrome (Figs. 9A and B)

It is an autosomal dominant hereditary condition with hamartomatous polyps in the bowel and pigmented lips. They often look like hyperplastic

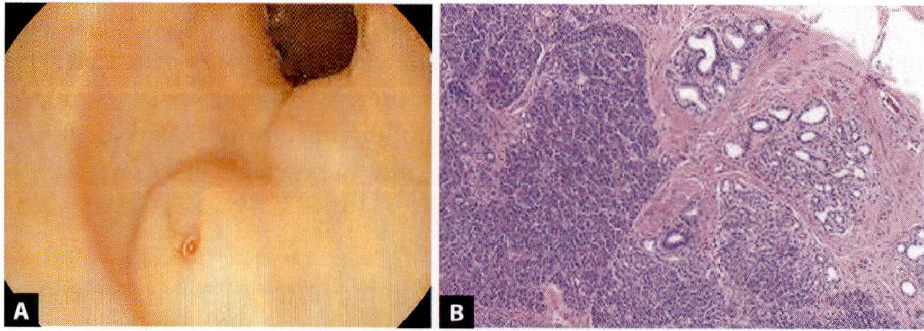

Figs. 8A and B: Ectopic pancreas.

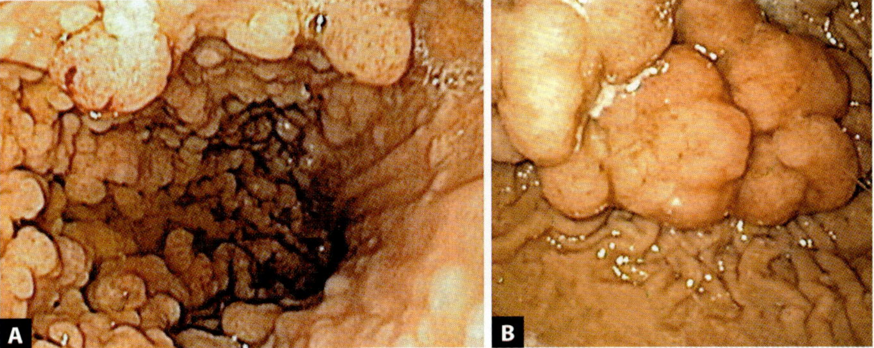

Figs. 9A and B: Peutz–Jeghers polyps and syndrome.

polyps and any polyp larger than 2 cm needs to be excised. We need to look for small bowel and colonic polyps in such cases.

- *Juvenile polyposis syndrome* ***(Figs. 10A and B)***: It is yet another autosomal dominant condition presenting typically with a solitary lesion in the distal stomach and it carries high malignant potential.

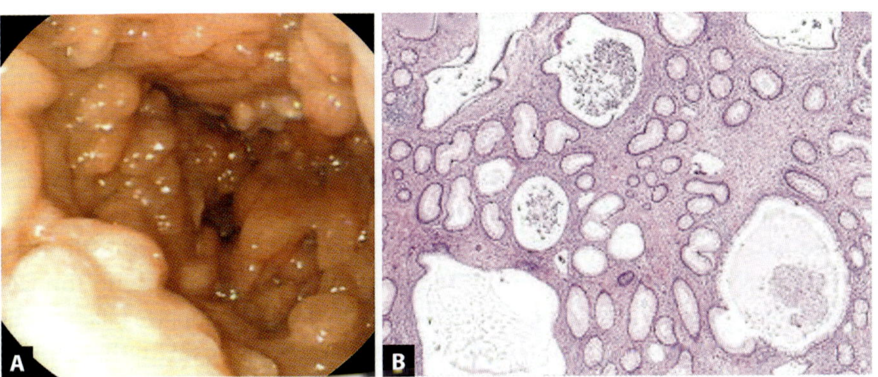

Figs. 10A and B: Juvenile polyposis syndrome.

NEUROENDOCRINE TUMORS (FORMERLY CALLED CARCINOIDS) (FIGS. 11A AND B)

They are commonly present as submucosal tumors with central ulceration in the fundus and body of the stomach. They arise from enterochromaffin-like (ECL) cells and stain with chromogranin A. There are four types of neuroendocrine tumor (NET).

1. *Type 1:* Seen as a cluster of lesions in the proximal stomach in cases of pernicious anemia.
2. *Type 2:* Often seen in the case of multiple endocrine neoplasia type 1 (MEN1) syndrome/Zollinger–Ellison syndrome as multiple lesions in the fundus and body of the stomach.

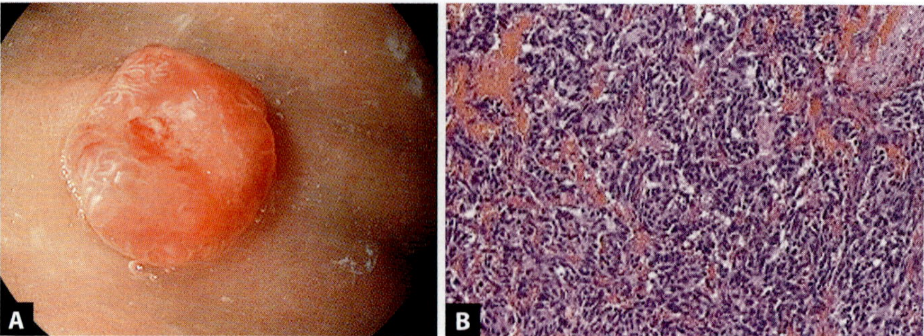

Figs. 11A and B: Neuroendocrine tumor.

3. *Type 3:* Solitary lesion in the stomach and has high malignant potential with lymphatic spread if it is >2 cm. Hence endoscopic resection is recommended.
4. *Type 4:* Large solitary lesion seen in the elderly person in any part of the stomach. It has the worst prognosis due to high malignant potential. Biopsy of surrounding mucosa is paramount in all cases of NET to assess the prognosis and treatment!

CARCINOMA STOMACH (FIGS. 12A TO C)

Locally Advanced Gastric Cancers

- Carcinoma stomach should be suspected in patients with new onset dyspepsia with alarm symptoms such as anorexia, significant weight loss, GI bleeding, vomiting, and dysphagia.
- Endoscopy will show the polypoidal, ulcerative, or ulceroinfiltrative tumor. Note the exact site, size, and extent both proximally to the OG junction and distally to the pyloric opening. Multiple biopsies (six to eight bites) from the edge of the lesion are recommended using either spiked biopsy forceps or multibite biopsy forceps.
- In the case of linitis plastica, the biopsy report often comes back as a false negative, and hence deeper biopsy or endoscopic US-guided biopsy is recommended.

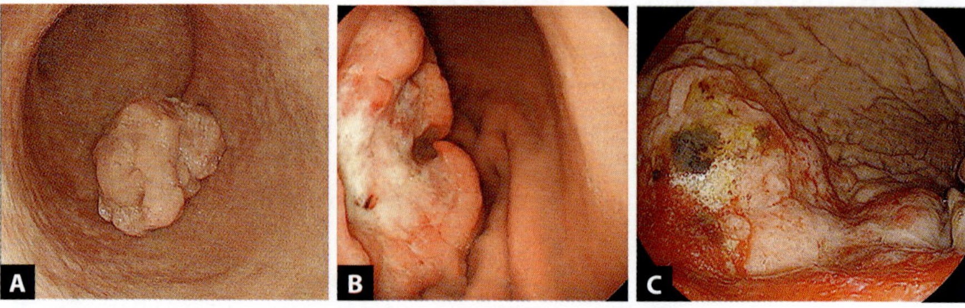

Figs. 12A to C: Carcinoma stomach.

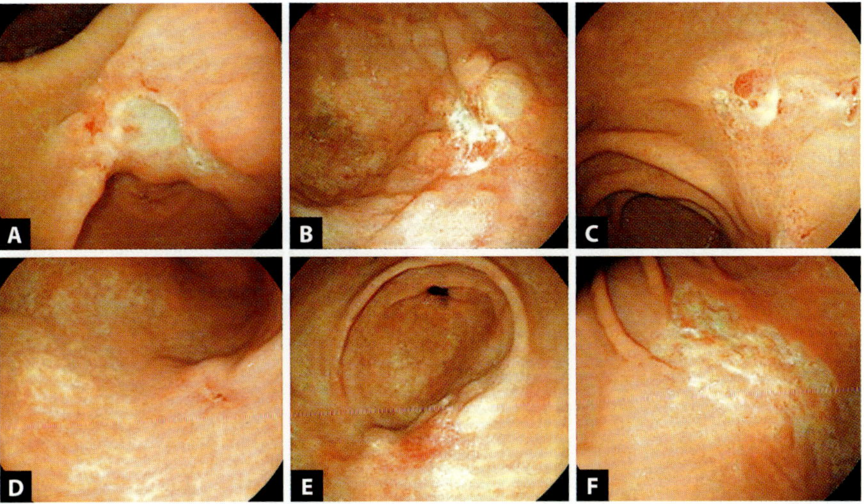

Figs. 13A to F: Early gastric cancers.

Early Gastric Cancers (Figs. 13A to F)

Early gastric cancers are uncommon, but we should look for them in all cases of endoscopy.

- Early gastric cancer is defined as gastric cancer occurring in the gastric mucosa and confined to the mucosa and submucosa irrespective of lymph node metastasis.
- The use of mucolytic and defoaming agents is strongly recommended because improved visibility of the mucosa leads to the detection of early gastric cancer. Use of intravenous (IV) Buscopan is optional.
- Sufficient time (>10 minutes) should be allowed for detailed inspection of gastric mucosa.
- HD magnification endoscopy with image enhancement modality is preferable for early diagnosis of gastric cancer. Chromo endoscopy using indigocarmine is also beneficial and it helps to clearly delineate the tumor margin.
- We need to look for mucosal surface irregularity (S) and microvascular pattern irregularity (V) to suspect cancer. (VS classification) **(Fig. 14)**.
- Paris classification of early gastric cancer divides these lesions into elevated, flat, and depressed lesions of variable size. A biopsy should be done to confirm whether it is differentiated or undifferentiated gastric cancer.
- Atrophy, intestinal metaplasia, nodularity, enlarged fold, and gastric xanthoma are endoscopic findings related to the risk of gastric cancer.

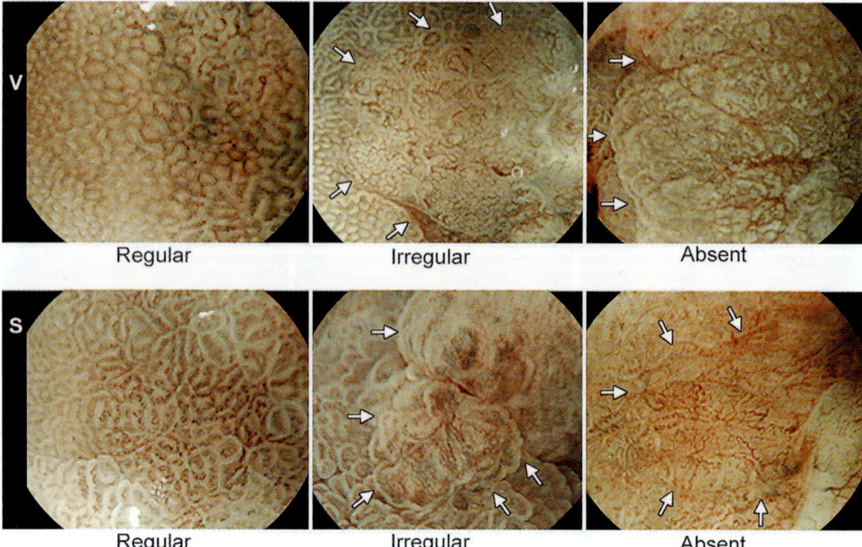

Fig. 14: VS classification. Microvascular pattern (V) is classified as regular/irregular/absent; microsurface pattern (S) is classified as regular/irregular/absent. (←: demarcation line).

2. ROLE OF THERAPEUTIC ENDOSCOPY IN UPPER GASTROINTESTINAL TUMORS

ENDOTHERAPY FOR BARRETT'S ESOPHAGUS

Cap Endoscopic Mucosal Resection

Barrett's esophagus with dysplasia requires endotherapy. Nodular lesions would be dealt with endoscopic mucosal resection (EMR) **(Figs. 15A and B)** or endoscopic submucosal dissection (ESD) **(Figs. 16A to D)**. Flat areas and residual lesions can be tackled with various endotherapeutic modalities namely radiofrequency ablation (RFA), argon plasma, and cryotherapy. EMR can be done by two different techniques. Cap EMR

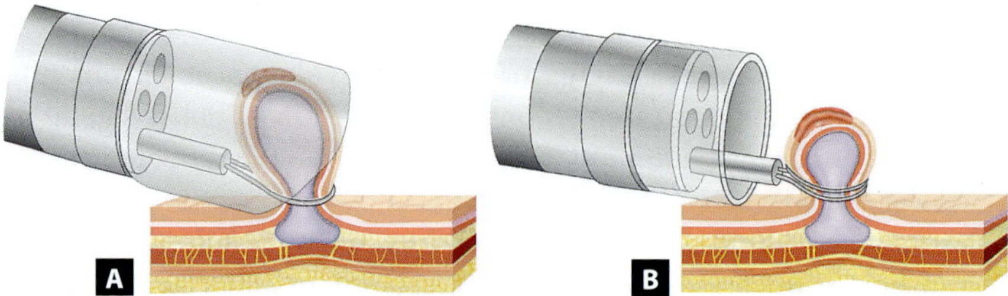

Figs. 15A and B: Cap endoscopic mucosal resection.

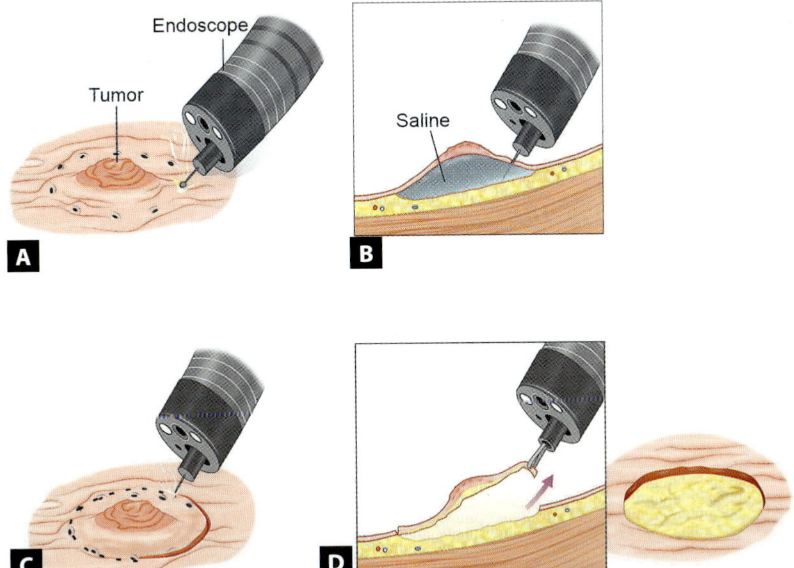

Figs. 16A to D: Endoscopic submucosal dissection.

involves submucosal saline injection followed by suction of the lesion into the transparent cap and snare excision. Band EMR is a slightly different method akin to the banding of varices **(Figs. 17A to D)**. The Duette multiband mucosectomy device has a barrel of preloaded bands attached to the endoscope's tip. BE is sucked into the barrel and bands are applied. This will be followed by snare excision of BE engulfed by the bands using endocut.

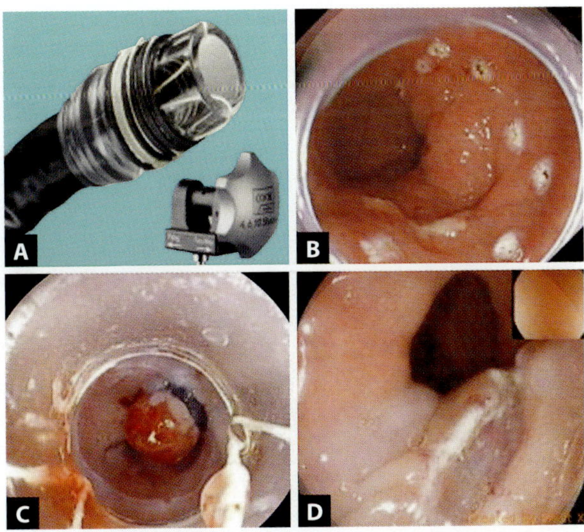

Figs. 17A to D: Band endoscopic mucosal resection (EMR).

Endoscopic Submucosal Dissection

Endoscopic submucosal dissection has five distinct steps namely lesion marking, submucosal injection and mucosal incision, submucosal dissection, en-bloc excision, and specimen fixation for biopsy.

Steps of ESD:

- *Lesion marking **(Fig. 18)**.*
- *Submucosal injection **(Fig. 19)**.*
- *Submucosal dissection **(Fig. 20)**.*
- *En-bloc excision of lesion **(Fig. 21)**.*
- *Specimen **(Fig. 22)**.*

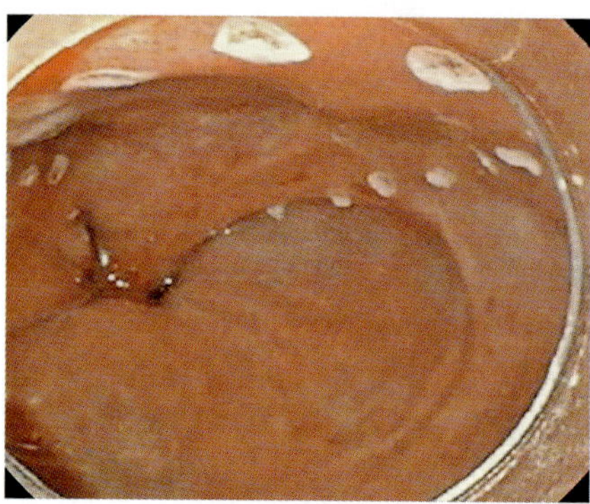

Fig. 18: Lesion marking.

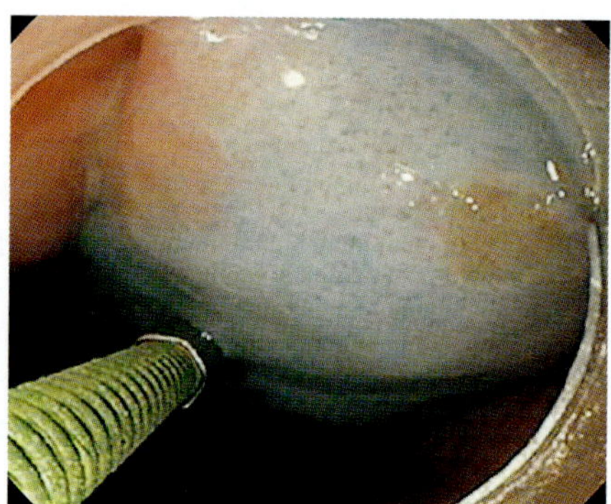

Fig. 19: Submucosal injection.

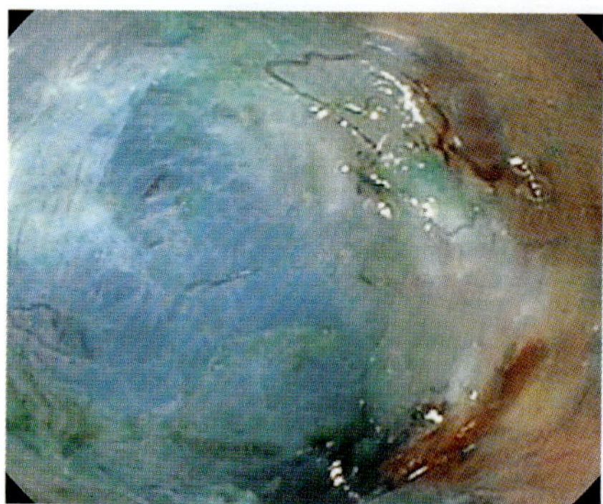

Fig. 20: Submucosal dissection.

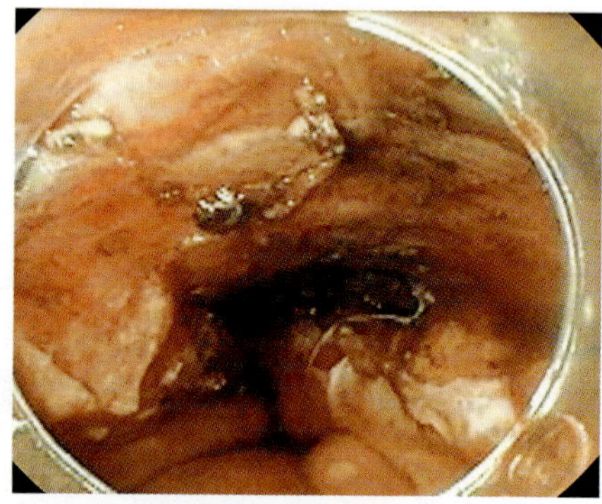

Fig. 21: En-bloc excision of lesion.

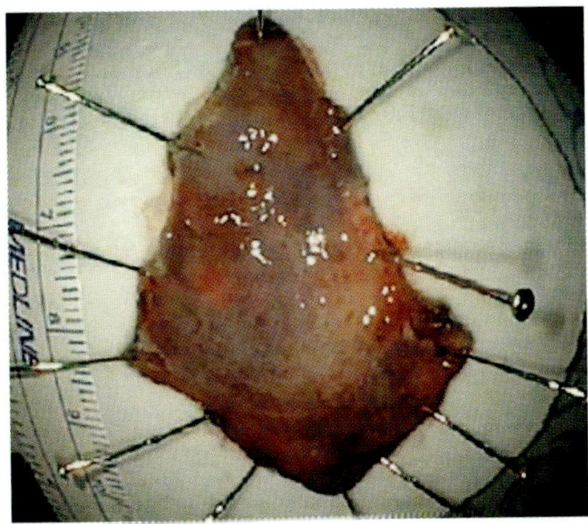

Fig. 22: Specimen.

ENDOSCOPIC MANAGEMENT OF LEIOMYOMA (FIGS. 23A TO D)

Tumors located strictly in the submucosal layer (second layer in EUS) are managed via EMR or ESD. On the other hand, tumors involving the muscularis propria (fourth layer in EUS) should undergo endoscopic full-thickness

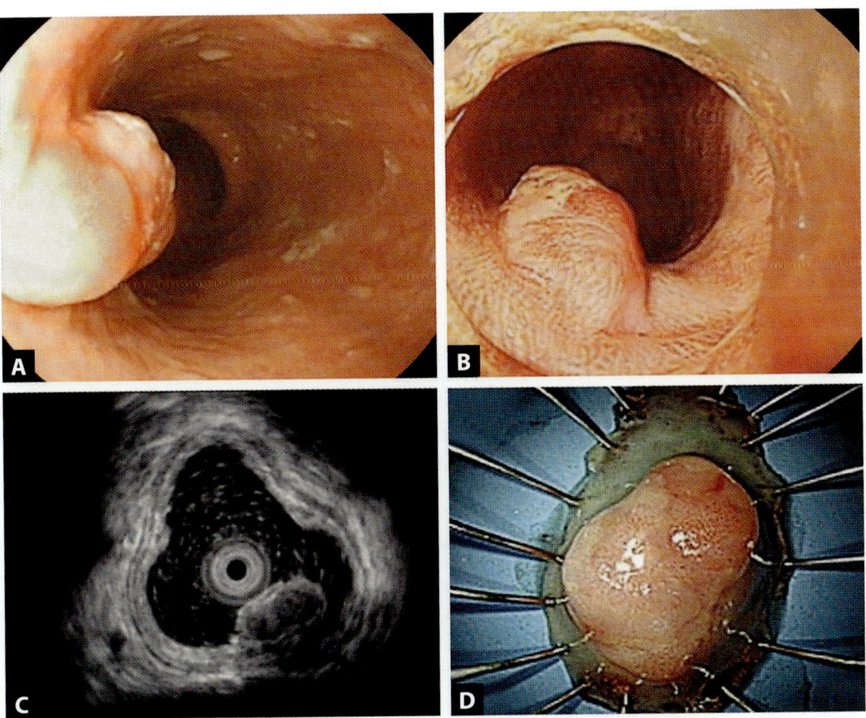

Figs. 23A to D: Endoscopic management of leiomyoma.

resection (EFTR) or submucosal tunneling endoscopic resection (STER). Based on the tumor size, location, and extension, an algorithm can be used to help with the surgical treatment of benign esophageal tumors.

ENDOSCOPY LAPAROSCOPY COOPERATIVE SURGERY FOR GASTRIC GASTROINTESTINAL STROMAL TUMOR (FIGS. 24A AND B)

We now live in the era of third-space endoscopy with great therapeutic potentials. Gastric GIST requires local excision with a 1–2 cm clear margin. Combined endoscopy and laparoscopic approach will enable the resection of gastric lesions safely with the preservation of gastric reservoir function. It can be done in two ways **(Figs. 24A and B)**.

Endoscopic submucosal dissection can be done while laparoscopic assistance ensures we can detect serosal breach early and proceed to laparoscopic suturing if needed. In the case of laparoscopic sleeve resection, endoscopic inspection is very reassuring that we are not encroaching either the pyloric canal or cardia too much.

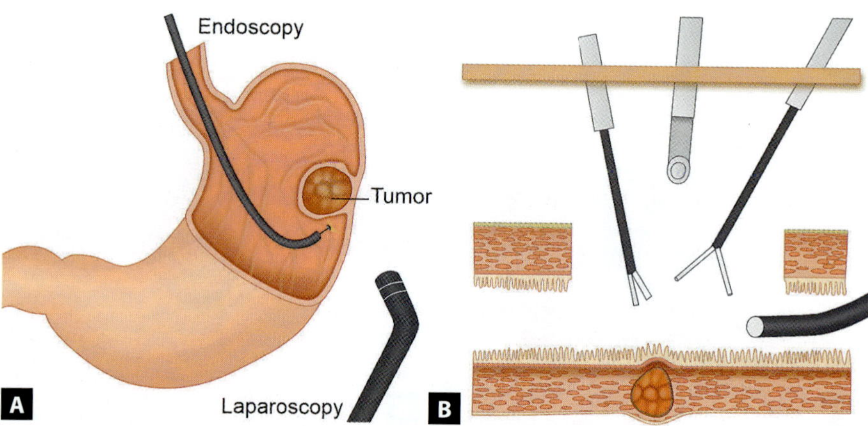

Figs. 24A and B: (A) Endoscopic excision of gastrointestinal stromal tumor with laparoscopic assistance; and (B) Laparoscopic sleeve resection of gastric gastrointestinal stromal tumor (GIST) with endoscopic assistance.

ENDOSCOPIC POLYPECTOMY FOR GASTRIC POLYPS

Tools Required

- Injection needle
- Various sizes of snare
- Roth net for retrieval
- Erbe diathermy and suction unit

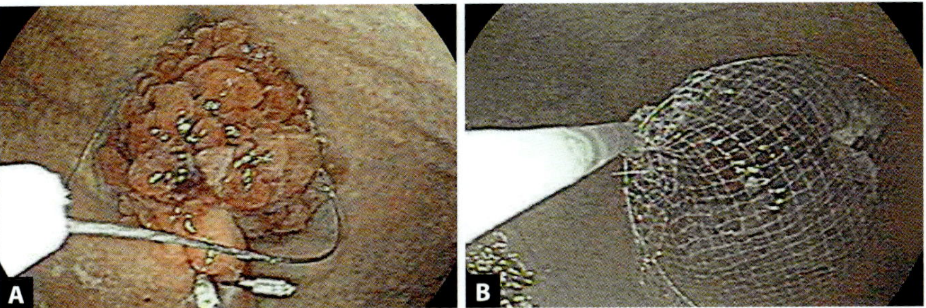

Figs. 25A and B: Key steps of polypectomy.

Key Steps (Figs. 25A and B)

- Check endoscopy to evaluate the polyp and clean the stomach.
- If sessile lesion or polyp with a thick stalk, then inject the base of the polyp with 1 in 100,000 dilute adrenaline mixed with methylene blue by using a 23 G 160 cm injection needle.
- Appropriately sized snare is taken, and a marking is made in its handle to note the exact point of complete closure of polypectomy wire around the stalk before initiating diathermy. We need to avoid cold snaring.
- Bring the polyp in the lower left quadrant for the upper GI Olympus endoscope with a 7 o'clock trajectory. Pass the snare through the access channel in the closed position
- Open the snare enough to encircle or garland the polyp and gently close it till you see the marking on the handle. Initiate the endocut Q mode for snare polypectomy.
- By the big wheel being turned toward you (Toe Up position), we ensure the pedicle is lifted well and the chance of transmural thermal damage is minimized.
- Once the polyp is completely cut, look for hemostasis.
- Exchange with a Roth net to catch the polyp lying in the fundus and retrieve it for histological examination.
- Broad-based sessile polyp warrants either EMR or ESD.

Complications

- Postpolypectomy bleeding
- Small risk of perforation

ROLE OF ENDOSCOPIC SUBMUCOSAL FOR GASTRIC LESIONS

- *Indication:* For any dysplastic lesion >20 mm or early cancer >15 mm, ESD is the preferred technique.
- *Tools:*
    - Injection needle

    - Hyaluronic acid solution for creating a submucosal cushion
    - Transparent hood
    - Various types of IT knife
    - Coagulation grasper
    - ERBE diathermy
    - Hemoclips
- *Key steps of ESD in gastric lesions* **(Figs. 26A and B)**:

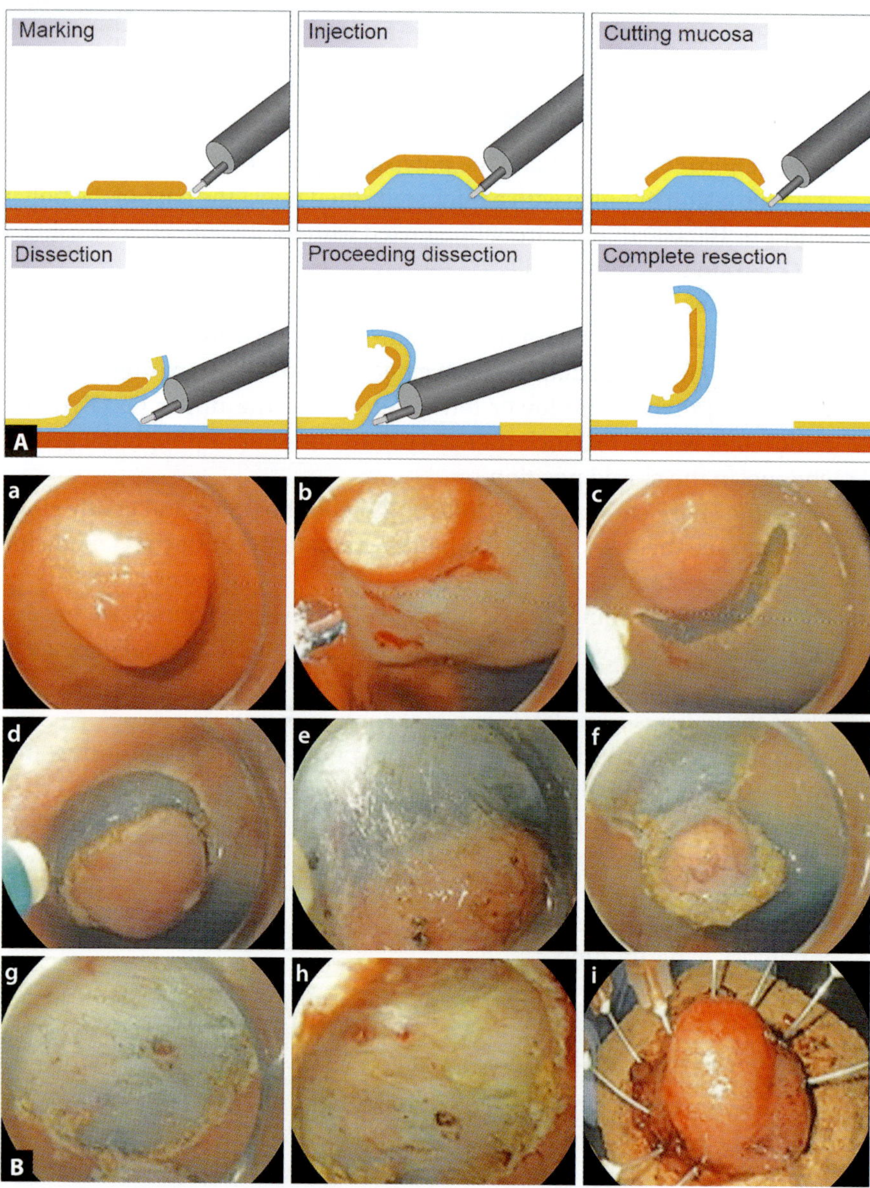

Figs. 26A and B: Endoscopic submucosal dissection steps.

- Spray the target area with indigo carmine to delineate the margin of the lesion.
- Mark the incision lines all around with a flex knife to create diathermy dots.
- Inject the submucosal plane with the hyaluronic solution with glycerol with dilute adrenaline to create a good lift.
- Mucosa is incised with a flex knife on the distal part of the lesion to start with.
- Submucosal dissection is done with an IT knife (endocut I with effect: 4, cut duration: 2, and cut interval: 3), and hemostasis is achieved using coagulation grasper.
- En-bloc excision is done and sent for histological examination.
- Keep the patient on PPI and sucralfate to facilitate healing of the raw area.

- *Complications:*
  - Bleeding
  - Perforation

ENDOSCOPIC SAVARY DILATATION (FIGS. 27A AND B)

- *Indication:*
  - Benign strictures like corrosive stricture, peptic stricture, anastomotic stricture, or postradiation stricture.
  - *Malignant stricture*: Esophageal carcinoma
- *Caution*: Midesophageal strictures are relatively easy to dilate while postcricoid strictures and lower esophageal strictures could be challenging and ideally need an image intensifier, preoperative imaging with barium swallow, and the presence of an experienced endoscopist.
- *Things required:*
  - *Savary-Gilliard dilators:*
    - Made up of polyvinyl chloride
    - The number denotes its diameter in mm
    - Available from 3 to 20 mm size
    - With smooth tapering end

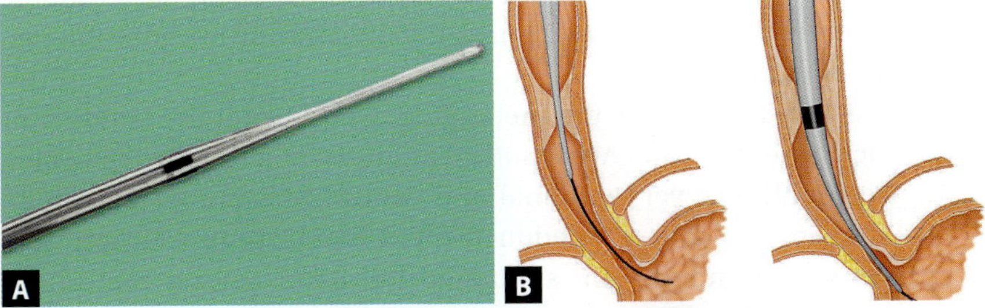

Figs. 27A and B: Endoscopic savary dilatation.

        - Has a hole through its shaft for rail-roading the guidewire.
        - Radio opaque markers at 5 cm intervals are helpful during imaging.
        - Very durable lifelong investment if maintained well!
    - Eder Puestow metal olive dilators are not used nowadays
    - Flexible tip metallic guidewire or Zebra guidewire
    - Controlled radial expansion (CRE) balloon and inflation device
    - Venous access/monitoring devices
    - Image intensifier
- *Procedure:*
    - *IV sedation/analgesics:* IV midazolam and tramadol in most of the cases would suffice. Consider IV ketamine or fentanyl also. Administer nasal oxygen. Monitor with a pulse oximeter and ECG. Give a single dose of antibiotic (IV cefotaxime 1 g).
    - Pass the endoscope and assess the site and nature of stricture. If the scope goes through the stricture area, then it means the stricture is >9 mm in diameter. Then you take note of nature and length of stricture. Tortuous stricture, strictures with diverticula, and stricture due to recent corrosive injury or radiotherapy are prone to false passage and perforation so be very careful. Anastomotic strictures are usually short and circumferential like a diaphragm and are often easy to dilate. If the scope is not going through the stricture, then consider passing metal guidewire under the image intensifier and proceed.
    - You could measure the size of the stricture with the use of biopsy forceps. Breath of an open biopsy forceps measures about 10 mm while every jaw is about 4–5 mm.
    - Guidewire should pass down easily or else consider C arm imaging. Measure the external length of the guidewire beyond the patient's mouth and be watchful. The length of the external section of the wire should not change following each dilatation. If it appears lengthened, then it is probable that the guidewire has slipped out of stricture. So, beware of this point, during each time of exchange of dilators. There should be coordinated action between the assistant and the endoscopist.
    - Choose the appropriate size of savary dilator. Usually start with the size tried during the last visit or size 10 if the scope has gone through the stricture.
    - Pass the dilator over the metal guidewire. Avoid any bending or buckling of the wire. Apply sufficient lubricant jelly over the dilator. We should use very minimal and controlled force for dilatation. So, keep both your arms adducted and kept close to the chest wall. Use your nondominant supinated left hand to pass the dilator gently inside while your dominant pronated right-hand guides it.

This ensures very gentle dilatation averting sudden thrust or jerky force risking perforation.
- If you start with size 10 then dilate up to three sizes upward, i.e., up to size 13. Follow the "Rule of Three" to avoid the risk of perforation. Resist the temptation and always under-dilate rather than over-dilate.
- Savary dilator exerts a linear force at the stricture. Hence if due care is not taken, there can be transmural laceration at the stricture site causing splitting or even perforation. If the patient complains of severe chest pain or any respiratory distress, then prepare to abandon the procedure.
- Perform a check gastroscopy to see the site of stricture and carefully pass the scope beyond into the stomach. Do not force your way. Do not overinsufflate with air.
- Be careful if you take a biopsy of the stricture following dilatation. It may be preferable to avoid a biopsy for a week.

- *Watch for:*
  - If the patient develops severe chest or abdominal pain, respiratory distress, or subcutaneous emphysema, consider the possibility of perforation. If so, consider the admission of the patient for close observation. Do an X-ray chest or CT chest with oral contrast. Most cervical perforations and small perforations in the thoracic esophagus would normally settle down with conservative treatment of IV PPI, antibiotics, IV fluids, and nil oral for 2–3 days. Large perforation in the thoracic esophagus merits surgical consultation to decide about either deployment of a fully covered self-expanding stent or surgery. Perforation is better averted than treated!
- *Options for refractory stricture:*
  - Consider injection of corrosive stricture site with 0.2 mL of triamcinolone in each of the four quadrants before dilatation.
  - Deployment of removable fully covered self-expanding metal stent (SEMS).
  - Use of removable self-expanding plastic stent (SEPS).
  - Use of biodegradable stent (Ella stent).
  - Surgery

ENDOSCOPIC CONTROLLED RADIAL EXPANSION BALLOON DILATATION (FIGS. 28A TO D)

- *Indication:*
  - Benign and malignant esophageal stricture
  - Pyloric stenosis (use a pyloric balloon)
  - Benign and malignant colonic stricture
  - To dilate the ampulla of Vater during endoscopic retrograde cholangiopancreatography (ERCP)

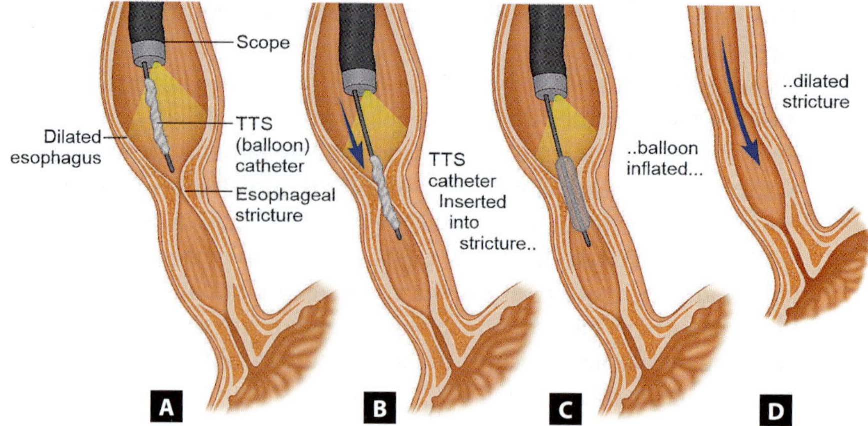

Figs. 28A to D: Endoscopic controlled radial expansion balloon dilatation. (TTS: through-the-scope)

- *Things required:*
  - CRE balloons with various diameters and lengths are available
  - Inflation device, e.g., Alliance Gun
  - Silicone gel
  - Image intensifier (optional)
- *Procedure:*
  - *IV sedative/analgesic:* IV midazolam and tramadol in most cases would suffice. consider IV ketamine or fentanyl also. Administer nasal oxygen. Monitor with Pulse oximeter and ECG. Give a single dose of antibiotic (IV cefotaxime 1 g)
  - Pass the endoscope and assess the site and nature of stricture.
  - CRE balloons are through the telescope dilators (TTS) and hence dilatation is done under endoscopic guidance and is relatively easy to perform and safe too.
  - It is available with its short guidewire which can be pushed in and out of the balloon catheter with the help of a plunging handle. The guidewire is initially guided through the stricture before the passage of the balloon.
  - CRE balloon exerts a radial force at the stricture site and expands to the predetermined diameter at the given pressure (psi). So read the attached label to know the diameter of the balloon for the given pressure.
  - Consider keeping various sizes and lengths of balloons. 10, 12, 15 mm diameter and 6–8 cm length balloons are normally preferred for esophageal dilatation
  - Place a few drops of silicone gel at the biopsy channel and pass the deflated CRE balloon.

- Once the balloon tip exits the distal end of the scope, pass the guidewire through the stricture and then pass the balloon gently over the guidewire. There should not be any undue resistance. Once three-fourths of the balloon has gone through and only 2–3 cm of the balloon is seen above the stricture, start inflating the balloon.
- The endoscopy should be close to the balloon and the balloon catheter should be held firmly or fixed at the biopsy channel with your right index finger and thumb to avoid the balloon popping out or sliding down beyond the stricture during dilatation.
- Proceed with gradual stepwise dilatation using the saline-filled inflation device. One may be able to appreciate the nature of stricture thanks to the transparency of the balloon.
- Deflate the balloon slightly and try to gently push the scope through stricture keeping the balloon as a guide.
- Completely deflate the balloon and gently remove it or else remove the scope with the balloon as one unit and then deflate to remove the balloon. CRE balloon is disposable but could be reused if ethylene oxide (EtO) is sterilized and maintained well.

ENDOSCOPIC STENT DEPLOYMENT (FIGS. 29A TO D)

- *Indication:*
  - All malignant tracheoesophageal fistula.
  - Inoperable or recurrent midesophageal carcinoma with severe dysphagia (careful case selection in cases of upper and lower third tumors).
- *Things needed:*
  - Savary dilators of all sizes
  - Flexible tip metal guidewire and stiff Zebra guidewire.
  - CRE balloon and inflation device.
  - Injection needle and contrast for internal marking.
  - Safety pins with tapes for external markings.
  - Various lengths of esophageal SEM stents (4 cm longer than the length of the tumor).
  - Image intensifier
- *Procedure:*
  - Patient is lying in a supine position with their head turned to the left side.
  - In the presence of an anesthetist for conscious sedation and analgesic administration. IV propofol with fentanyl or IV ketamine/antiemetic/IV antibiotic (injection cefotaxime 1 g).
  - Perform diagnostic endoscopy. Note the exact site and length of the malignant stricture. Note the size and location of any fistulous communication with the airway.

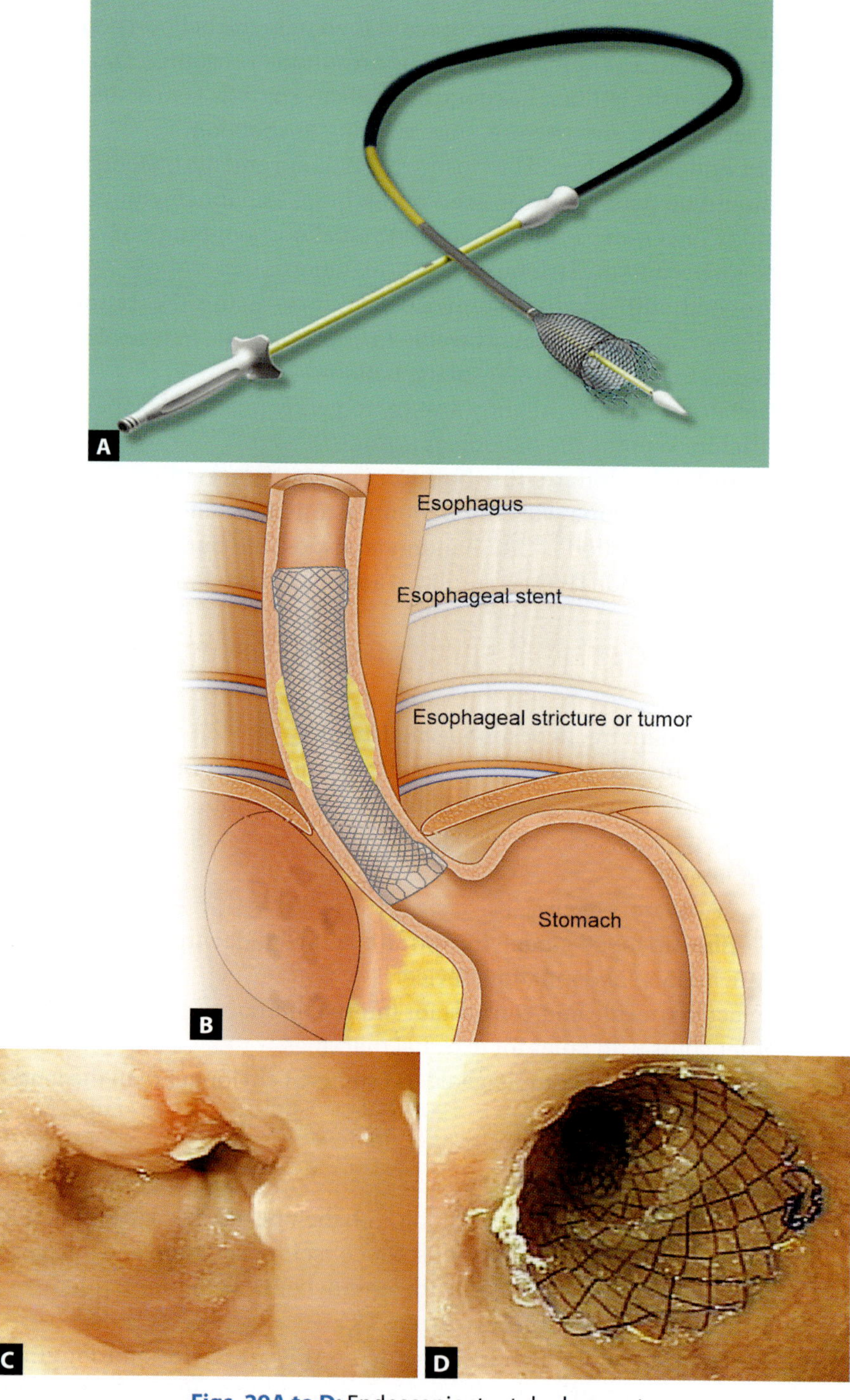

Figs. 29A to D: Endoscopic stent deployment.

- CRE balloon dilatation or guidewire-directed Savary dilatation may be necessary just to let the scope pass down to assess the distal end of the tumor and its distance from LES. Do not over-dilate to avoid stent migration later. Examine the stomach and duodenum and do the J maneuver to assess cardia to note any tumor extension.
- Pass a metallic guidewire with a flexible tip into the stomach while gently withdrawing the scope.
- Note the exact site of hiatus, the lower end of the tumor, the site of fistulous communication, the upper end of the tumor, and the location of the cricopharynx and keep external markers of safety pins over the patient's chest wall at all these sites and fix them securely with tape. Additional internal marking of the top and bottom end of the tumor is preferable by injecting urogram in 2–3 mL with the help of a 23 G sclerotherapy needle.
- Measure the length of the tumor with the help of endoscope markings or externally by using a measuring scale to note the distance between the external markers at the upper and lower end of the tumor.
- If the tumor is 10 cm in length, then choose a stent at least 4 cm longer. Stents are available as 10, 12, 15 cm, and even 20 cm. The length of the covered part of the stent and its diameter are clearly mentioned in the pack and this has to be verified always prior to unpacking.
- Take the correct size stent with its assembly, lubricate its distal part, and pass it over the guidewire.
- Ensure that all the markers are in place and the guidewire is in a satisfactory position.
- Pass the stent assembly over the guidewire until it reaches beyond the distalmost marker.
- Most of the stents have a very simple deployment system by gradually pulling back the outer sheath. (Except Ultraflex stent which needs just unraveling of thread around the stent assembly)
- Keep your arms by the side and hold the stent assembly with your right hand close to your chest and start gently pulling back the outer sheath using your left hand which will start moving towards your chest. Avoid the temptation of pushing the stent assembly unit with your right hand. Keep it still, close to the chest wall!
- Monitor the whole process of deployment closely with the help of an image intensifier.
- Ensure initial distal release of the stent and then the gradual proximal opening of the stent exactly at the preferred sites by constant reference to the external and internal markers. One could also re-sheath a partially deployed stent and repeat the deployment again if not satisfied.
- Once deployment is complete, perform an endoscopy to see the site of the proximal end of the stent and ensure that is well above the tumor

and the fistula and not reaching the cricopharynx. Do not try to go down any further or else you risk stent migration.

- *Look for:*
  - Correct position by postoperative chest X-ray.
  - *Any perforation:* X-ray chest prior to oral fluids.
- *Dietary instruction:*
  - Liquid diet for 1 week till the stent expands completely and snugly fits at the site of stricture.
  - Semi-solid diet and mashed vegetables after that time including cooked rice, idly, half-boiled, or scrambled eggs.
  - Avoid chapattis, mutton, chicken pieces, or vegetables with thick skin to avoid stent blockage.
  - Regular intake of effervescent drinks such as soda, sprite, or 7-up juices helps to wash down the food debris at the end of each meal.
  - Avoid lying flat soon after eating.
- *Treatment advice:* Chemoradiation can be resumed 1 week after stent deployment
- *Challenging situations:*
  - *Upper esophageal cancer:* It will be challenging to deploy a stent for carcinoma upper esophagus above 18 cm level from incisor teeth. Also, choose a low-profile proximal stent (Niti-S Conio stent) or a proximal release system stent.
  - *OG junction cancer:* Severe reflux and vomiting will be bothersome after stenting. Stents with antireflux valves are available but of no real benefit. Advise the patient to eat less at night and lie down with head up position while sleeping.
  - *Pyloric and duodenal cancer:* We recommend endoscopy-guided stent deployment under vision using a 7F assembly unit that passes through the access channel!
- *Complications following stenting:*
  - Stent obstruction due to food bolus
  - *Tumor in-growth:* In case of uncovered stent.
  - *Tumor over-growth*: If the stent is not of the correct length.
  - *Stent migration*: Due to over-dilatation of stricture before deployment or faulty deployment of the stent.

ENDOSCOPIC RESCUE FOR SURGICAL COMPLICATIONS

As an endoscopic surgeon, you could come to rescue a sick patient with an anastomotic leak, infected fluid collection, or post-operative anastomotic site bleeding.

- *Leaks and fistula following upper GI surgery:*
  - Leaks are not uncommon after upper GI surgery. Sleeve gastrectomy has a leak rate of 1–2% and following esophagectomy, it could be up to 8–26%.

- In a clinically stable patient, after clinical and radiological evaluation, we need to consider endoscopic rescue employing defect closure, drainage, or diversion.
- Perforation or fistula can be closed by an OTSC device (Ovesco) or suturing can be attempted using an Apollo suturing device. Ovesco clip is a biocompatible nitinol clip with a bear-trap shape design **(Figs. 30A and B)**. It is mounted on a cap installed at the tip of the endoscope allowing full-thickness closure of GI defects up to 2 cm in size. The review reported an overall success rate of 51.5% in the case of fistulae and 66% for anastomotic leaks

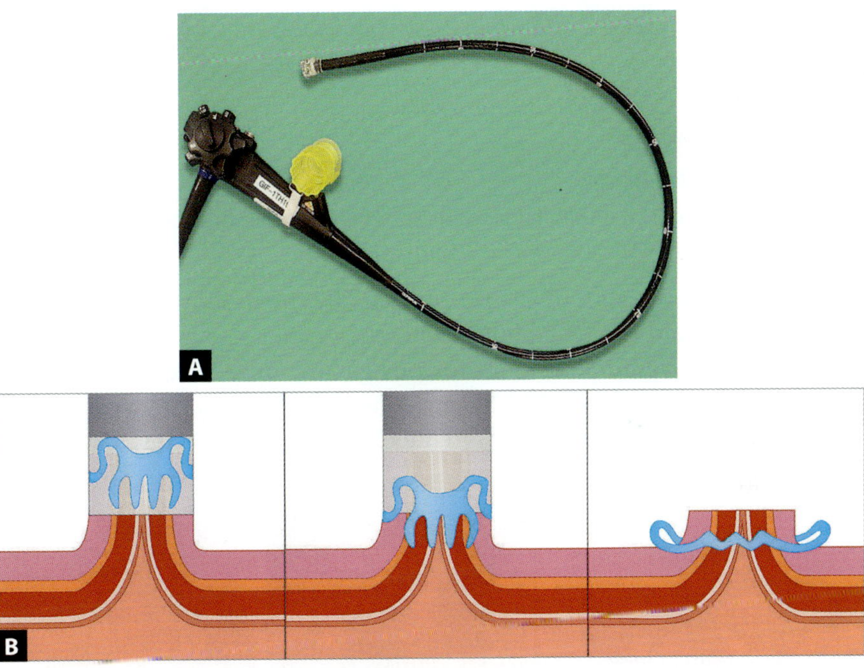

Figs. 30A and B: Ovesco suturing device.

- The Apollo overstitch system has been successfully used for a growing variety of indications, including sleeve gastroplasty in obese patients, transoral outlet reduction after bariatric surgery, and stent anchorage to avoid migration and closure of mucosal defects after endoscopic resections.
- Endoscopy-guided internal drainage by use of double pigtail stents are also found useful in sleeve gastrectomy leaks.
- Endoscopic sponge application with vacuum drainage would facilitate closure of the fistula by drainage of the infected fluid collection **(Figs. 31A and B)**.

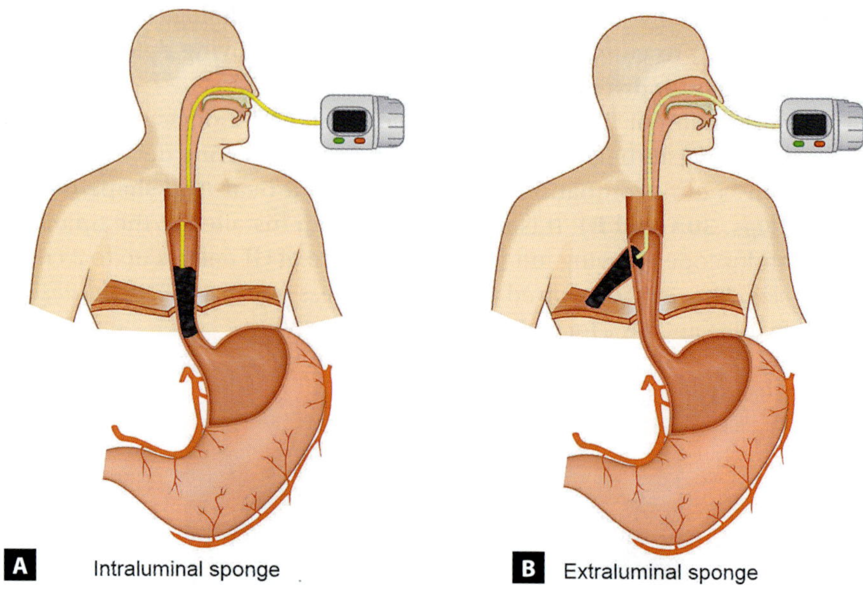

Figs. 31A and B: Endoscopic sponge—vacuum drainage.

- Finally, diversion of gastric contents by the deployment of a mega stent would rescue a patient with a leak after sleeve gastrectomy, or a fully covered SEM stent for postgastrectomy leaks. Hanaro fully covered metal stent, Niti-S Beta Stent, or SX Ella Seal Stent can also be considered, as they have less tendency for migration **(Figs. 32A and B)**.

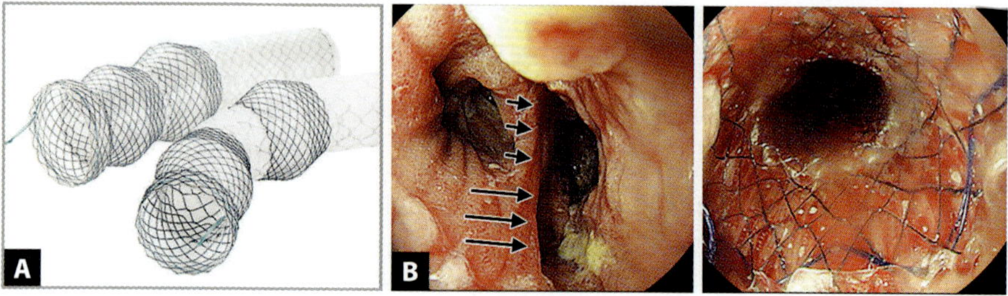

Figs. 32A and B: Stent deployment for post-gastrectomy leak.

- *Anastomotic stricture* ***(Figs. 33A to D)****:* Post-RYGB stricture can be dilated using an endoscopic CRE balloon for symptomatic relief **(Figs. 33A to D)**. A 15 mm CRE balloon is used with an inflation device for this purpose.
- *Anastomotic site bleeding* ***(Fig. 34)****:* Diagnostic endoscopy with hemoclip application of an active bleeding site could be very rewarding. We should avoid any diathermy energy over the staple lines as it might risk an anastomotic leak later!

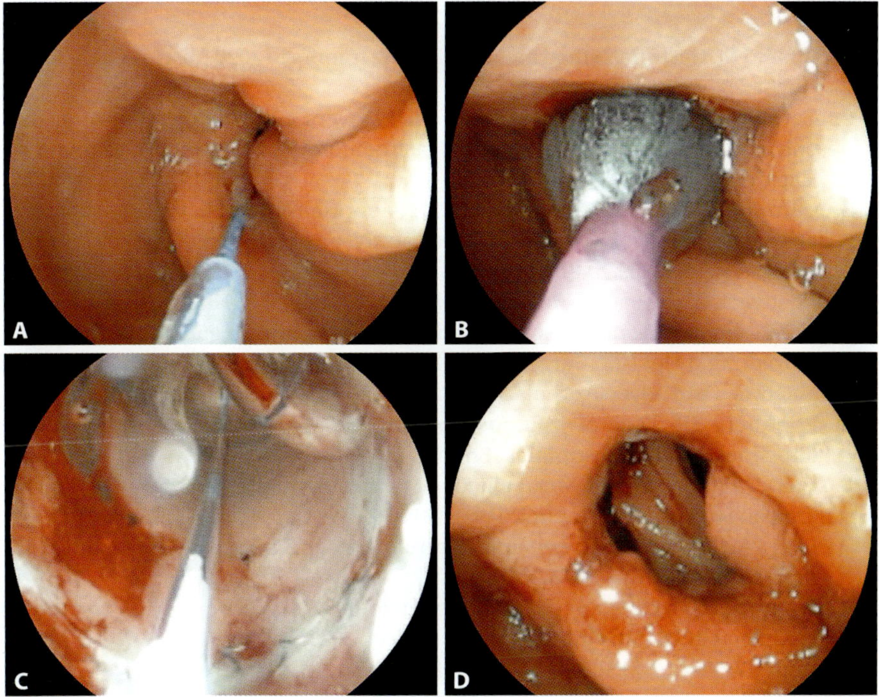

Figs. 33A to D: Anastomotic stricture.

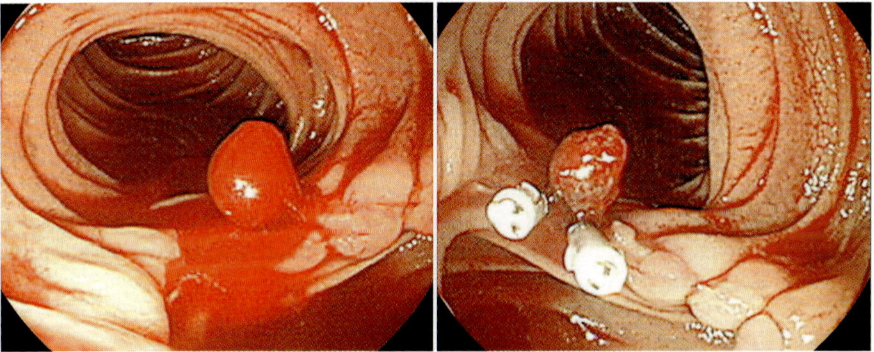

Fig. 34: Anastomotic site bleeding and hemoclip application.

CONCLUSION

Endoscopy is an essential tool for upper GI surgeons, and it has enormous diagnostic and therapeutic potential. Early upper GI cancers can be effectively managed by endotherapy. Endoscopy could become a lifesaving tool in certain postsurgical complications.

The endoscopy skillset is not optional but essential for every upper GI surgeon.

SUGGESTED READING

1. Ahmed M. Gastrointestinal neuroendocrine tumors in 2020. World J Gastrointest Oncol. 2020;12(8):791-807.
2. Carmack SW, Genta RM, Graham DY, Lauwers GY. Management of gastric polyps: a pathology-based guide for gastroenterologists. Nat Rev Gastroenterol Hepatol. 2009;6(6):331-41.
3. Carmack SW, Genta RM, Schuler CM, Saboorian MH. The current spectrum of gastric polyps: a 1-year national study of over 120,000 patients. Am J Gastroenterol. 2009;104(6):1524-32.
4. Chadwick G, Groene O, Markar SR, Hoare J, Cromwell D, Hanna GB. Systematic review comparing radiofrequency ablation and complete endoscopic resection in treating dysplastic Barrett's esophagus: A critical assessment of histologic outcomes and adverse events. Gastrointest Endosc. 2014;79(5):718-31.e3.
5. Friedberg SR, Lachter J. Endoscopic ultrasound: Current roles and future directions. World J Gastrointest Endosc. 2017;9(10):499-505.
6. Halpern AL, McCarter MD. Palliative Management of Gastric and Esophageal Cancer. Surg Clin North Am. 2019;99(3):555-69.
7. Jang J-Y. The Past, Present, and Future of Image-Enhanced Endoscopy. Clin Endosc. 2015;48(6):466-75.
8. Japanese Gastric Cancer Association Japanese gastric cancer treatment guidelines 2018 (5th edition) Gastric Cancer. 2021;24(1):1-21.
9. Kim KY, Tsauo J, Song H-Y, Kim PH, Park J-H. Self-Expandable Metallic Stent Placement for the Palliation of Esophageal Cancer. J Korean Med Sci. 2017;32(7):1062-71.
10. Lalor PF, Tucker ON, Szomstein S, Rosenthal RJ. Complications after laparoscopic sleeve gastrectomy. Surg Obes Relat Dis. 2008;4(1):33-8.
11. Leeds SG, Burdick JS. Management of gastric leaks after sleeve gastrectomy with endoluminal vacuum (E-Vac) therapy. Surg Obes Relat Dis. 2016;12(7):1278-85.
12. Niland B, Brock A. Over-the-scope clip for endoscopic closure of gastrogastric fistulae. Surg Obes Relat Dis. 2017;13(1):15-20.
13. Salinas A, Baptista A, Santiago E, Antor M, Salinas H. Self-expandable metal stents to treat gastric leaks. Surg Obes Relat Dis. 2006;2(5):570-2.
14. Shaheen NJ, Falk GW, Iyer PG, Souza RF, Yadlapati RH, Sauer BG, et al. Diagnosis and Management of Barrett's Esophagus: An Updated ACG Guideline. Off J Am Coll Gastroenterol ACG. 2022;117(4):559-87.

Expert's Comment

As a surgeon treating malignancies of the upper gastrointestinal (GI) system, I regard endoscopy as an essential extension of my office—indispensable for both diagnosis and treatment. With the remarkable advancements in technology, upper GI endoscopy today allows us to differentiate between benign and malignant lesions with up to 97% accuracy using digital chromoendoscopy. This has been particularly valuable in conditions such as Barrett's esophagus, improving early detection and survival outcomes in malignancies.

Another breakthrough has been the integration of artificial intelligence (AI) in endoscopy, which enables us to distinguish between benign and malignant polyps with over 90% accuracy. Similarly, the advent of third-space endoscopy has revolutionized the management of upper GI malignancies, especially through techniques like endoscopic submucosal dissection (ESD)/endoscopic mucosal resection (EMR) for early esophageal and gastric cancers.

From a therapeutic perspective, endoscopic dilation has proven highly effective in managing postoperative and postradiation strictures, while endoscopic stent deployment has dramatically reduced mortality in postoperative leaks—from 15–20% to <3%. Beyond salvage therapy, stenting also serves as a cornerstone in palliation for inoperable malignancies of the esophagus and stomach.

In this context, the IAGES Endoscopy Book, authored by Professor Dr S Easwaramoorthy, will be a true jewel for surgeons. It provides knowledge and vision for the future of endoscopy, empowering us to deliver safer and more effective care for our patients.

Dr K Govindaraj
Trichy

CHAPTER 10

Steps of Colonoscopy: Planning, Preparation, and Procedure

Chapter Outline

- Indications for Colonoscopy
    - Diagnostic Colonoscopy
    - Screening Colonoscopy
    - Surveillance Colonoscopy
    - Therapeutic Colonoscopy
- Contraindications
- Caution
- Bowel Preparation
- Informed Consent
- Patient Information Leaflet
- About the Hardware of Colonoscope
- About the Colonoscopy Room Layout
- Preprocedure Patient Checklist
- Instrument Checklist
- Medication and Monitoring during Colonoscopy
- Single or Two-Person Colonoscopy
- Understanding Basic Colonoscopic Anatomy
- 10 Key Steps of Colonoscopy
    - Examination of Anal Canal and Rectum
    - Sigmoid Navigation
    - Descending Colon
    - Reaching Splenic Flexure
    - Travel Through the Transverse Colon
    - Reaching Hepatic Flexure
    - Right Colon Down to Cecum
    - Terminal Ileum
    - Cecum to Rectum Withdrawal
    - Retroflex in Rectum
- Top 10 Tips for a Successful Colonoscopy
- Ancillary Measures for Difficult Colonoscopy
    - Colonoscopy after Colonic Resections
    - Colonoscopy Through Colostomy

Keywords: Diagnostic colonoscopy, bowel preparation, colonoscopy steps

INTRODUCTION

Colonoscopic examination is indicated in various lower gastrointestinal (GI) disorders, both for diagnostic and therapeutic purposes. Unlike upper GI endoscopy, it is technically more demanding to navigate the whole colon and hence takes longer to become competent in the art of colonoscopy. This chapter outlines the planning, preparation, and procedure with several useful practical tips.

INDICATIONS FOR COLONOSCOPY

Diagnostic Colonoscopy

- All cases of bleeding per rectum (PR)
- Anemia due to occult GI blood loss
- Persistent diarrhea
- To investigate constipation
- To evaluate the colon showing some abnormality in imaging

Screening Colonoscopy

Screening for colonic polyps/cancers in risk groups (family history of colonic polyposis or cancer colon).

Surveillance Colonoscopy

- Long duration of inflammatory bowel disease (IBD) (>10 years)
- Postpolypectomy cases
- Postoperative colonic cancer cases

Therapeutic Colonoscopy

For various therapies, e.g., polypectomy, hemostasis, dilatation, and stenting.

CONTRAINDICATIONS

- *Absolute contraindication*:
  - Acute abdomen, e.g., suspected viscus perforation
  - Toxic megacolon
- *Relative contraindication*:
  - Avoid for 3 months after myocardial infarction
  - Avoid during pregnancy with a past history of miscarriage
  - Avoid during acute diverticulitis

CAUTION

- In case of severe IBD with large ulcers, postradiation strictures, postoperative cases with fixed loops of bowel (for fear of perforation)

- In cases of cirrhosis with ascites or a patient on peritoneal dialysis, because of the risk of bacterial peritonitis.
- Careful in patients with pacemakers and implantable defibrillators not to use diathermy indiscriminately.

BOWEL PREPARATION (FIG. 1)

- Mechanical bowel preparation using a balanced electrolyte solution containing polyethylene glycol is a common practice. Several commercial preparations are available (Peglec, Golytely) **(Fig. 1)** but use one you are familiar and happy with. Avoid the ones that are unpalatable and make the patient vomit. Magnesium salts or sodium picosulphate are also useful. Avoid mannitol because of the risk of an explosion hazard.
- Advise the patient to be on a low-residue diet for 2 days and a liquid diet on the previous day.
- Ask the patient to take the 2 L of prepared solution (polyethylene glycol) over a period of 2 hours in the early morning and report to you once they have passed 5–10 times of clear watery motion.
- Slate the procedure in the early afternoon as a day case. Admit if the patient is a high-risk case or needs major therapeutic intervention.
- Split dosing of bowel preparation is also beneficial. In such a case, ask the patient to take 1 L of the mixed-up solution in the previous day's evening and take only clear liquids afterward. The remaining 1 L can be consumed in the early morning to ensure a clean bowel.
- Water, tender coconut, green tea, or black coffee, and fruit juices can be consumed up to 1–2 hours prior to colonoscopy and do not pose any trouble in bowel preparation.
- Explain to them the importance of a clean bowel for a safe and successful procedure
- A chronically constipated patient may require an additional dosage.

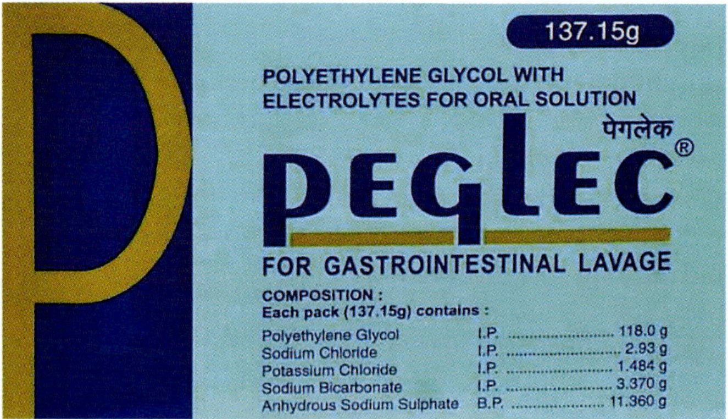

Fig. 1: Peglec powder.

- A patient with an obstructed left-sided colonic tumor or stricture may not succeed in clearing the bowel, and it may even be hazardous. So, instead, give a phosphate enema to evacuate the distal bowel, and then you may proceed to a limited colonoscopy **(Fig. 2)**.
- In the case of IBD with severe diarrhea, bowel preparation may not always be necessary.
- In a patient with a defunctioning colostomy, pass a catheter into the distal stoma opening and flush the bowel with saline or tap water, followed by a phosphate enema **(Fig. 3)**.
- In a bleeding patient, Ryle's tube-aided lavage or colonoscopy in an unprepared bowel can be considered. A good irrigation and suction system is invaluable during such cases.

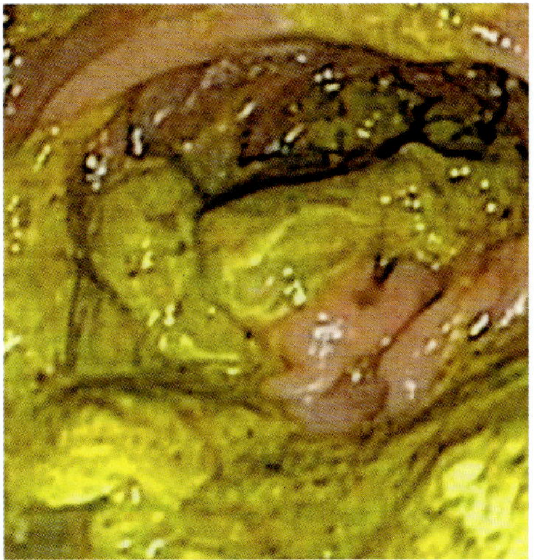

Fig. 2: Unprepared distal bowel.

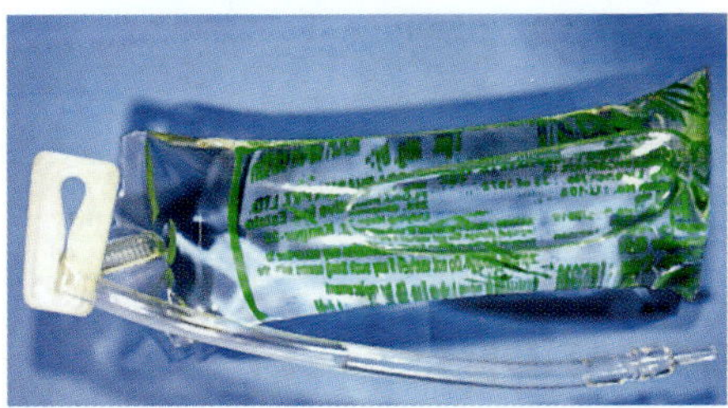

Fig. 3: Sodium phosphate enema.

INFORMED CONSENT

Written informed consent is paramount for moral and ethical reasons, and also to prevent any medicolegal consequences.

- Consent should ideally be taken by the colonoscopist himself/herself.
- Ensure that the patient is competent to give consent. Obtain consent from parents or spouses for young children, and unconscious or mentally disturbed patients.
- Consent should be given voluntarily by the patient after receiving sufficient information regarding the colonoscopy procedure, namely why it is done, how it is done, what the benefits and risks of the procedure are, any alternatives to colonoscopy, and the possibility of performing any additional procedures if needed **(Fig. 4)**.
- Give a "Patient information leaflet" written in simple and easy-to-follow language with all the details regarding the colonoscopy procedure
- The patient should be encouraged to ask questions and clarify any doubts.
- The patient should sign with their name and address in bold letters with the date and time.
- The consent form should also have the name and signature of the colonoscopist and a witness (next of kin).

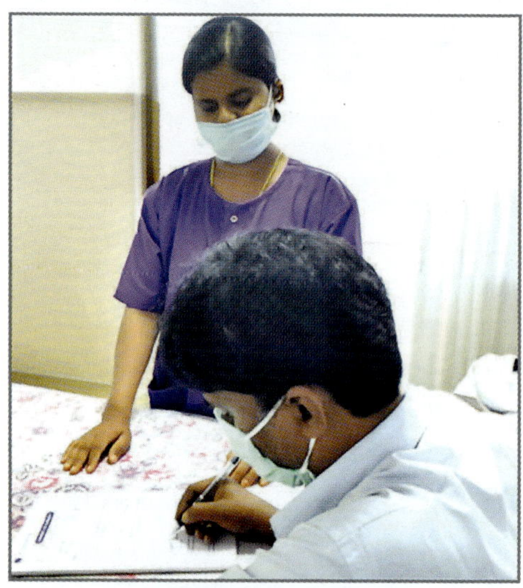

Fig. 4: Informed consent.

PATIENT INFORMATION LEAFLET

1. *Why do I need a colonoscopy?*
   Obviously, your symptoms suggest the possibility of large gut pathology, and hence your doctor asked you to undergo a colonoscopy.
2. *What is a colonoscopy?*
   Your doctor would use a video colonoscope, which would allow him to see inside of large gut and rectum to look for any abnormality.

3. *What is a video colonoscope?*
   A colonoscope is a long, slim, flexible tube with a tiny camera chip at its tip. This allows us to take video or pictures of the interior of your large gut in fine detail and help in the diagnosis.
4. *When does one need a colonoscopy?*
   Patients with bleeding rectum, changes in bowel habits, and unexplained abdominal pain, anemia, unexplained weight loss, and a family history of colonic polyps or cancer would require this novel investigation.
5. *Is there any alternative to colonoscopy?*
   Though ultrasound (US) abdomen, computed tomography (CT) abdomen, and barium enemas can be considered, they have several limitations. They won't be as useful as a colonoscopy.
6. *How is a colonoscopy done?*
   - You will be given 2 L of bowel cleansing fluid to drink [e.g., polyethylene glycol (Peglec)] over a period of 2 hours. This means you will be having >5–10 times of motion to clean the large gut sufficiently to enable the surgeon to have a good look inside your gut.
   - Your blood pressure (BP) and pulse, and body weight will be checked and the nurse will ask you and note down your other medical illnesses, previous abdominal surgery, any medication, and any history of allergies. Kindly bring all your medical prescriptions and investigation reports, and films.
   - You will be changed to a hospital gown, and a Venflon needle may be placed on the back of your hand if any injection is to be given.
   - You will be asked to sign the informed consent form. You could ask any relevant questions.
   - You will be administered oxygen by a nasal cannula and asked to lie down in the examination couch on your left side. You may be given injections to calm you down to ease the discomfort of the procedure. You could sleep, but often you would be awake and able to converse with the surgeon during the whole procedure and watch the screen to look at any abnormality noted.
   - At first, the surgeon will perform an examination of your back passage with his creased right index finger to examine your rectum and anus and then start a colonoscopic procedure by gently inserting the scope tip into your back passage.
   - As he puts in the air to distend the large gut to enable smooth navigation of the scope, you may feel a bit bloated and uncomfortable. But if it becomes very painful, let the surgeon know so that he can think of some remedial measures.
   - Colonoscopy usually takes about 20–30 minutes. So, try to relax and lie still, and concentrate on your breathing while the surgeon completes the procedure.

- The procedure is usually recorded, and any abnormality noted will also be taken as still images for reporting and printing.
- Additional procedures such as biopsy and removal of any abnormal tissue might be done as and when required.

7. *What happens after the procedure?*
    - Once the colonoscopy is over, you will be taken to a recovery area to recuperate. You may want to get to the toilet for few more times to pass motion or flatus to ease the tummy, and it is quite expected.
    - You will be allowed to take liquids 30 minutes after and solids 1 hour after the procedure.
    - You may feel drowsy if sedation was given, and in that case, you will not be able to drive your car or ride a motorbike for a day.
    - You may be asked to get admitted if any therapy was given.
    - If any biopsy was done, then the specimen will be sent to the histology lab and the results will take a few days.
8. *Are there any risks with the procedure?*
    - Colonoscopy is a reasonably safe procedure
    - You may feel a bit bloated and have the urge to pass flatus or feces soon after the examination
    - If you have severe abdominal pain, kindly inform the medical personnel.
    - Some unexpected complications could rarely happen to 1 in 500 patients such as heart or chest difficulties, bleeding, and perforation in the gut. If any of the problems happen, then you may have to stay in the hospital and even require surgery in rare instances.
9. *When should you contact us?*

    If you have persistent abdominal pain, bleeding rectum, or fever, then do not hesitate to contact the hospital.

    You will be given an appointment with a doctor to discuss the result of the colonoscopy and all other reports and decide about further therapy.

ABOUT THE HARDWARE OF COLONOSCOPE

- The insertion section is longer, and wider, but more flexible than gastroscopes. Standard colonoscopes are 130 cm long, while long colonoscopes with 160–180 cm lengths are also available. It has an 11–13 mm outer diameter with a 3.2–3.8 mm channel for accessories.
- The compact but complex design of the Insertion section allows for the best combination of flexibility, column strength, and torque ability.
- The distal 40 cm insertion section is more flexible as it is covered by the soft outer polymer. The proximal portion (50–160 cm) is a bit stiffer due to the hard resin covering. Colonoscopes with variable stiffness have a tensioning wire that runs the length of the insertion section. The amount

of tension in this wire is controlled by rotating a knob at the top end of the insertion section just below the control head.

- Note the size of the channel and where it exits at the scope tip. It is usually 3.2 mm in diameter. When you pass a biopsy forceps through the access channel, see where it comes out in the picture seen in the monitor. Imagine the monitor like a big clock with the top middle of the monitor as 12 o'clock and the bottom middle at 6 o'clock. The biopsy forceps will be seen exiting at the 5 o'clock position. This is very important to understand for the successful conduct of various therapeutic interventions. So, treat the monitor like a clock! It is always better to rotate the scope to bring any colonic lesion to the bottom half of the monitor so tissue sampling or endotherapy would be easy to perform.
- Variable stiffness colonoscopes are also available. They are armed with a twisting control unit at the junction of the control head with the insertion section. It enables stiffening of the shaft of the scope to avoid relooping of the bowel.

ABOUT THE COLONOSCOPY ROOM LAYOUT (FIG. 5)

- Large, spacious, well-ventilated room with optional C-arm X-ray facility for monitoring scope position. Magnetic imaging is nowadays available, e.g., a scope guide by Olympus.
- Patient lying in the left lateral position **(Fig. 6)**.
- Endoscopist standing to face the patient's back and viewing the ergonomically placed monitors.
- One assistant at the head end of the patient to administer drugs and to monitor the patient.
- Another staff member to assist the endoscopist with the procedure and help with accessories.

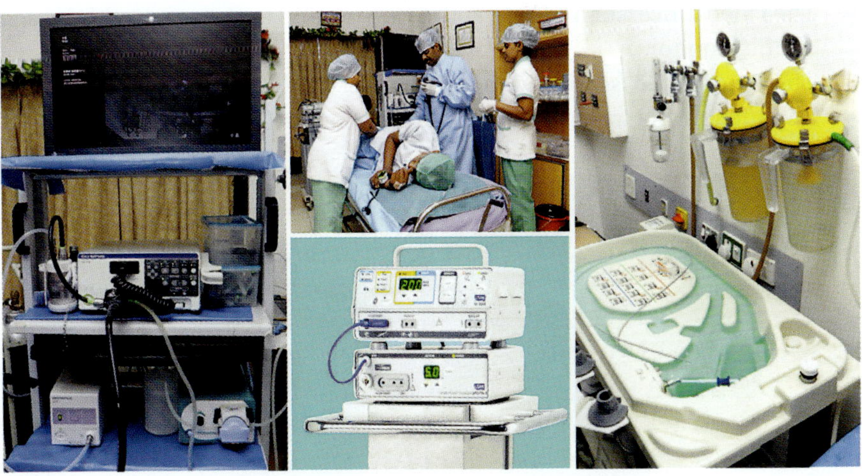

Fig. 5: Colonoscopy room layout.

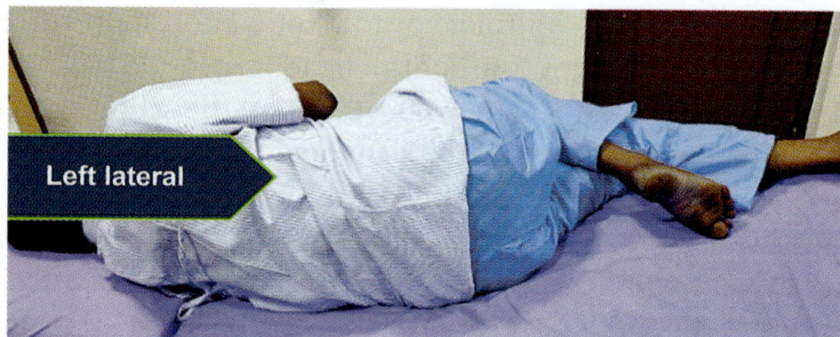

Fig. 6: Left lateral position.

- Energy sources and irrigation, and suction system.
- Facility for image and video recording and printing.

PREPROCEDURE PATIENT CHECKLIST

- Check for indication of colonoscopy
- Look for any comorbidity such as ischemic heart disease (IHD)/diabetes mellitus (DM)/hypertension (HT).
- *Drug history:* Warfarin, aspirin, clopidogrel, and diabetic and hypertensive drugs
- Any history of (H/O) drug allergy.
- Previous abdominal surgery and pacemaker insertion.
- Bowel preparation is adequate as per the inquiry.
- Documentation of vital signs and blood reports.
- Informed consent form signed.

INSTRUMENT CHECKLIST

- Clean, disinfected, and leak-tested colonoscope is ready for use.
- The video processor and light source are on, and the image display is seen on the monitor.
- The water bottle is full, and the air pump is working.
- The suction and irrigation system is functioning **(Figs. 7A and B)**.

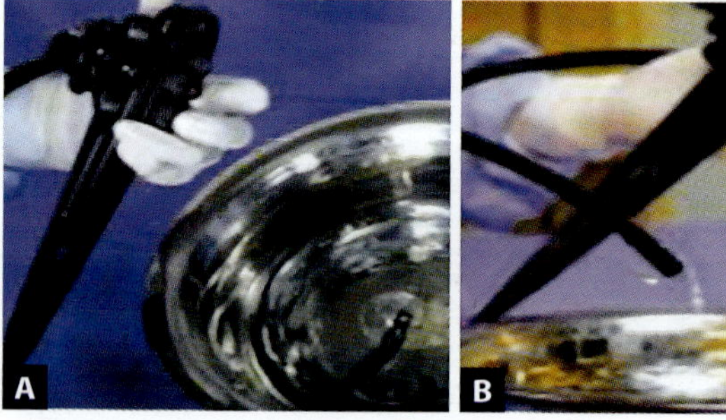

Figs. 7A and B: Checking air and water feeding.

MEDICATION AND MONITORING DURING COLONOSCOPY

- Conscious sedation, along with analgesics, is the common practice
- Use midazolam along with fentanyl, pethidine, or tramadol. Intravenous (IV) propofol can also be used **(Fig. 8)**.
- No sedation colonoscopy requires an understanding patient and a skillful. It is only practiced in a few centers.
- Rational use of antispasmodic drugs like IV 20 mg of hyoscine N-butylbromide (Buscopan) is often helpful, and we routinely use it.
- We administer 2 mg of midazolam, 50 mg of tramadol, and 20 mg of Buscopan IV bolus for all our adult patients routinely.
- Give prophylactic antibiotics in needy high-risk patients (infective endocarditis protocol). Give a single IV dose of gentamicin (120 mg) with amoxicillin 1 g and a further oral dose of amoxicillin (500 mg) 6 hours later.
- Use of CO_2 instead of air during colonoscopy minimizes pain, especially in patients with diverticular disease or IBS.
- Ensure venous access catheter, nasal O_2, electrocardiogram (ECG) monitoring, and pulse oximetry.
- Be alert about the patient's pain intensity and restlessness.
- Avoid rash or undue force during colonoscopy. Be gentle and always be watchful.

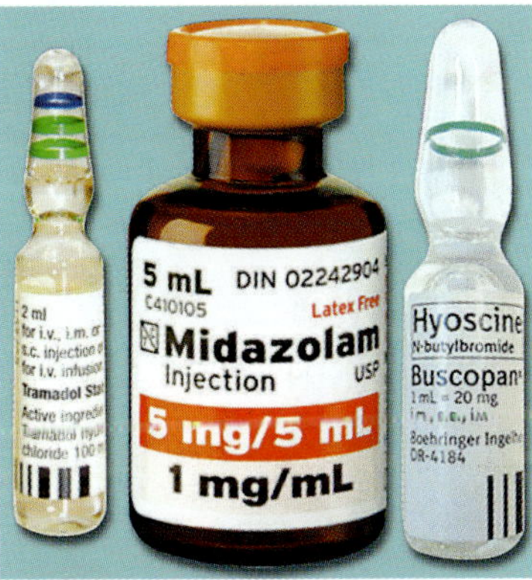

Fig. 8: Medication given during colonoscopy.

SINGLE OR TWO-PERSON COLONOSCOPY

Single-person colonoscopy means the surgeon himself controls the wheels and buttons with his left hand and holds the moving shaft with his right hand. We strongly recommend this technique **(Fig. 9)**.

Hold the shaft about 20–25 cm from the anal verge using a gentle finger grip. Hold the shaft of the scope gently like a pen with a piece of gauze and avoid gripping the scope like a tennis racket **(Figs. 10A and B)**.

Two-person colonoscopy means the surgeon takes control of the control head with both his hands while his assistant manipulates the shaft **(Fig. 11)**.

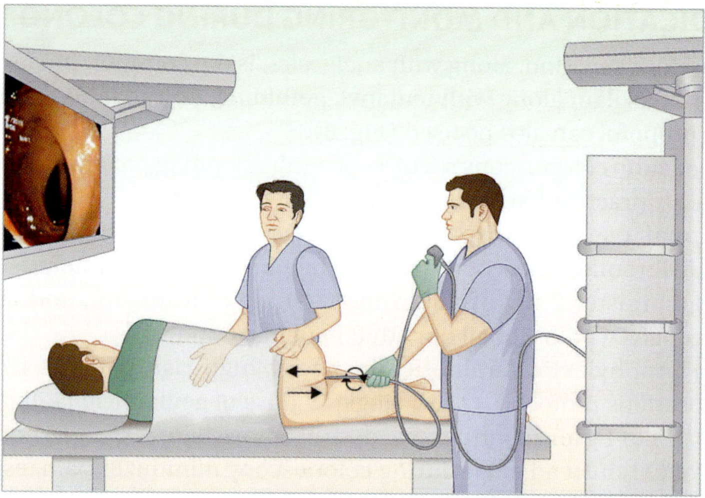

Fig. 9: Single-person colonoscopy.

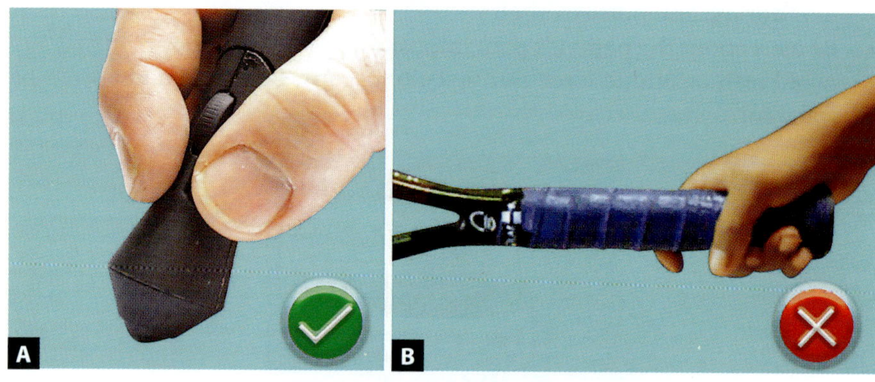

Figs. 10A and B: Handling of colonoscopy.

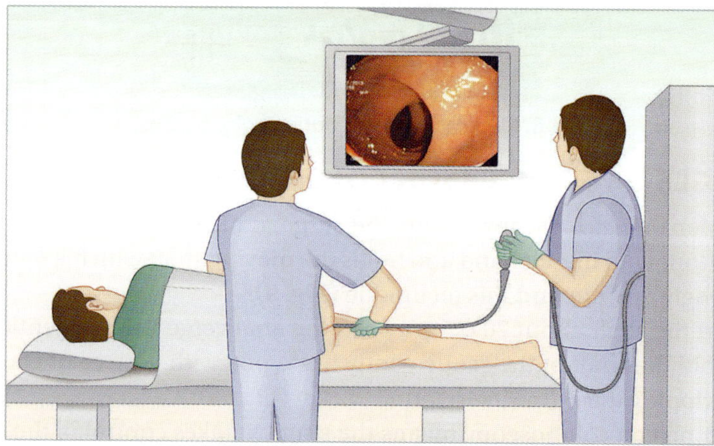

Fig. 11: Two-person colonoscopy.

UNDERSTANDING BASIC COLONOSCOPIC ANATOMY

- *Rectum* **(Fig. 12)**:
  - Dentate line forms the boundary between the anal canal and the rectum
  - Rectum has smooth and reflective mucosa
  - More prominent vascular patterns compared to the rest of the colon
  - Crescent-shaped rectal valves of Houston
  - 15 cm length
- *Sigmoid colon* **(Fig. 13)**:
  - Composed of tortuous bowel with round or oval-shaped lumen and shiny, smooth surface.
  - Looping can occur due to its mobility.
- *Descending colon* **(Fig. 14)**:
  - Runs mostly straight for 20–30 cm and has an oval-shaped lumen.
  - The bottom half of the lumen may be filled with fluid.
  - Bluish discoloration of the spleen heralds the arrival of the splenic flexure.
- *Transverse colon* **(Fig. 15)**:
  - Characteristic triangular lumen with pronounced haustrations.
  - Bluish discoloration due to the liver is appreciable at the hepatic flexure.
- *Ascending colon and cecum* **(Figs. 16 and 17)**:
  - Widest part and usually triangular lumen and thin wall.
  - Note the curved, thick, yellowish ileocecal fold, often with an indentation at its center.
  - Cecal pole with appendicular opening is recognized as a crow's foot due to converging taenia.

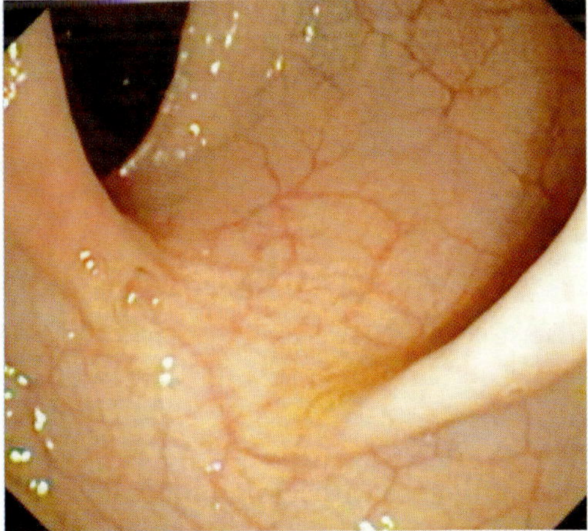

Fig. 12: Rectum.

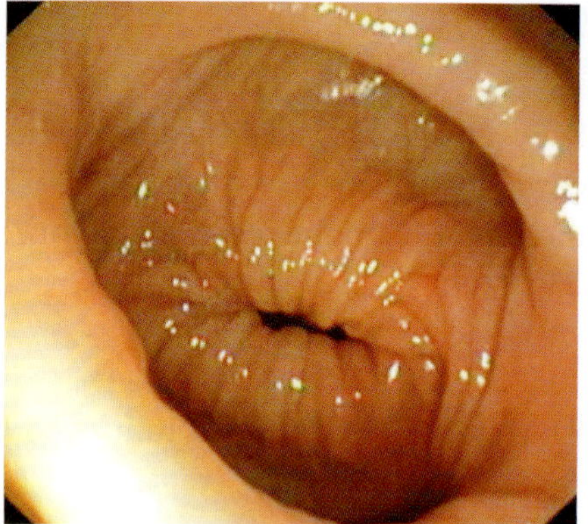

Fig. 13: Sigmoid colon.

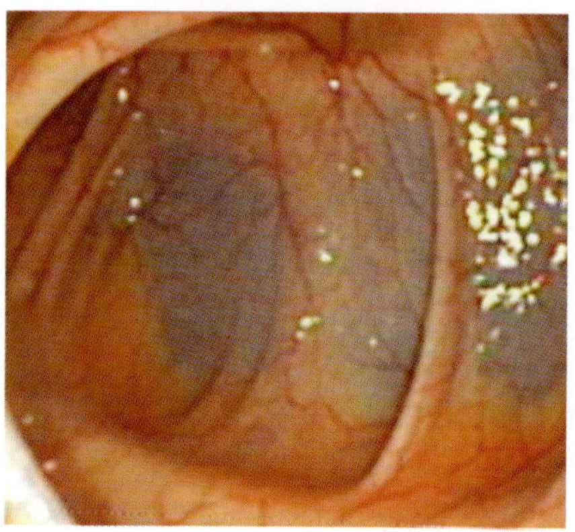

Fig. 14: Splenic flexure.

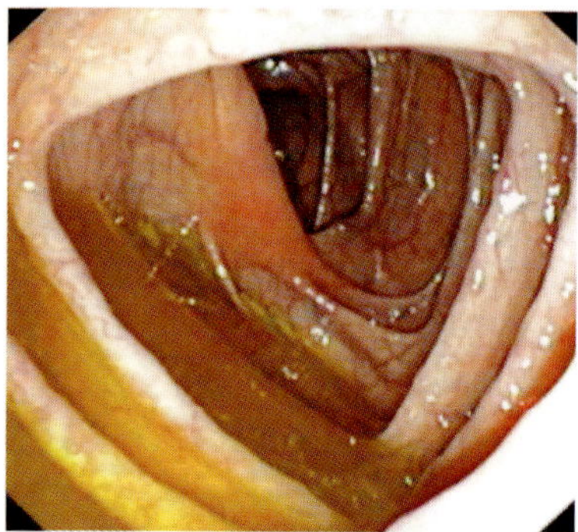

Fig. 15: Transverse colon.

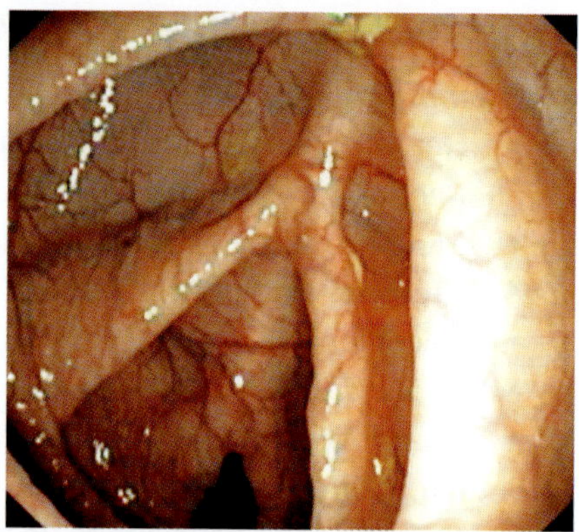

Fig. 16: Ascending colon.

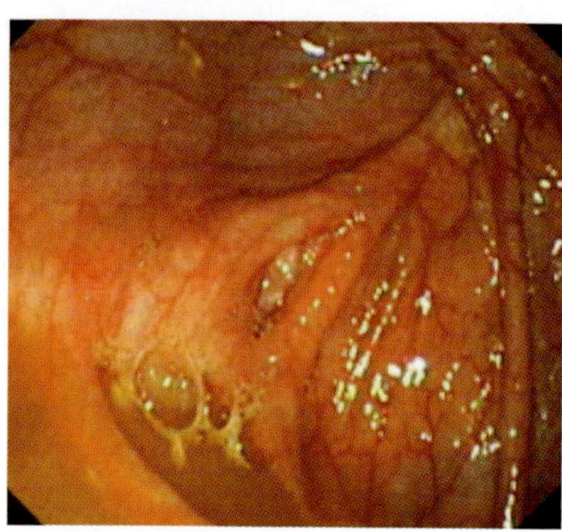

Fig. 17: Cecal pole.

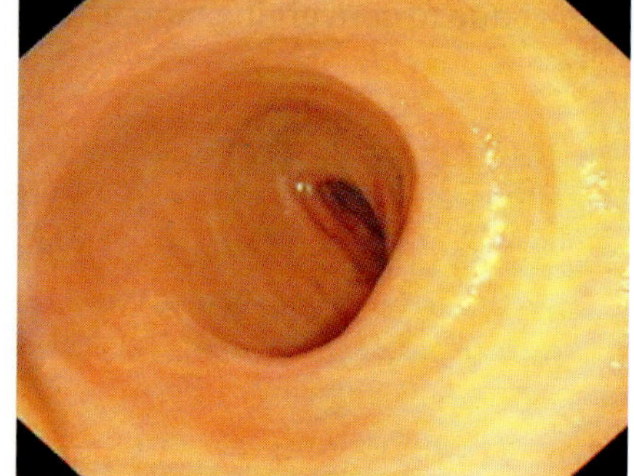

Fig. 18: Terminal ileum.

- *Terminal ileum **(Fig. 18)**:*
  - Velvety granular mucosa with less prominent vascular pattern.
  - May have some prominent lymphoid follicles.

10 KEY STEPS OF COLONOSCOPY

Examination of Anal Canal and Rectum

- Inspect the anal region for any skin tags, external piles, fistula, and fissure or prolapse rectum.
- Use 2% xylocaine jelly and lubricant for rectal examination and feel for sphincter tone, luminal pathology such as growth and polyps, and prostate. Also, look for any evidence of malena or fresh blood on the finger stalls **(Fig. 19)**.
- Finger-guided insertion of the well-lubricated colonoscope through the anal sphincter **(Fig. 20)**.

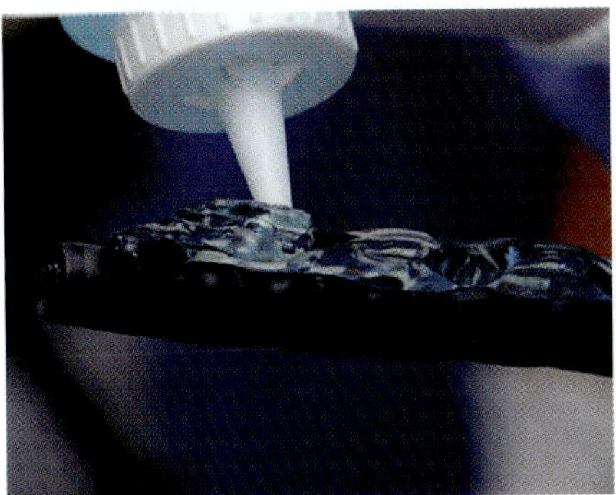

Fig. 19: Lubricant application in colonoscopy.

Fig. 20: Inserting the colonoscope.

- Liberal lubrication of the bending section is the key to the smooth insertion of the colonoscope.
- Visualize the lumen of the rectum and insufflate and proceed to the rectosigmoid junction at 15 cm from the anal margin.
- Upper rectum is examined on the way in, while the lower rectum is better visualized on the way out (retroflexion of colonoscope)
- Air leakage due to a lax sphincter would be a challenge. Apply a cotton pad to the perineal body and press against the colonoscopy to minimize air leakage in such cases.
- Anticipate the difficult rectosigmoid junction in young and thin patients with previous pelvic surgery or radiotherapy. Gentle torque steering and repeated small jiggling movements would help to cross the acute rectosigmoid angle.

Sigmoid Navigation (Fig. 21)

- Be slow and gentle with minimal insufflation.
- Right-hand torque steering is the key to successful navigation.

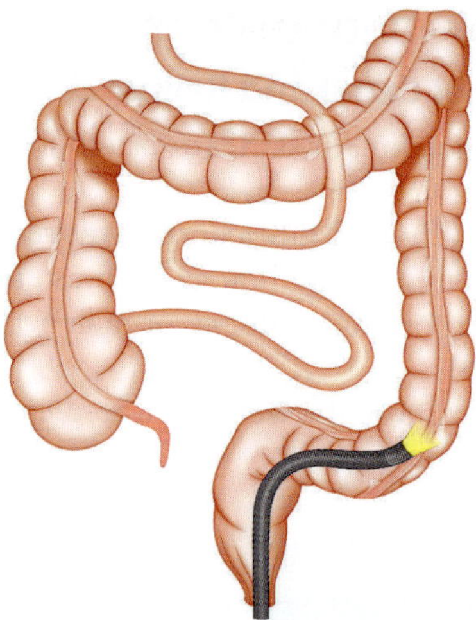

Fig. 21: Sigmoid navigation.

- Keep the lumen at the center or the top right corner of the monitor.
- Pass the sigmoid colon under vision and reach the sigmoid descending colon junction.
- Presumed directions of bends are shown by the shadowing and also by the direction of the taenia coli **(Figs. 22A to C)**.

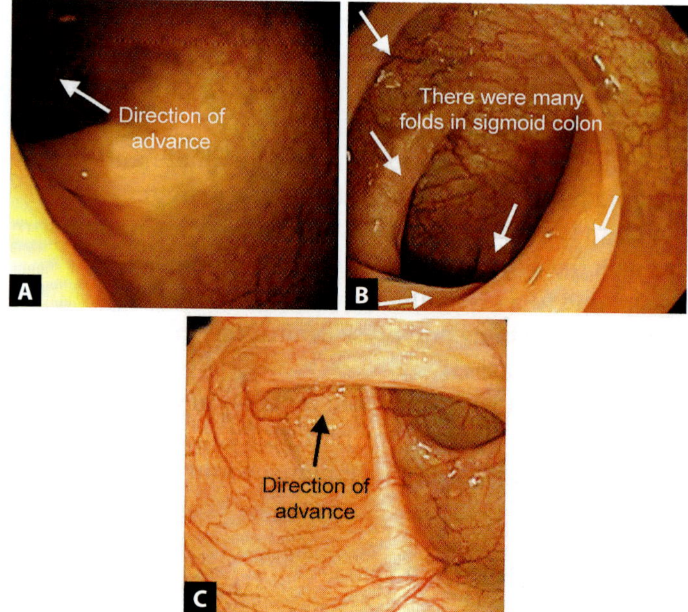

Figs. 22A to C: Inside view of sigmoid navigation.

- Repeated "pull-backs" would help. So, prepare to take "One step forward but two steps backward" **(Fig. 23)**.

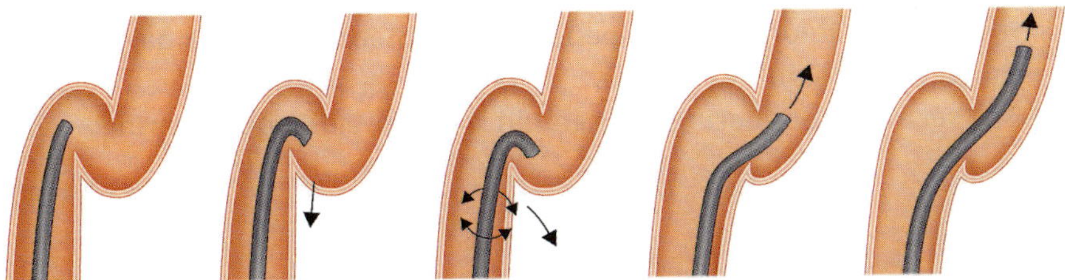

Fig. 23: Tips in navigating sigmoid.

- *Suspect bowing or looping of the scope*:
    - If there is no 1:1 progress of the scope inside
    - If there is any paradoxical movement
    - Stiffness of control wheels
    - Onset of severe pain
- Recognize N-loop formation due to the acute angle at the sigmoid descending colon junction. Pull back, suck, and apply suprapubic external pressure **(Figs. 24 and 25)**.

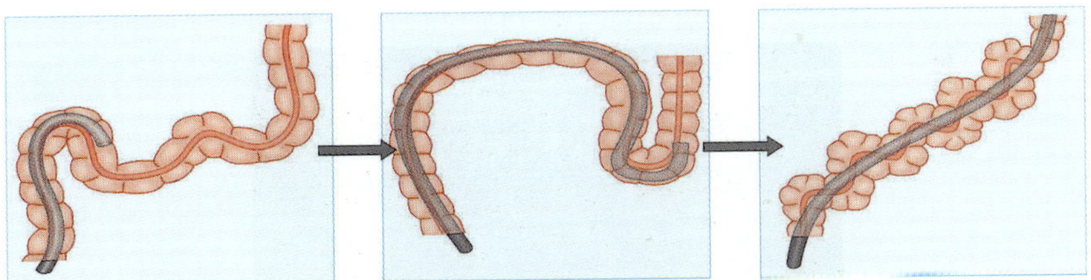

N loop
Pullback/Suctions/Suprapubic pressure

Fig. 24: N loop reduction.

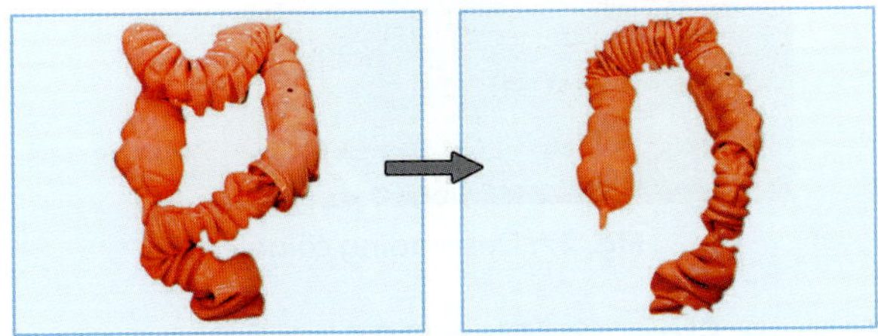

Before/after loop reduciton

Fig. 25: N loop reduction.

- Suspect alpha loop formation **(Fig. 26)** when the scope passes through the descending colon relatively easily and reaches the splenic flexure with a 90 cm mark in the scope. Reduce the loop in the sigmoid by counterclockwise torque, pressure on the lower abdomen, and repeated pullback.
- A successful colonoscopy depends on the smooth and sleek navigation of the sigmoid colon.
- The secret of conquering the sigmoid is clockwise torque steering!

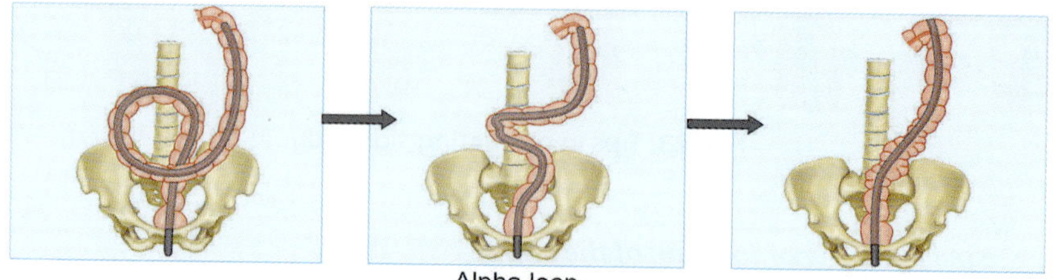

Fig. 26: Alpha loop reduction.

Descending Colon

Descending colon is relatively straight and oval in shape, and with evenly spaced haustrations, and often you notice a typical fluid level. Try not to suck the fluid and navigate above the fluid levels with minimal insufflations **(Fig. 27)**.

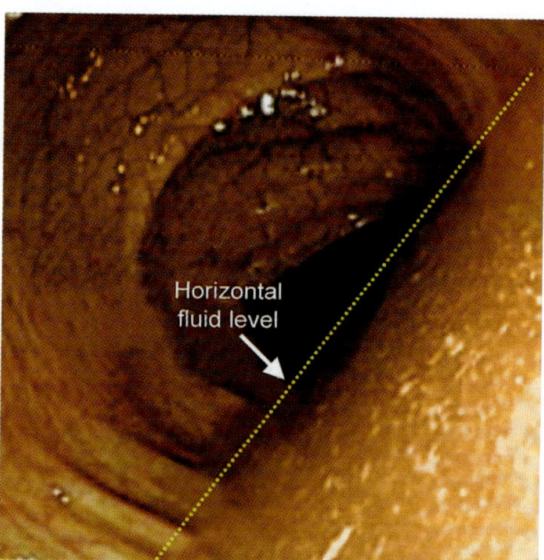

Fig. 27: Descending colon.

Reaching Splenic Flexure (Figs. 28A and B)

- A visible fold in the lumen on the other side of this segment (usually at 9 o'clock in the monitor) and the appearance of bluish coloration of the spleen indicate that we have reached the splenic flexure.

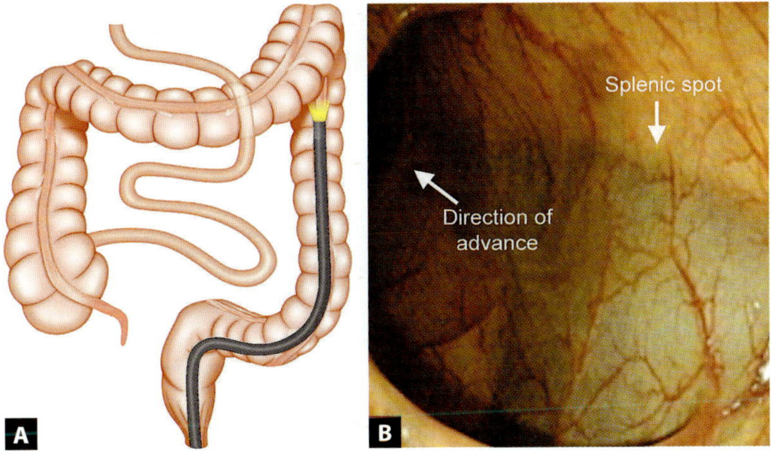

Figs. 28A and B: Reaching the splenic flexure.

- Fluid around the flexure may hinder navigation. So, suck or surf above the fluid to cross the flexure.
- If the lumen is not clearly seen, follow the course of the taenia coli to cross the bend or consider changing the patient to the right lateral position to obliterate the acute angle at the flexure **(Figs. 29A and B)**.

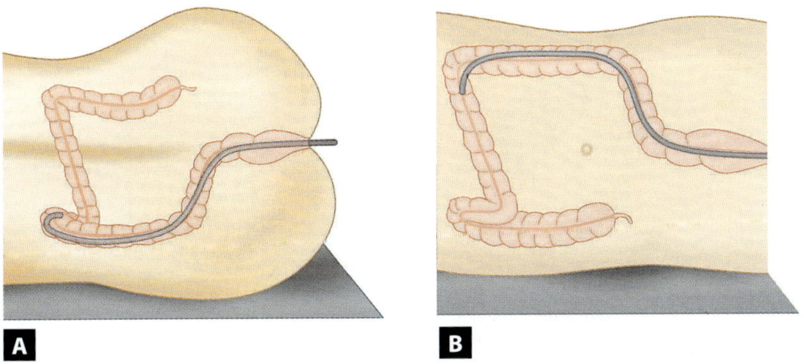

Figs. 29A and B: (A) Left and (B) right lateral position.

- Ask the patient to breathe in deeply to bring the left dome and hence the splenic flexure down.
- If the scope is straight with no looping in sigmoid, the splenic flexure is usually reached with a 40 cm mark in the scope.

Travel Through the Transverse Colon (Figs. 30A and B)

- The transverse colon is triangular in shape and with evenly spaced haustrations.

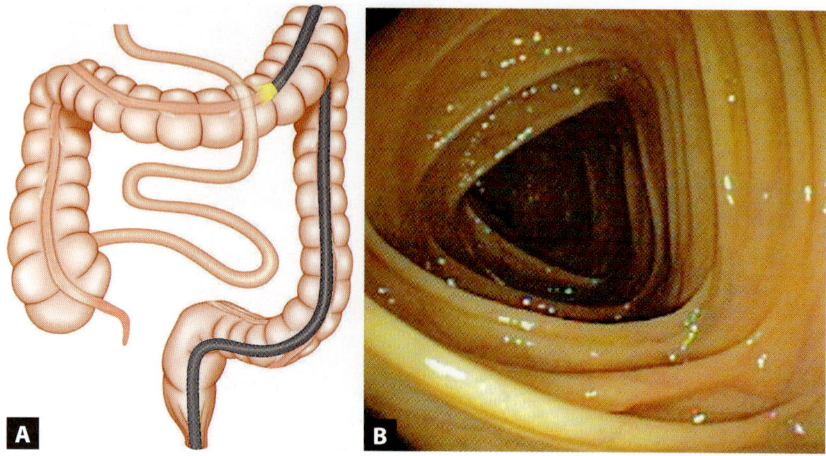

Figs. 30A and B: Traveling transverse colon.

- Proceed to hepatic flexure by using a combination of advancing/withdrawing and external hand pressure.
- Occasionally, a gamma loop may form due to redundant transverse colon and may need anticlockwise torque with pull back of the scope for correction **(Fig. 31)**.

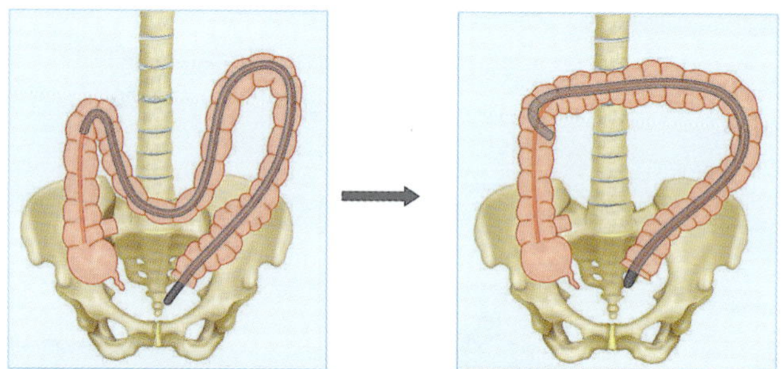

Gamma loop: Pullback/anticlockwise torque central abdominal upward pressure

Fig. 31: Gamma loop reduction.

Reaching Hepatic Flexure (Figs. 32A and B)

- Hepatic flexure is noted by the sharp angling of the lumen. Again, by advancing/withdrawing the scope, changing the patient to supine or even right lateral position, and external hand pressure, we should reach the ascending colon.
- At times, ask the patient to breathe in and hold so as to bring the hepatic flexure down along with diaphragm movement and thereby aiding successful passage.

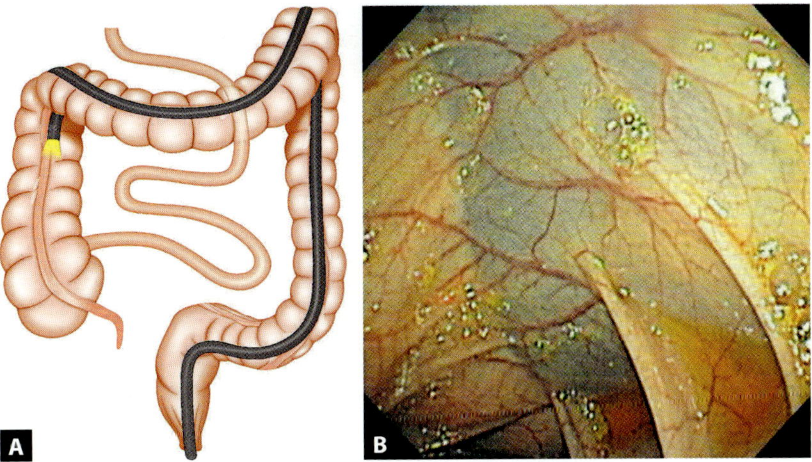

Figs. 32A and B: Reaching hepatic flexure.

- Intermittent suction and withdrawal of the scope often leads to paradoxical forward movement of the scope tip and helps to reach the hepatic flexure! **(Fig. 33)**.
- Remember that an air-distended colon is a long colon, while suction helps to shorten the colon and aids in easy intubation of the right colon!

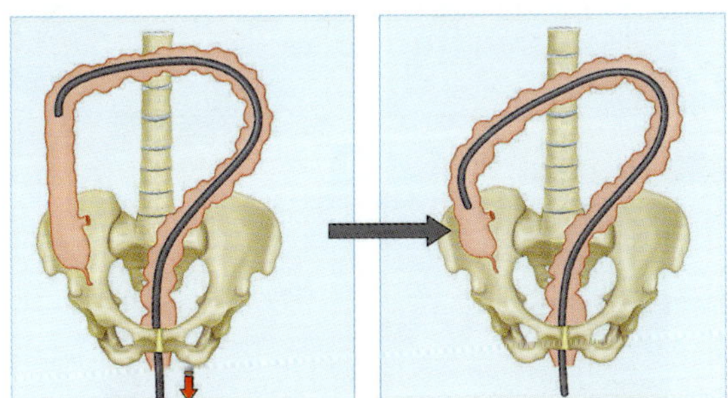

Fig. 33: Suction and withdraw the scope.

Right Colon Down to Cecum (Figs. 34A and B)

- The cecum is identified by the typical crow's foot appearance due to three converging taenia (Mercedes Benz Sign). Appendix opening is usually seen at its center as a semicircular opening.
- Cecum is reached with a 60 cm level in a shortened straight scope.
- The ileocecal fold is seen as a thick lipomatous shiny fold just above the cecum and is usually seen in the bottom half of the monitor **(Figs. 35A to C)**.
- A 90–95% cecal intubation rate is the anticipated standard we should strive to achieve.

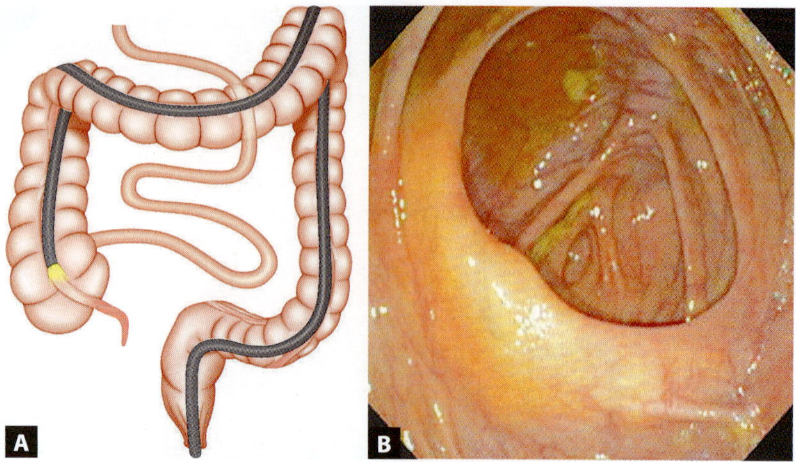

Figs. 34A and B: Reaching cecum.

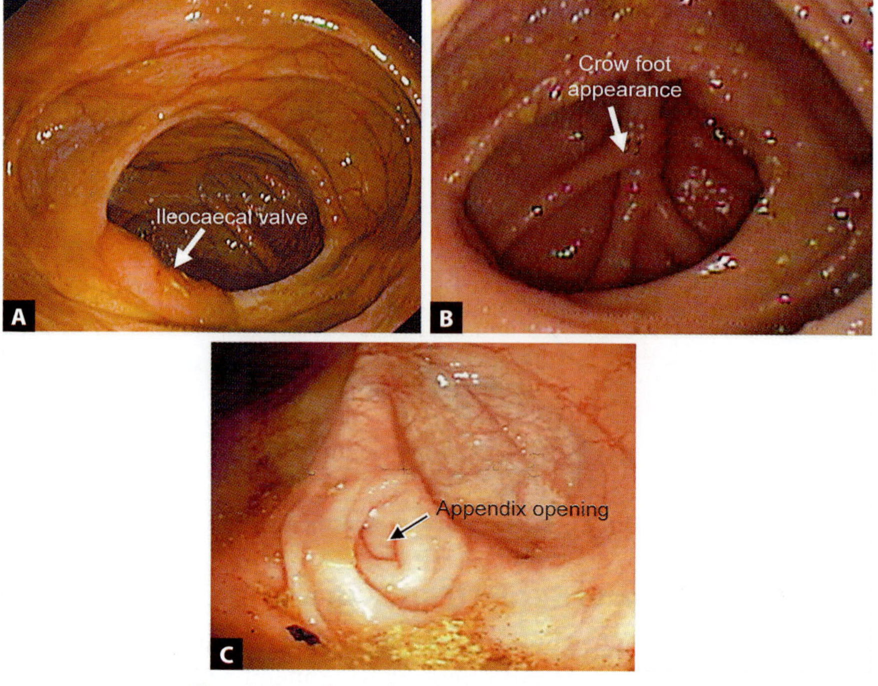

Figs. 35A to C: Landmarks to confirm the cecum.

Terminal Ileum

- The bow and arrow sign **(Fig. 36)** is often helpful to locate the ileocecal valve. Locate the appendix orifice. Imagine the appendix lumen as a bow, and an imaginary arrow is shot from it. Its direction would be normally pointing toward the ileocecal valve, and hence angulate the scope in that

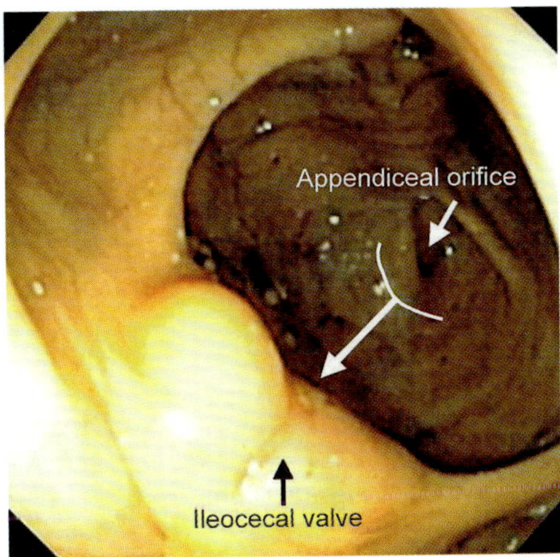

Fig. 36: Bow and arrow sign.

direction (Turn the big wheel away from you) and pull the scope back to reach the proximal lip of the ileocecal valve. Gently insufflate **(Fig. 37)**.

- Various types of ileocecal valve can be seen volcano like, wide mouthed or slit like with thin or thick lips. It is usually found hidden just below the lipomatous thick ileocecal fold.

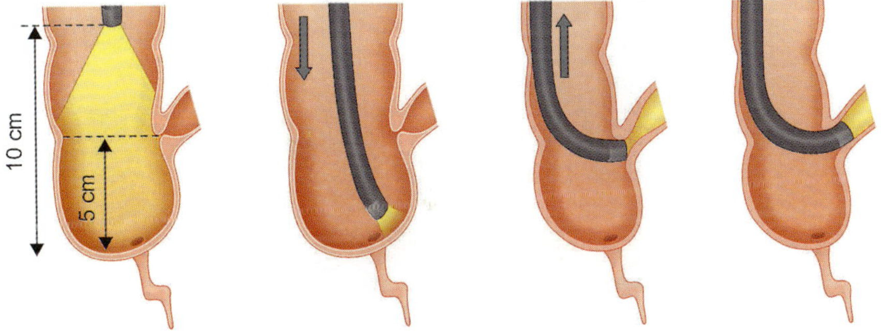

Look down, pullback, and insufflate

Fig. 37: Ileal navigation.

- Normally ileocecal valve would be seen at the 6–7 o'clock position in the monitor. Shifting the patient to the supine position can also bring the valve to a favorable position for intubation. We should be able to intubate the ileum with downward deflection of the big wheel and anticlockwise torque of the scope while withdrawing the scope from the cecal pole **(Fig. 38)**.

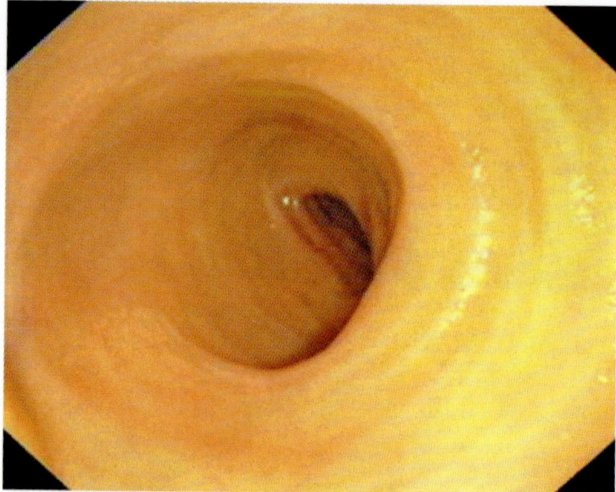

Fig. 38: Ileum.

- Frothy small bowel secretion greets you at the valve, and the granular appearance of the mucosa confirms successful intubation of the ileum. At times, a biopsy forceps can be inserted into the ileum and used as a guide to pass the scope through **(Fig. 39)**.
- Examine at least 2 feet of the terminal ileum to look for any lesions.

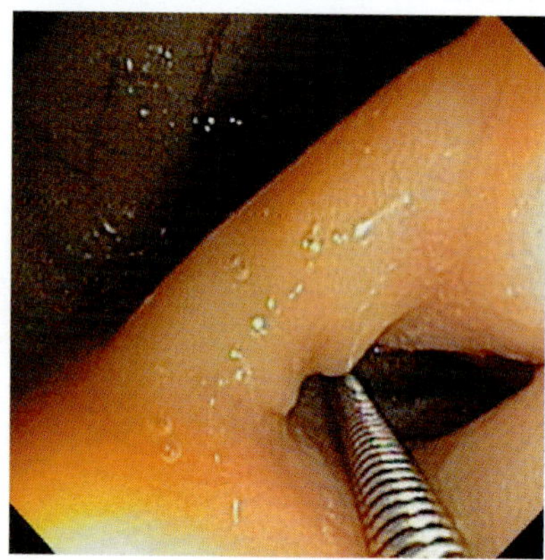

Fig. 39: Navigating the ileum with a guidewire.

Cecum to Rectum Withdrawal

- Do a slow withdrawal of the scope from the cecum to the rectum, taking care to look for blind spots like the area behind the haustral folds and flexures.
- On withdrawal, the cecum is found at 60 cm, the splenic flexure at 40 cm, and the sigmoid colon at 30 cm level **(Figs. 40A to D)**.
- A minimum of 6 minutes is to be spent on the withdrawal so as not to miss any small flat lesions.

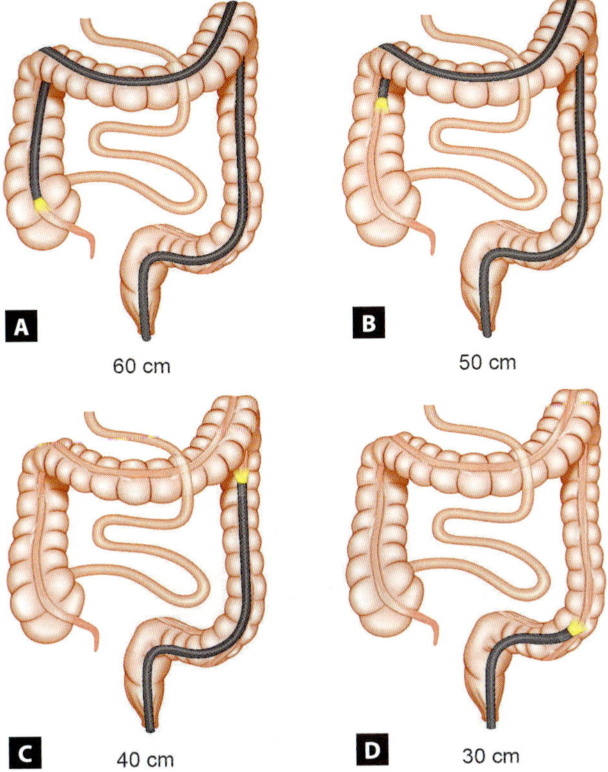

Figs. 40A to D: Scope length in withdrawal.

- *Beware of the following blind spots while performing a colonoscopy:*
  - Ileocecal valve
  - Behind haustral folds
  - Inner fold of hepatic flexure
  - In the pool of fluid near the splenic flexure
  - Behind the rectal valves of Houston

Retroflex in Rectum (Figs. 41A and B)

- Retroflex the scope in the rectum to look for any lower rectal lesions and piles.
- Turn both small and big wheels fully toward you when the scope is in the mid rectum, and then push the scope in and rotate all around to have a panoramic view of the lower rectum and pectinate line **(Fig. 42)**.
- Avoid this step in patients with diseased rectum, like IBD, for want of distensibility.
- Document all the findings with relevant pictures and discuss with the patient and relatives regarding the final diagnosis and further management.

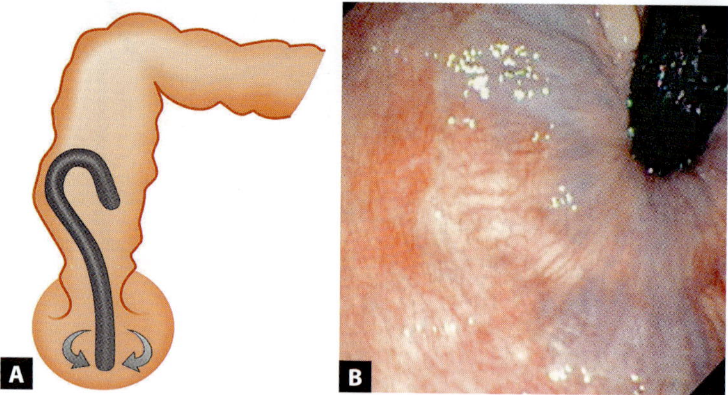

Figs. 41A and B: Retroflexion.

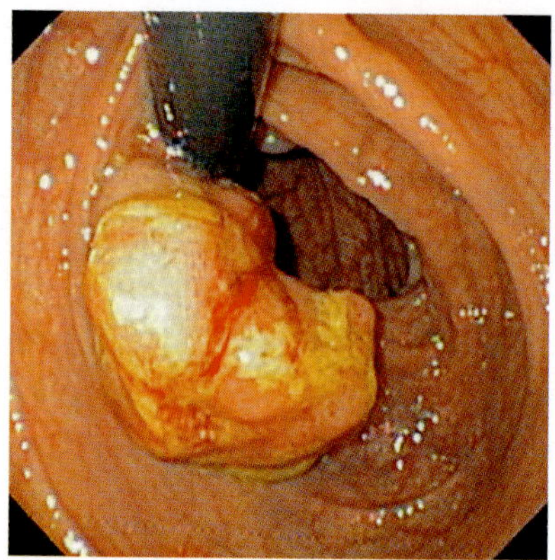

Fig. 42: Growth at the dentate line.

TOP 10 TIPS FOR A SUCCESSFUL COLONOSCOPY

1. *Be slow and gentle:*
   - Do not be in a hurry, as loops tend to form and the patient becomes uncomfortable.
   - Remember the rabbit and turtle story! Be slow and steady to win the race!
2. *Minimal insufflation:*
   - Minimal air insufflation to distend the bowel should suffice.
   - Distension makes the bowel loops longer and more tortuous, and hence the procedure becomes more difficult.
3. *Straight scope:* Ensure that the scope is straight with one-to-one movement.
4. *Art of torque steering:* Clockwise twisting of the shaft of the insertion tube while pushing the scope aids in easy navigation.

5. *Keep the lumen at the center or the top right corner of the screen:* Steering the scope in such a way as to keep the lumen in view.
6. *Loop recognition and reduction* **(*Fig. 43*)**:
    - N loop, alpha and reverse alpha loops, and gamma loop formation are well appreciated if we use the C arm or scope guide.
    - We should know all the tricks to reduce the loops and proceed further with the least discomfort to the patient
7. *One step forward and two steps backward:* To undo loops and to avoid blind entry around a corner, never hesitate to withdraw the scope to orient and then proceed again. Repeated such maneuvers help in proper navigation.
8. *Benefit of abdominal wall pressure:* External hand pressure by your assistant does help to contain the loop and seamless progression
9. *Importance of change of position:* Though the whole procedure can be done in the left lateral position in most cases, at times, patient position change would help us to get through some tough angles.
10. *Success with suction:* Periodic suction of the bowel lumen will not only decompress the bowel but also shorten the bowel to make navigation easy.

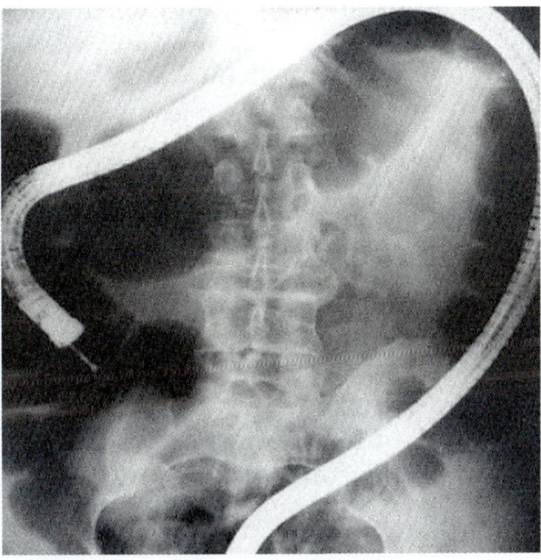

Fig. 43: Loop recognition with C arm.

ANCILLARY MEASURES FOR DIFFICULT COLONOSCOPY

- *External abdominal pressure* **(Figs. 44A to C)**:
    - Suprapubic pressure to prevent sigmoid loop formation.
    - Epigastric upward pressure to prevent transverse colon loop formation.
    - Pressure on the right lateral wall to aid passage of the scope through the hepatic flexure and the ascending colon.

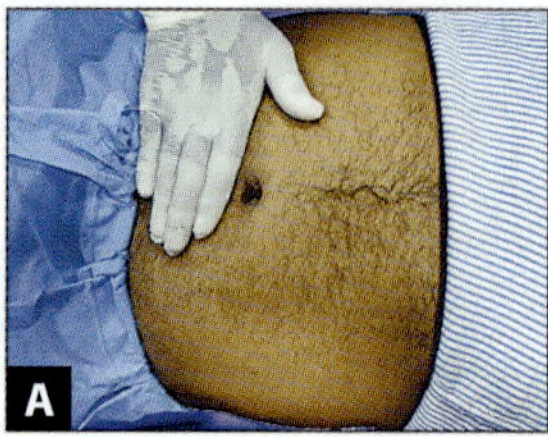

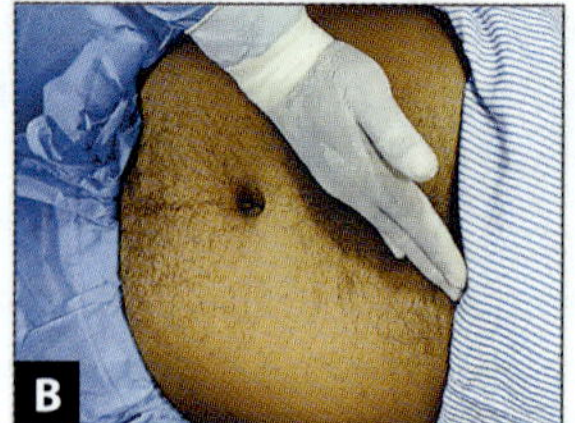

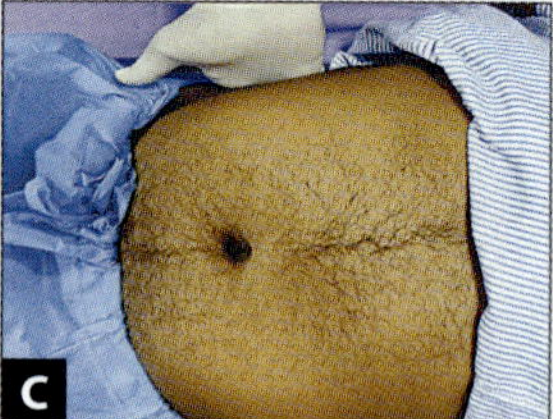

Figs. 44A to C: External abdominal pressure. (A) Suprapubic pressure for sigmoid; (B) Upper abdomen pressure for transverse colon; (C) Right loin pressure for ascending colon.

- *Change of position of the patient* **(Fig. 45)**:
  - Routinely patient is lying left lateral during the start of the procedure.
  - In case of difficulty at the sigmoid-descending colon or at the splenic flexure, consider turning the patient to supine or even right lateral for easy passage.
  - Passage across the hepatic flexure and down through the ascending colon could be aided by the right lateral position.
- *Successful suction:* Suction decompression of the colon helps in easier intubation, especially in the proximal part. Air-distended colon is wider and longer, while a decompressed colon is shorter and could easily be crossed.
- *Breath-holding technique:* Breath holding on deep inspiration brings both colonic flexures down, making them less acute and easier to navigate.

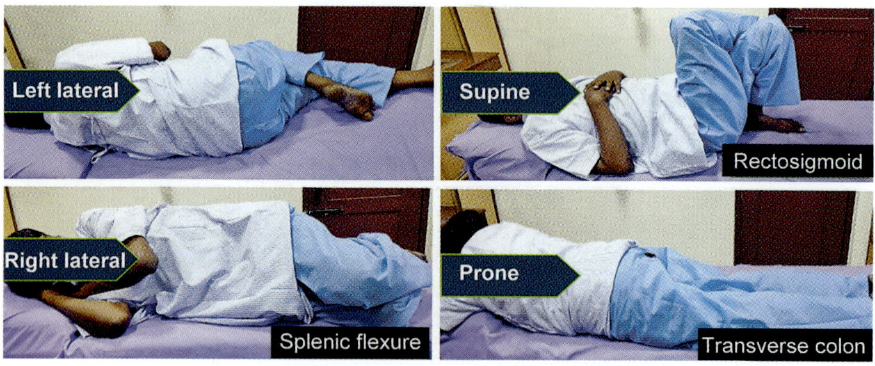

Fig. 45: Change of position of a patient.

- *Water infusion colonoscopy* ***(Fig. 46)****:*
  - CO_2 colonoscopy is relatively pain-free, but on occasion, we could consider water infusion using an irrigation pump.
  - As it keeps the sigmoid bends less acute, an underwater colonoscopy is able to pass through the bends more efficiently.

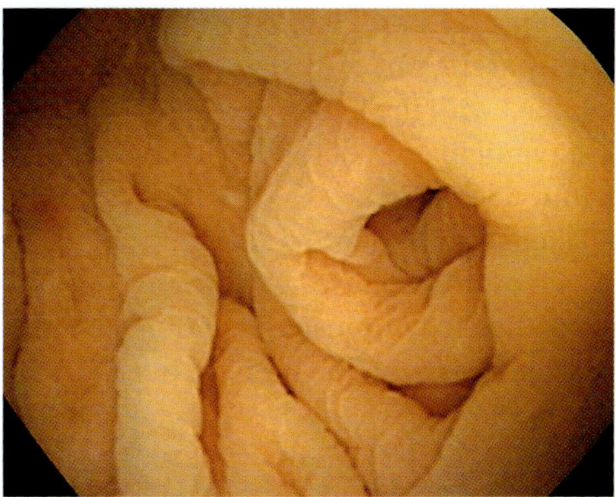

Fig. 46: Water infusion colonoscopy.

- *Variable stiffness colonoscope:*
  - Distal 60 cm of insertion section can be stiffened by turning a knob just below the access channel in certain versions of colonoscope. It makes the distal part of the insertion section stiffer and hence helps in easy navigation and prevents loop formation.
- *Scope guide:*
  - Loop formation during colonoscopy is uncomfortable for the patient, and it will also hinder cecal intubation.
  - Though fluoroscopy is useful to know the shaft position, radiation risks deter its routine use.
  - The scope guide (Olympus) works on the principle of magnetic resonance and clearly depicts the scope shaft position, thereby helping the surgeon for the loop recognition and loop reduction. The addition of the hand probe helps us to apply the abdominal pressure at the exact place to prevent loop formation.
  - Scope pilot-NCU-7000 is a navigation system technology by Pentax designed to provide a three-dimensional (3D) live representation of the colonoscope shape and position inside the patient's large bowel.
- *CO_2 colonoscopy:*
  - Instead of room air, use CO_2 for colonoscopy.
  - Absorbed from the colon 160 times faster than nitrogen and 12 times faster than oxygen (main component of air), CO_2 is transported via the bloodstream to the lungs and rapidly exhaled.
  - This ensures less pain, and also there is no risk of explosion during any diathermy use
  - Well tolerated and safe even in patients with chronic obstructive pulmonary disease (COPD).
  - It is also very easy to set up with the help of a dedicated CO_2 insufflator (Olympus).

- *Cap colonoscopy* **(Figs. 47A and B)**:
  - Putting a transparent cap at the scope tip keeps the mucosa from coming in contact with the lens.
  - Helps in better anticipation of turns and also minimizes the chance of loop formation.
  - Better and faster cecal intubation rate with this technique makes you wonder why we should not use cap colonoscopy routinely!
- Also consider a pediatric colonoscope, a double balloon colonoscope, a gastroscope, an enteroscope, or even an overtube in cases of difficult colonoscopy.

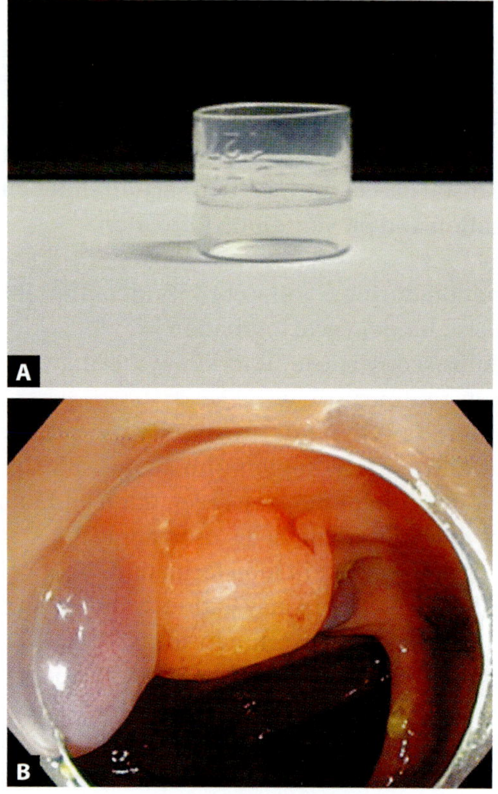

Figs. 47A and B: Cap colonoscopy.

Colonoscopy after Colonic Resections

- Surveillance colonoscopy is usually done 1 year after resection of the carcinoma colon.
- After sigmoid resection, the colon is straighter and shorter, and after right hemicolectomy, you reach the ileo-transverse anastomosis fairly easily.

- Staple line or suture line with granuloma or characteristic white scar should be recognized. Recognize the type of anastomosis (End-to-end or end-to-side, or side-to-side). Look for any stenosis or local recurrence. Look for any polyps.

Colonoscopy Through Colostomy (Fig. 48)

- It can be done both through end and loop colostomy stomas.
- Inspect and perform digital palpation of the stomal opening prior to inserting the colonoscopy.
- Parastomal hernia would make the examination challenging at times.
- Air leakage is a constant problem, and hence, keep a cotton pad around the scope at the stomal opening.

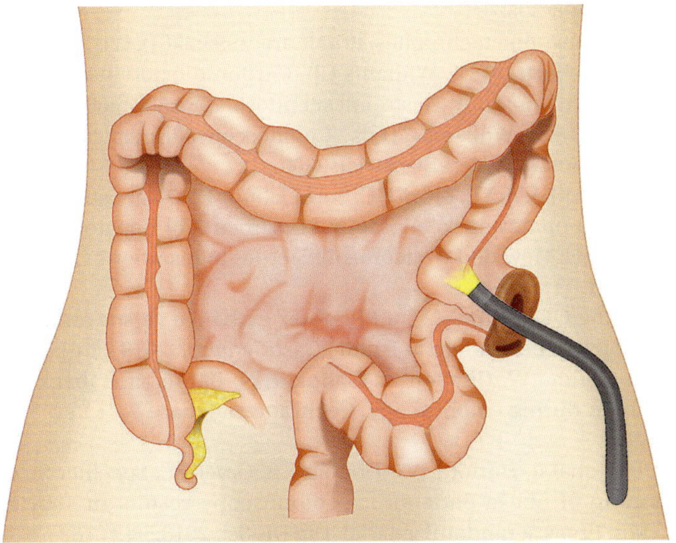

Fig. 48: Colonoscopy through colostomy.

KEY MESSAGES

- Good bowel preparation is the key for a successful colonoscopy.
- Key steps for successful navigation during colonoscopy.
- Repeated pullback
- Clockwise torque steering
- Secrets for consistent cecal intubation
- Practice, practice, and practice

SUGGESTED READING

1. Church JM. Ancillary colonoscope insertion techniques. An evaluation. Surg Endosc. 1993;7(3):191-3.

2. Cohen LB, Wecsler JS, Gaetano JN, Benson AA, Miller KM, Durkalski V, et al. Endoscopic sedation in the United States: results from a nationwide survey. Am J Gastroenterol. 2006;101(5):967-74.
3. Cooper GS, Kou TD, Rex DK. Complications following colonoscopy with anesthesia assistance: a population-based analysis. JAMA Intern Med. 2013; 173(7):551-6.
4. Corporaal S, Kleibeuker JH, Koornstra JJ. Low-volume PEG plus ascorbic acid versus high-volume PEG as bowel preparation for colonoscopy. Scand J Gastroenterol. 2010;45(11):1380-6.
5. DiPalma JA, Wolff BG, Meagher A, Cleveland Mv. Comparison of reduced volume versus four liters sulfate-free electrolyte lavage solutions for colonoscopy colon cleansing. Am J Gastroenterol. 2003;98(10):2187-91.
6. Dominitz JA, Baldwin LM, Green P, Kreuter W, Ko CW. Regional variation in anesthesia assistance during outpatient colonoscopy is not associated with differences in polyp detection or complication rates. Gastroenterology. 2013;144(2):298-306.
7. Hopper WJ. Insertion techniques. Prim Care. 1995;22(3):411-31.
8. Hussein AM, Bartram CI, Williams CB. Carbon dioxide insufflation for more comfortable colonoscopy. Gastrointest Endosc. 1984;30(2):68-70.
9. In: Waye JD, Rex D, Williams C (Eds). Colonoscopy: Principles and Practice, 2nd edition. New Jersey: Wiley-Blackwell; 2009.
10. Jeong SH, Lee KJ, Kim YB, Kwon HC, Sin SJ, Chung JY. Diagnostic value of terminal ileum intubation during colonoscopy. J Gastroenterol Hepatol. 2008;23(1):51-5.
11. Jung Y, Lee SH. How do I overcome difficulties in insertion? Clin Endosc. 2012; 45(3):278-81.
12. Liu Y, Huang QK, Dong XL, Jin PP. Water exchange versus air insufflation for colonoscopy: A meta-analysis. Saudi J Gastroenterol. 2018;24(6):311-6.
13. Singh H, Poluha W, Cheung M, Choptain N, Baron KI, Taback SP. Propofol for sedation during colonoscopy. Cochrane Database Syst Rev. 2008;2008(4): CD006268.
14. Uddin FS, Iqbal R, Harford WV, Dunbar KB, Cryer BL, Spechler SJ, et al. Prone positioning of obese patients for colonoscopy results in shortened cecal intubation times: a randomized trial. Dig Dis Sci. 2013;58(3):782-7.
15. Walsh CM, Ahmad A, Saunders BP, Cohen J, Cotton PB, Williams CB. Practical gastrointestinal endoscopy. In: Peter B (Ed). Cotton and Williams' Practical Gastrointestinal Endoscopy: The Fundamentals, 8th edition. New Jersey: Wiley Blackwell; 2023.
16. Wernli KJ, Inadomi JM. Anesthesia for colonoscopy: too much of a good thing? JAMA Intern Med. 2013;173(7):556-8.
17. Williams C. Position changes during colonoscopy: opening a can of worms? Gastrointest Endosc. 2007;65(2):270-1.

Expert's Comment

Colonoscopy is a complex procedure that requires a deep understanding and has a long learning curve.

It is also difficult to describe complex colonoscopy techniques in easy and understandable language. This chapter describes the colonoscopy procedure in a very crisp manner with nice illustrations.

As a surgeon, we are well versed with digital rectal examination (DRE) and it helps us a lot. After the DRE, just gently put the colonoscope into the rectum, and your colonoscopy journey will start. As we know, surgeons will not stop at the rectum but rather try to insert the scope further and end up at the cecum.

Once we understand how to navigate the tortuous colon with wheel movements and torque of the insertion section, make early diagnosis of various loop formations, and pass the scope gently with minimal insufflation, we will slowly but surely become a master colonoscopist.

Practice, practice, and practice is the mantra of the art of colonoscopy.

Avoid undue force and blind push; you will conquer the colon. Perspire till you perform a perfect 100 plus cases to know all the tips and tricks as described in this chapter by the author.

Professor Easwaramoorthy is a global star in the field of endoscopy and an academic leader. His effort for endoscopy training for surgeons is exceptional.

I am proud to be a member of his academic group.

Dr Masfique Ahmed Bhuiyan
Bangladesh

11

CHAPTER

Atlas of Colonoscopic Pathology

Chapter Outline

- Common Pathology
  - Diverticular Disease
  - Polyps
  - Polyposis Syndrome: More than 100 Polyps
  - Malignant Tumors
  - Submucosal Tumors
  - Inflammatory Bowel Diseases
  - Vascular Malformations
  - Solitary Rectal Ulcer
  - Melanosis Coli
  - Piles

Keywords: Diverticular disease, carcinoma colon, colonic polyps, Kudo's classification, and colitis

INTRODUCTION

Detailed history and systematic clinical examination should precede colonoscopy. Good bowel preparation, conscious sedation, minimal air, or preferably CO_2 insufflation ensures a satisfactory colonoscopic examination. Use of high-definition (HD) colonoscopy with magnification and image enhancement facilities would certainly be beneficial in identifying the lesions. The examination should be through both during insertion and also during withdrawal of the scope. We should describe the findings using standard medical terminology. This chapter enumerates common pathologies seen during colonoscopy.

COMMON PATHOLOGY

Diverticular Disease (Figs. 1 to 4)

- Variable number of pseudodiverticula, often with stool impaction or prominent nearby vessels
- Diverticular openings are oval or circular, while the colonic lumen appears slit-like or half-moon shaped.

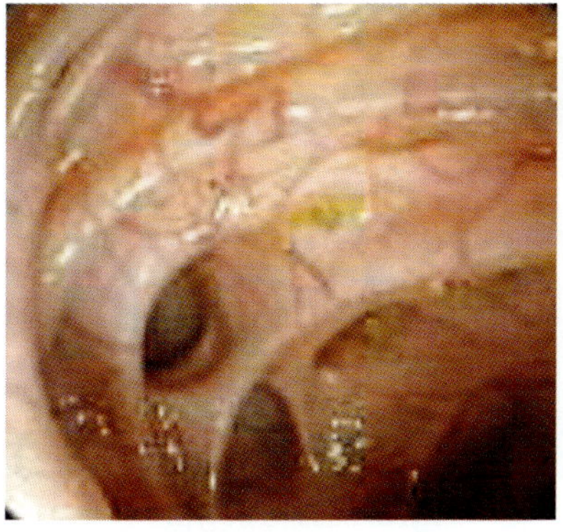

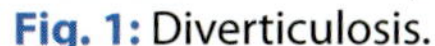

Fig. 1: Diverticulosis.

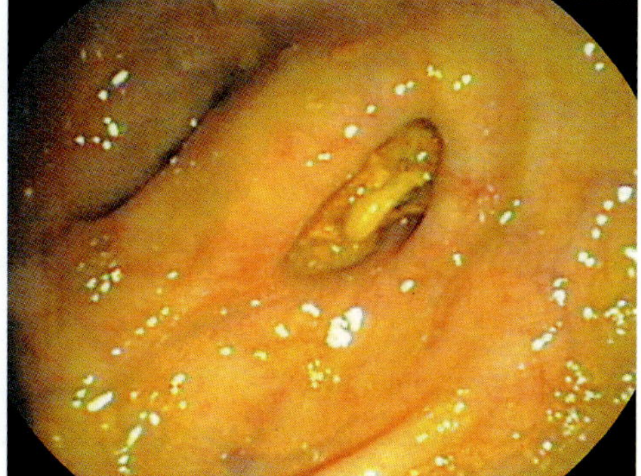

Fig. 2: Diverticulum with fecal impaction.

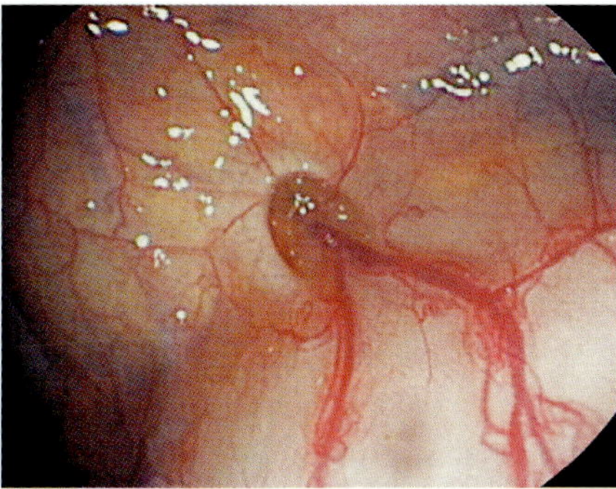

Fig. 3: Diverticulum with a vessel.

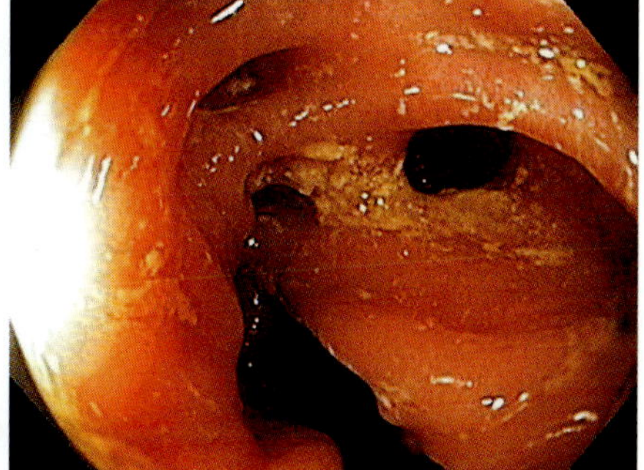

Fig. 4: Slit-like colonic lumen.

- Narrowing of bowel lumen due to circular muscle hypertrophy
- Evidence of inflammation, stricture, or bleeding and even fistula

Polyps (Figs. 5 to 7)

Adenomatous Polyps

- Morphologically, it could be sessile or pedunculated polyps of variable size and with smooth or lobular contour.
- Histologically, it could be tubular, tubule-villous, or villous adenoma.
- These are considered as precancerous lesions and, hence, need removal.
- Magnification images, chromoendoscopy, and narrow-band imaging (NBI) help to characterize the lesions.
- As per the Paris classification, there are three types of polyps, namely **(Fig. 7)**:
    - *Type I: Protruded lesions:*
        - *Ip:* Polypoidal
        - *Is:* Sessile

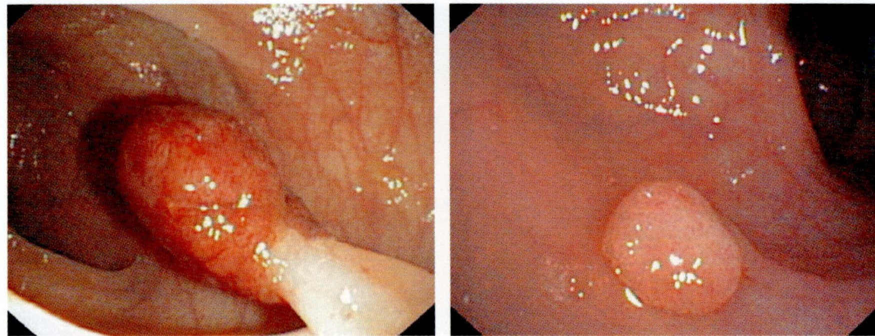

Fig. 5: Pedunculated polyp.

Fig. 6: Sessile polyp.

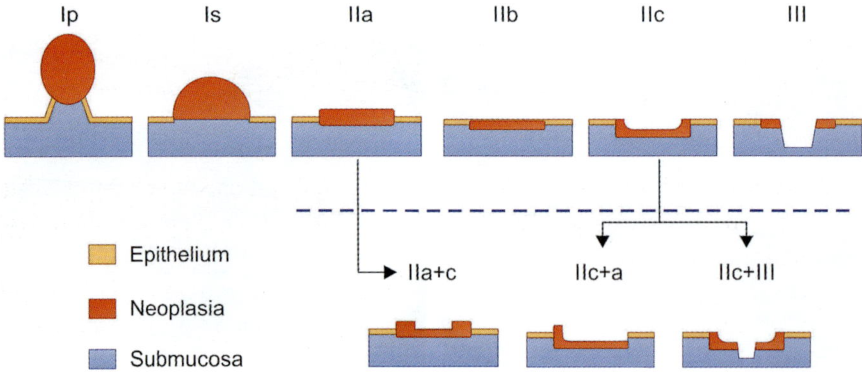

Fig. 7: Paris classification.

- *Type II: Superficial lesions:*
    - *IIa:* Flat elevated
    - *IIb:* Flat
    - *IIc:* Flat depressed
- *Type III: Excavated or ulcerated lesions*

- *Kudo's pit pattern classification* ***(Fig. 8)****:* It classifies the polyps according to the form of the pit pattern. There are five different types of polypoidal lesions as follows. The risk of malignancy differs accordingly to Kudo's type.
    i. Round pits
    ii. Stellar pits
    iii. Tubular pits
    iv. Gyrus-like pits
    v. Nonstructured pits
- Types I and II are considered non-neoplastic polyps, and III–V are neoplastic polyps. Type V is very suspicious of malignancy.
- Presence of deformation, friable surface, depression at the center, ulceration, or undue bleeding are signs of probable malignant transformation.

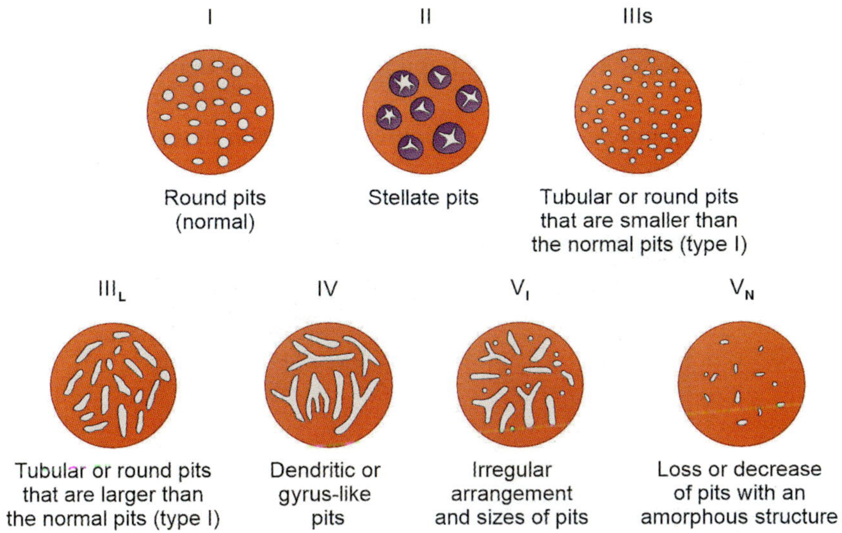

Fig. 8: Kudo's classification.

- *Lateral spreading tumor (LST):* These are defined as superficial tumors >1 cm. It will present with granular or nongranular surfaces as newly recognized entities.
- NICE classification (Narrowband Imaging International Colorectal Endoscopic classification) is also applicable based on color, vessels, and surface pattern using NBI.

Hyperplastic Polyps (Fig. 9)

- Sessile polyps <10 mm in diameter
- Same color as surrounding mucosa
- Use NBI to differentiate from adenomatous polyp
- Have round or stellar pit pattern

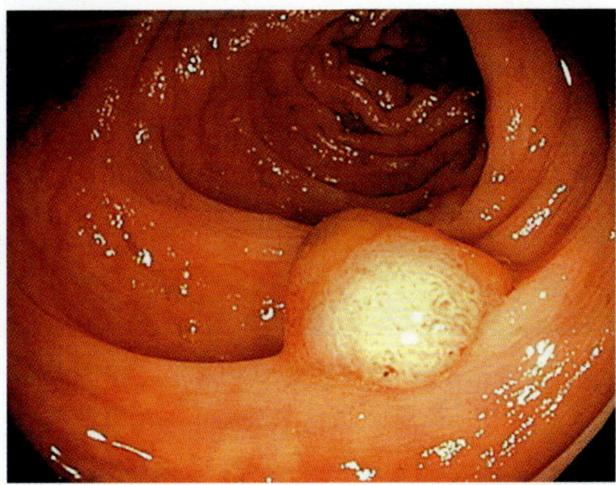

Fig. 9: Hyperplastic polyp.

Juvenile Polyp (Fig. 10)

- Usually presents as a solitary large friable pedunculated polyp in the rectum
- It is a hamartomatous polyp (mucinous retention cysts) amenable for snare polypectomy.

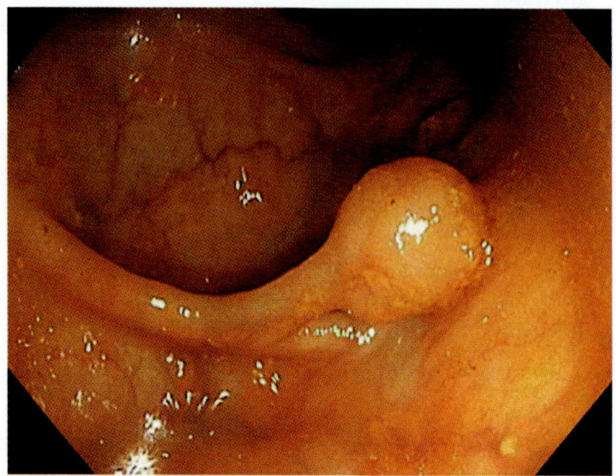

Fig. 10: Juvenile polyp.

Pseudopolyps (Fig. 11)

Inflammatory polyps are often seen in cases of inflammatory bowel disease (IBD) during remission.

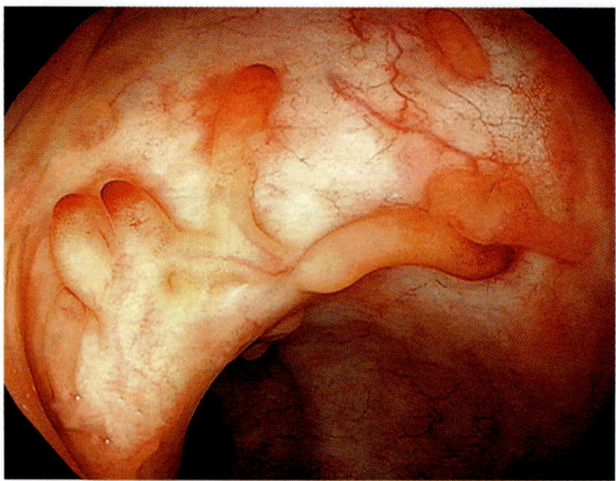

Fig. 11: Pseudopolyps.

Polyposis Syndrome: More than 100 Polyps

Non-neoplastic Polyposis Syndrome

- Peutz–Jeghers syndrome **(Figs. 12A to C)**
- Inflammatory polyposis

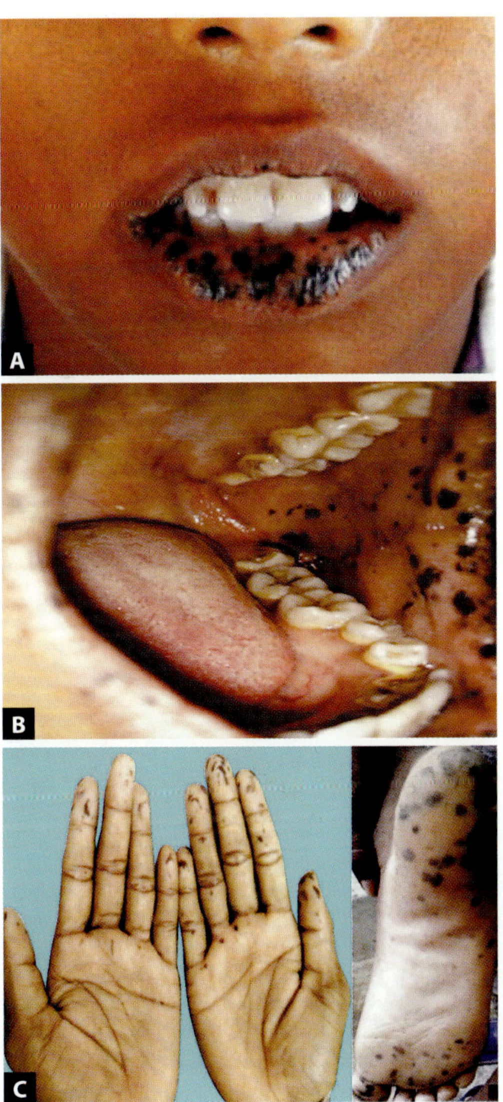

Figs. 12A to C: Peutz–Jeghers syndrome.

Neoplastic Polyposis Syndrome

- Familial adenomatous polyposis **(Figs. 13A to C)**
- Gardner syndrome
- Turcot syndrome

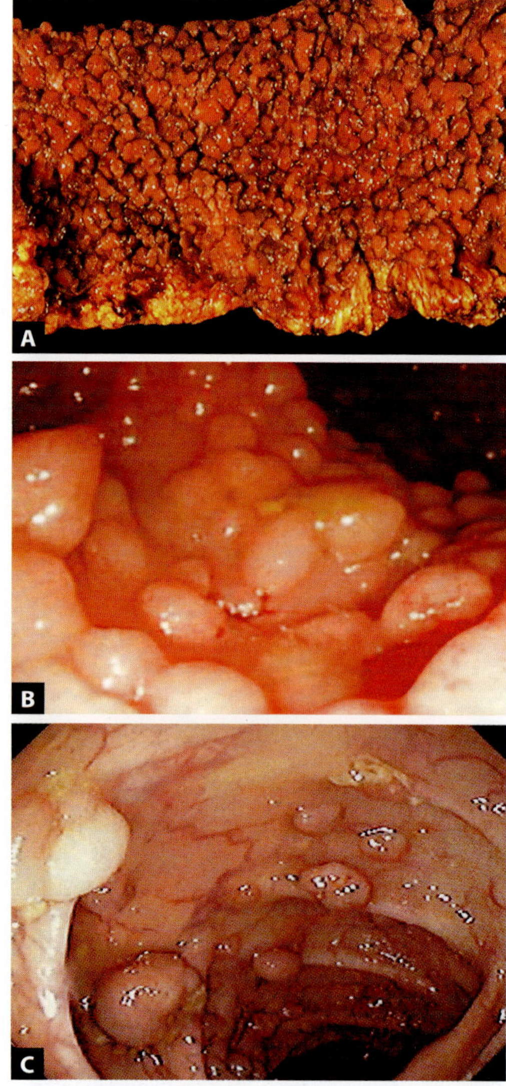

Figs. 13A to C: Familial adenomatous polyposis.

Malignant Tumors (Figs. 14A to D)

- Present as ulcerative lesion, polypoidal mass, annular growth, or even as flat elevated tumor

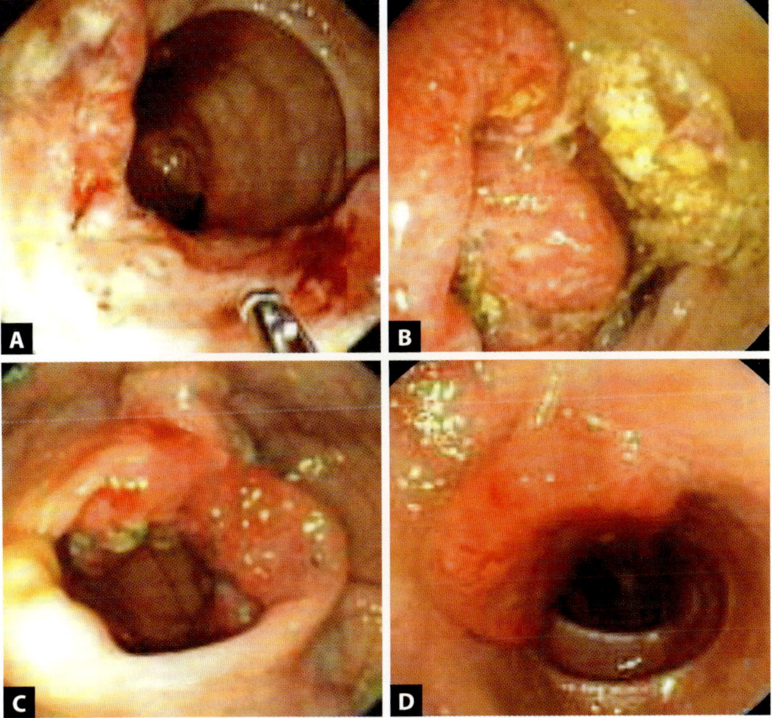

Figs. 14A to D: Different types of carcinoma colon.

- Note the site, size, and extent of tumor and degree of luminal obstruction
- Look for and document the evidence of any synchronous tumors or polyps
- Take multiple biopsies from the margins of the tumor and send for histopathological examination (HPE)
- CT abdomen is helpful for TNM staging.
- Endorectal US and MRI rectum are useful in T and N staging of carcinoma rectum.
- Rigid sigmoidoscopy is often done in case of carcinoma rectum to assess the lower limit of tumor from anal verge.

Submucosal Tumors (Figs. 15A to C)

Lipoma colon:

- *Lipoma:* Has yellowish hue and soft yielding nature on prodding with closed biopsy forceps (pillow sign)
- *Leiomyoma:* Appear as well-defined smooth firm tumor with reddish stretched mucosa
- *Carcinoid tumor:* Appear as firm pale yellow sessile rectal tumor with vascularized surface

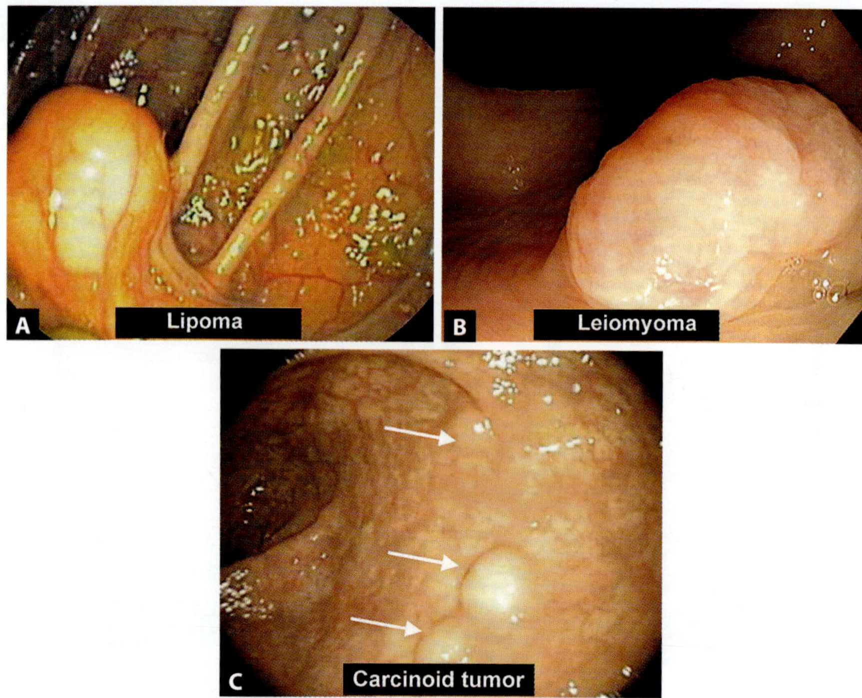

Figs. 15A to C: Submucosal tumors.

Inflammatory Bowel Diseases (Figs. 16A and B)

Ulcerative Colitis

- Starting from the rectum, it could involve a variable extent of the colon.
  - Rectum only (proctitis)
  - Rectum and sigmoid (distal proctocolitis)
  - Up to splenic flexure (left-sided colitis)
  - Up to cecum (total or pan proctocolitis)
  - Occasionally changes in terminal ileum (backwash ileitis)
  - Involving anal pouch (pouchitis)
- Look for and recognize the following findings and accordingly grade the colitis as mild, moderate, or severe **(Figs. 17A and B)**
  - Hyperemia, loss of vessel pattern, contact bleeding, ulcerations, and fibrinous exudates denote active colitis
  - Atrophic mucosa, loss of vessel pattern, loss of haustrations, and presence of pseudopolyps is seen in chronic colitis.
  - Areas of dysplasia or malignant change are seen in long-standing cases.
- Unlike Crohn's colitis, there are no skip lesions and no strictures.
- Assess with NBI and do multiple biopsies to document the type and severity of colitis and correlate with clinical presentation.

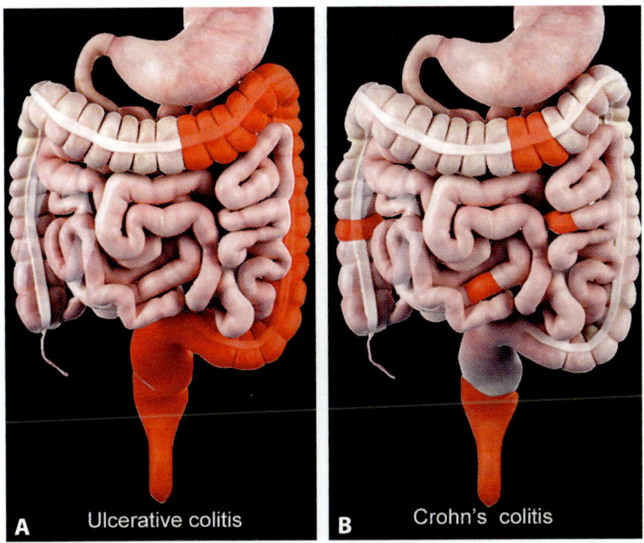

Figs. 16A and B: Inflammatory bowel diseases.

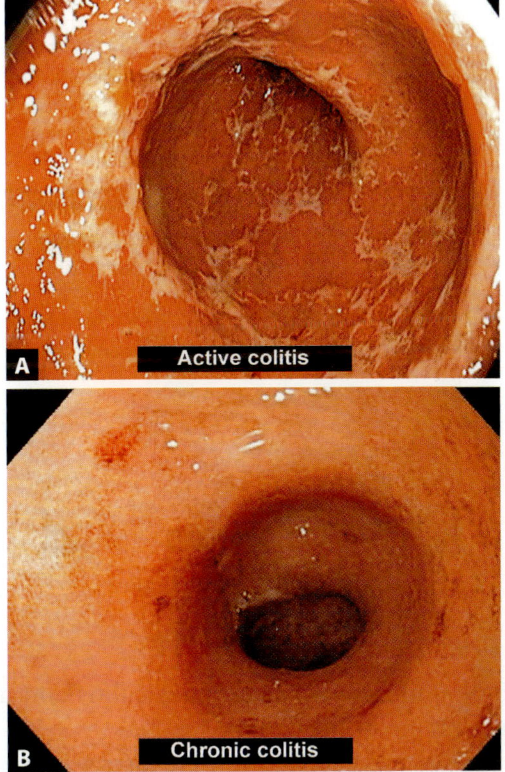

Figs. 17A and B: Ulcerative colitis.

Crohn's Colitis (Figs. 18A to C)

- The rectum is often spared. Discontinuous involvement of various lengths of colon with skip lesions.
- Active disease is often seen in the terminal ileum.
- Erythema, aphthous ulcers, contact bleeding, cobblestone mucosa, long serpiginous ulcers, pseudopolyps, and areas of fibrous stricture are the common findings.
- Perianal bluish skin tags and multiple anal fistulae may also be present.
- Stenosis or areas of cobblestone ulcerations may be observed in the terminal ileum following limited right hemicolectomy.
- Take multiple biopsies and document the severity and extent of colitis
- Plan for small bowel study with CT enterography to look for mass lesion, abscess, or fistula
- MRI may be beneficial in the presence of perianal disease with fistula-in-ano.

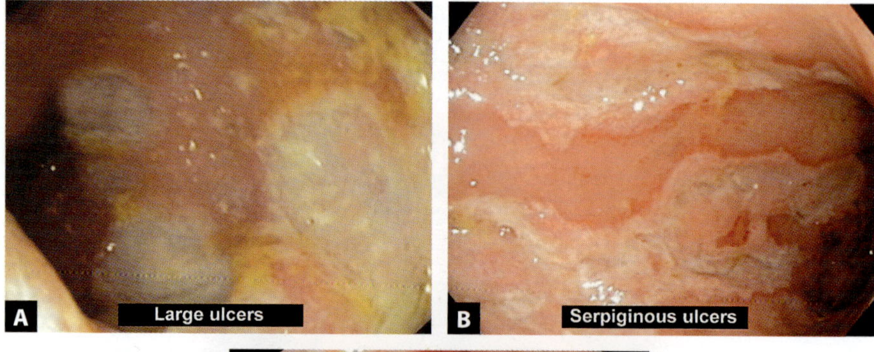

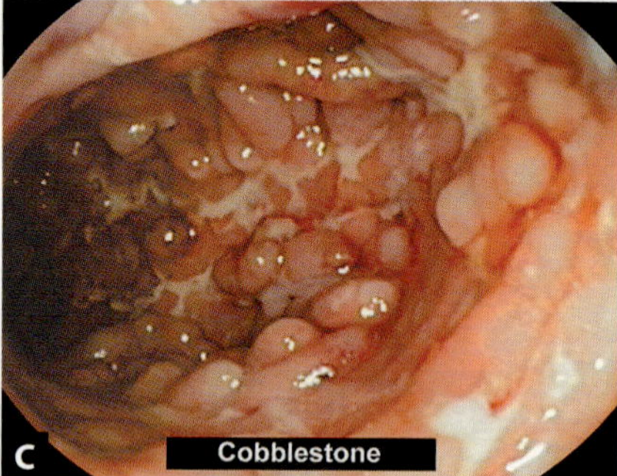

Figs. 18A to C: Crohn's colitis.

Indeterminate Colitis (Fig. 19)

- Has endoscopic findings of both Crohn's colitis and ulcerative colitis (UC), and biopsy is inconclusive.
- Avoid pouch surgery in such cases as a few cases might turn to be Crohn's disease.

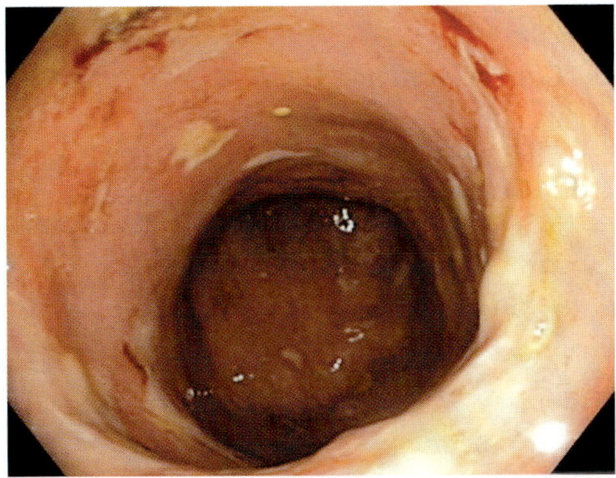

Fig. 19: Indeterminate colitis.

Tuberculosis of Large Intestine (Figs. 20A to C)

- Circumferential ulcerations, nodularity in the right colon with lesions predominantly in the cecal pole, and in the region of ileocecal valve
- Areas of luminal narrowing
- After the treatment with antituberculosis drugs, we may notice healing ulcers and deformed ileocecal valve and stricture in the right colon.

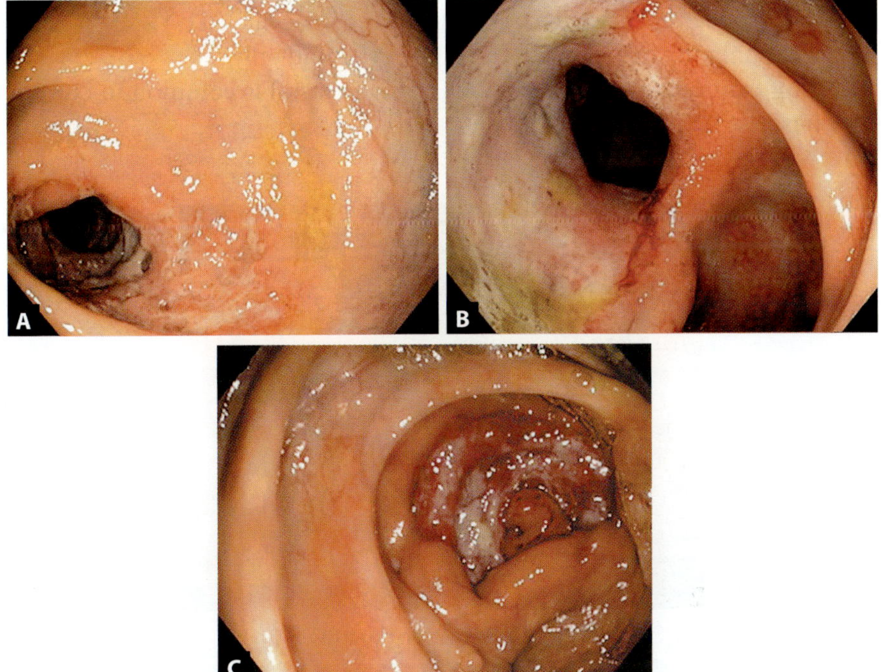

Figs. 20A to C: Colonic tuberculous ulcers.

Infectious Colitis (Fig. 21)

Due to amebiasis, *Campylobacter, Yersinia, Salmonella, Cytomegalovirus (CMV)*, and Rotavirus colitis

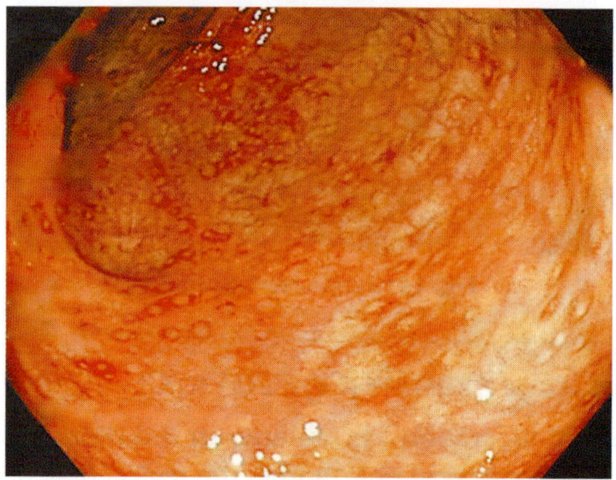

Fig. 21: Infectious colitis.

Radiation Colitis (Fig. 22)

- Often follows few years after pelvic radiotherapy for carcinoma cervix
- Mucosal edema, ulceration, and bleeding can occur.
- Predominantly in the rectum and lower sigmoid only
- Significant new vessel formation (telangiectasia) is common in chronic phase.

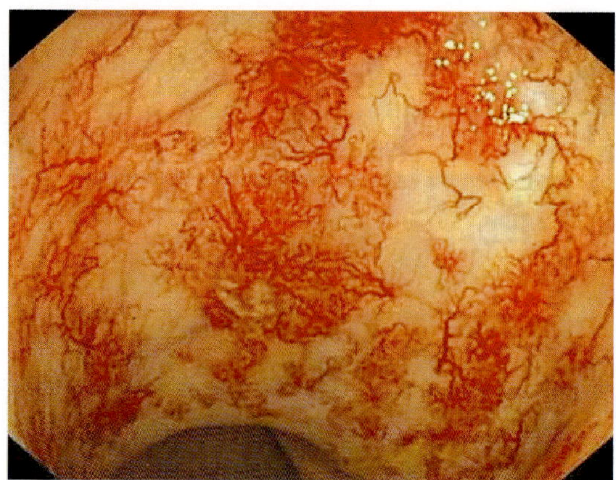

Fig. 22: Radiation proctitis.

Ischemic Colitis (Fig. 23)

- Left colon near the splenic flexure is the common site. The rectum is usually spared.
- Mucosal edema, ulcers, and necrosis leading to evidence of healing after a few days

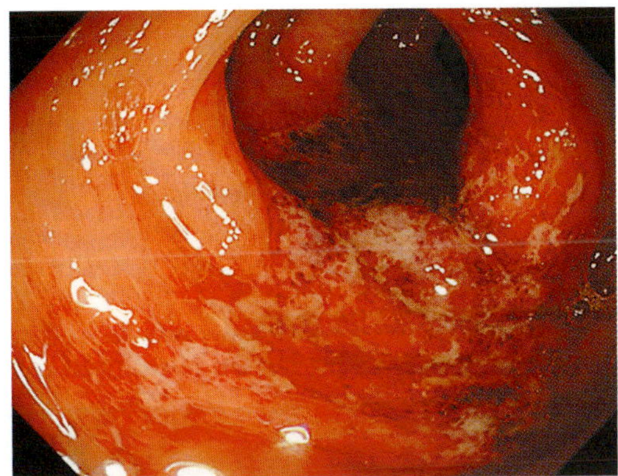

Fig. 23: Ischemic colitis.

Nonsteroidal Anti-inflammatory Drug Colitis (Fig. 24)

- Typically affects right colon and ileocecal valve
- Aphthous ulcers and broad deep ulcers can be seen with surrounding normal mucosa

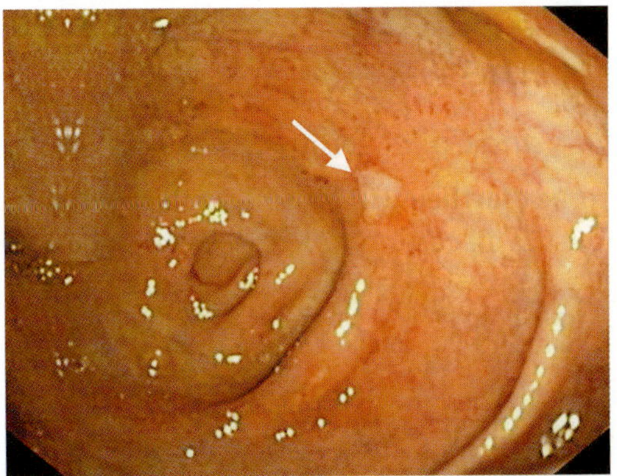

Fig. 24: Nonsteroidal anti-inflammatory drug (NSAID) colitis.

Diversion Colitis (Fig. 25)

- In the left colon, distal to transverse loop colostomy
- Erythema, ulcers as in cases of UC

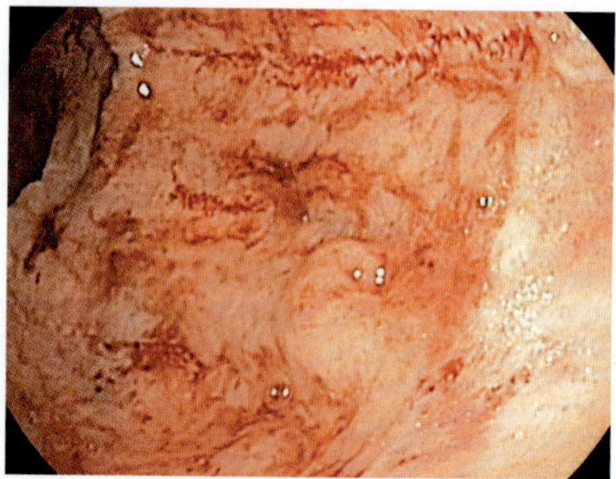

Fig. 25: Diversion colitis.

Pseudomembranous Colitis (Fig. 26)

- In cases of antibiotic induced-diarrhea
- Yellowish elevated plaques with underlying inflamed mucosa

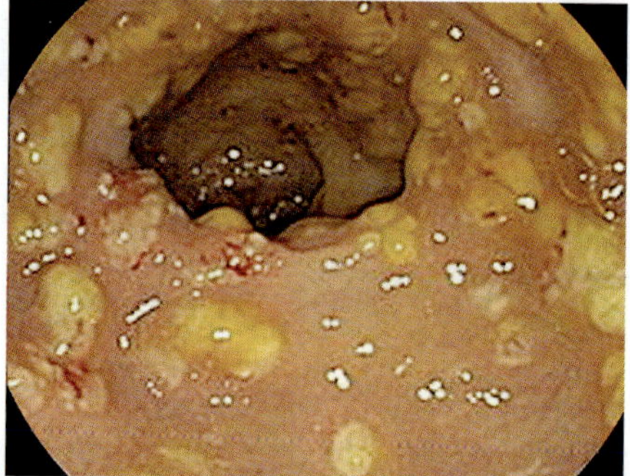

Fig. 26: Pseudomembranous colitis.

Microscopic Colitis and Collagenous Colitis (Fig. 27)

- Present as chronic diarrhea with normal colonoscopy
- So, biopsy is must in all cases of colonoscopy done for chronic diarrhea.

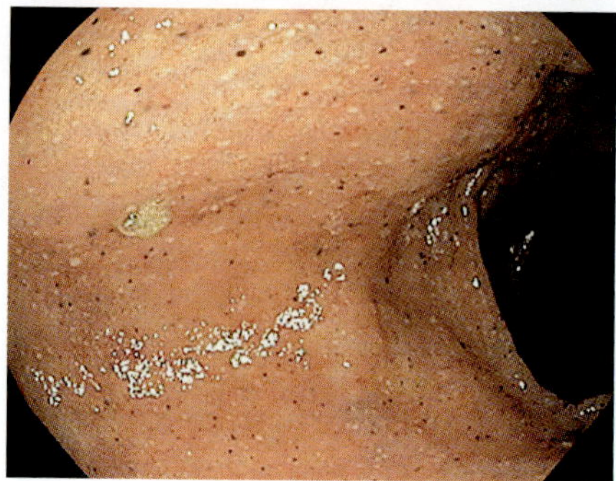

Fig. 27: Microscopic colitis and collagenous colitis.

Vascular Malformations

Angiodysplasia (Fig. 28)

- Mainly in right colon and frequently multiple
- Often, it could be an incidental finding.
- Look for active bleeding, adherent clot, or submucosal bleeding before blaming them as the source of lower gastrointestinal (GI) bleeding.
- Bipolar coagulation, argon plasma, or laser can be used to arrest any bleeding.

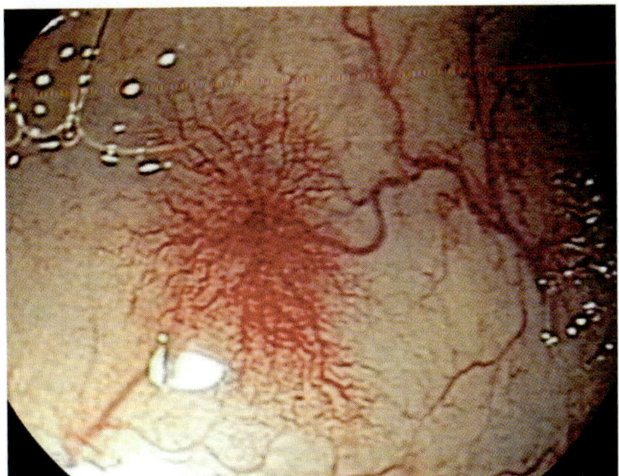

Fig. 28: Angiodysplasia colon.

Rectal Varix in Patients with Portal Hypertension (Fig. 29)

Tortuous, bluish, and submucosal vascular lesions are sometimes noted in patients with cirrhosis.

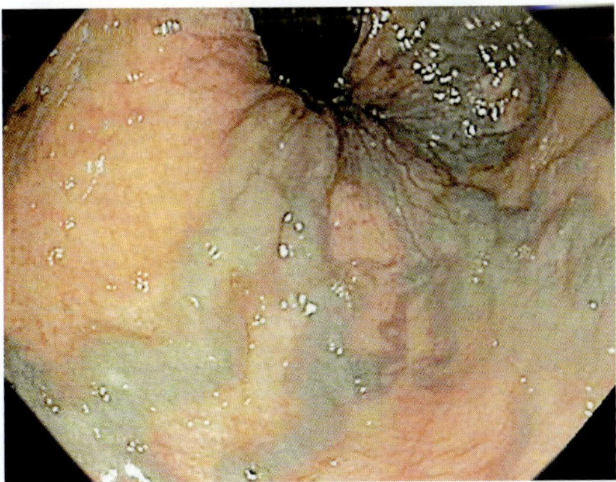

Fig. 29: Rectal varix in patients with portal hypertension (HT).

Solitary Rectal Ulcer (Fig. 30)

- Superficial ulcer 0.5–2 cm in diameter seen in the midrectum in the anterior rectal wall with surrounding normal mucosa
- May be with rectal or anal prolapse

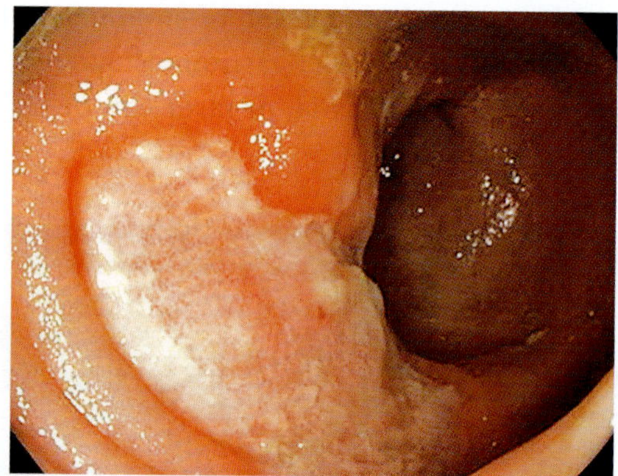

Fig. 30: Solitary rectal ulcer.

Melanosis Coli (Fig. 31)

- Seen in patients with laxative abuse
- Dark brownish reticulated mucosal pattern (leopard skin-like)

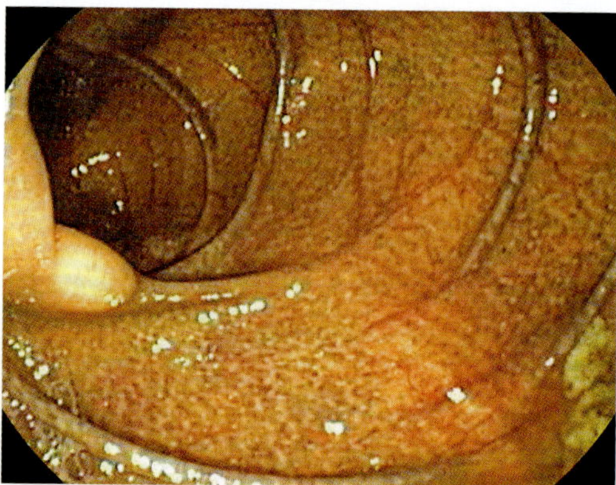

Fig. 31: Melanosis coli.

Piles

- Proctoscopy is the investigation of choice to evaluate for the presence of and grade of piles.
- Retroflexion of colonoscopy in the rectum will also exhibit the pile masses clearly **(Fig. 32)**.

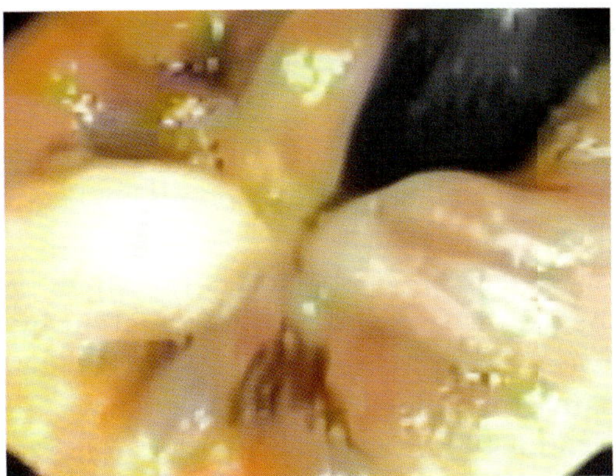

Fig. 32: Piles on retroflexion.

- Examine for associated fissure, skin tags, and any other coexisting colorectal tumor

CONCLUSION

Colonoscopic evaluation after good bowel preparation will aid us in recognizing all different pathologies in the colon. The availability of appropriate accessories helps us in all types of therapeutic interventions.

SUGGESTED READING

1. Brown WR, Tayal S. Microscopic colitis. A review. J Dig Dis. 2013;14(6):277-81.
2. Haycock A, Cohen J, Saunders BP, Cotton PB, Williams CB. Cotton and Williams' Practical Gastrointestinal Endoscopy: The Fundamentals. UK: Wiley Blackwell; 2008.
3. Kaltenbach T, Sandborn WJ. Endoscopy in inflammatory bowel disease: advances in dysplasia detection and management. Gastrointest Endosc. 2017;86:962-71.
4. Ponz de Leon M, Di Gregorio C. Pathology of colorectal cancer. Dig Liver Dis. 2001;33(4):372-88.
5. van den Broek FJ, Fockens P, van Eeden S, Stokkers PC, Ponsioen CY, Reitsma JB, et al. Narrow-band imaging versus high-definition endoscopy for the diagnosis of neoplasia in ulcerative colitis. Endoscopy. 2011;43(2):108-15.
6. Waye JD, Rex DK, Williams CB. Colonoscopy: Principles and Practice. USA: Wiley-Blackwell; 2009.
7. Yasutomi M, Baba S, Hojo K. Japanese classification of colorectal carcinoma. Tokyo: Kanehara & Co. Ltd.; 1997.

Expert's Comment

This is a very interesting "Atlas of Colonoscopy" compiled by Dr Easwaramoorthy. I appreciate that all the minute details about pathologies in the colon have been elaborated, and emphasis has been given on proper patient preparation.

In this atlas, we can see crisp images of colonic pathologies like inflammatory bowel disease and also information by which we can differentiate between Crohn's disease and ulcerative colitis endoscopically. Other inflammatory pathologies in the colon have been elaborated. Various manifestations of diverticular disease of the colon have been described with ample photographs.

Modern endoscopes with the capability of image enhancement and magnification are a great tool since they help in the characterization of lesions. For the characterization of polyps, all three classifications, namely Paris, Kudo, and NICE, are equally important.

In this atlas, we can see all the pathologies at a glance, and it would certainly be helpful in day-to-day practice. I appreciate the author for bringing this atlas to us.

Dr Vijay Borgaonkar
Chhatrapati Sambhajinagar

CHAPTER 12

10 Practical Points about Colonic Polyps

Chapter Outline

- Colonic Polyps are not Uncommon
- Colonic Polyps are Mostly Asymptomatic
- Colonic Polyps are Precancerous
- Good, Bad, and Ugly Polyps
- Diagnostic Modalities: Past, Present, and Future
- Advances in Endoscopic Imaging
- Treatment Modalities: Endoscopic, Laparoscopic, or Open Surgery
- Pathology Report Comes as Malignant Polyp: What is Next?
- Guidelines for Surveillance
- Primary Prevention of Polyps

Keywords: Adenomatous polyp, Kudo's classification, Sessile serrated adenoma, lateral spreading tumor, endoscopic submucosal dissection, endoscopic mucosal resection

INTRODUCTION

Polyps are the protuberant lesions often noticed on the surface of the colon during colonoscopy. Here are the 10 points for clinical practice regarding such lesions.

1. **Colonic polyps are not uncommon**
   - Colonic polyps are very common in western countries. Nearly one-third of people over 50 years harbor polyps. It is not uncommon here in India.
   - Magnification and image enhancement along with meticulous bowel preparation and careful examination of colon especially during withdrawal of colonoscope are paramount to identify such less perceptible lesions.
2. **Colonic polyps are mostly asymptomatic**
   - Polyps are usually discovered during colonoscopy done for other lower gastrointestinal (GI) ailments. They are also seen when screening colonoscopy is done in risk groups with family history of carcinoma colon, family history of familial polyposis, and in patient with long history of inflammatory bowel disease.

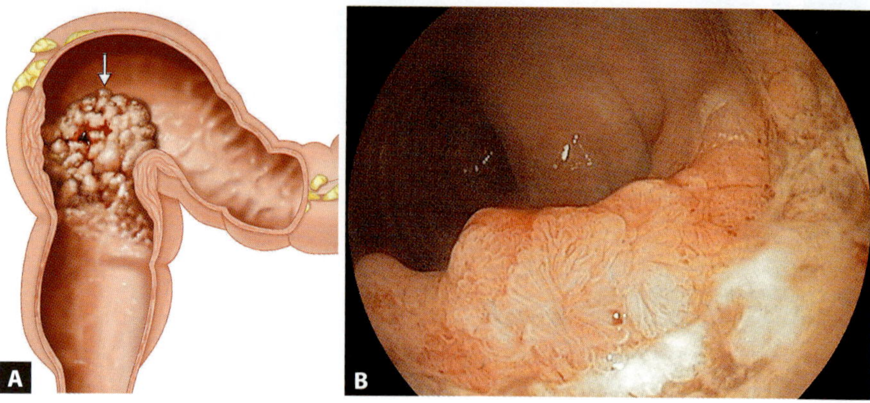

Figs. 1A and B: Villous adenoma.

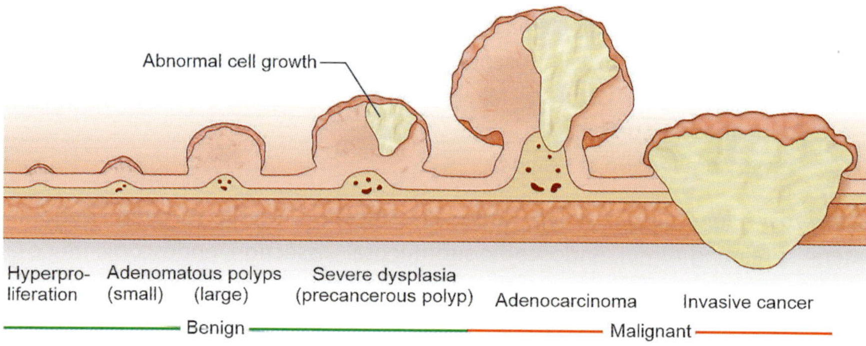

Fig. 2: Adenoma carcinoma sequence.

- Occasionally, polyps can present with bleeding PR (e.g., infantile polyp in a child) or mucus discharge (e.g., villous adenoma rectum in an elderly) **(Figs. 1A and B)**.
- Sessile serrated polyps are early precursor lesions in the serrated neoplasia pathway, which results in colorectal carcinoma with high levels of microsatellite instability. These usually occur in the right colon with more risk of lymphatic invasion. Careful colonoscopy is essential, so we do not miss such inconspicuous lesion.

3. **Colonic polyps are precancerous (Fig. 2)**

   Polyps have varying degrees of malignant potential. Adenoma carcinoma sequence is a well-established concept orchestrated by various genetic mutations (*APC* gene, K-ras, and p53). Removal of colonic polyps reduces the mortality due to colonic cancer.

4. **Good, bad, and ugly polyps (Figs. 3A to C)**
   - Morphologically, a polyp is classified as pedunculated or sessile depending on whether it contains a discrete stalk or not.

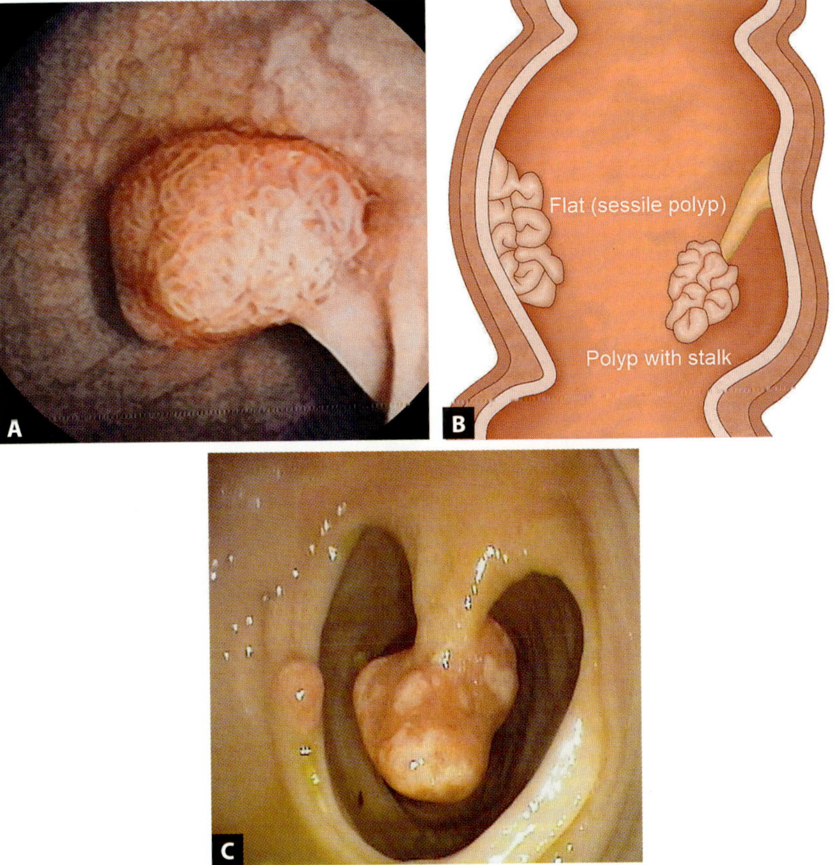

Figs. 3A to C: Sessile and pedunculated polyps.

Histologically, there are four types of colonic polyps namely (1) adenomatous, (2) hyperplastic, (3) harmartomatous, and (4) inflammatory **(Figs. 4A to D)**.

- Not all polyps behave badly. Hyperplastic polyps, infantile polyps and inflammatory polyps have very little risk of malignancy.
- While small pedunculated adenomatous polyps carry some risk, the risk is high for large pedunculated polyps >2 cm diameter and sessile villous polyps. These need special attention.

5. **Diagnostic modalities: Past, present, and future**
   - In the past, fecal occult blood and double-contrast barium enema were the tests used to detect polyps.
   - Currently colonoscopy is the test of choice which is both diagnostic and therapeutic. But, the disadvantages of colonoscopy are possible incomplete examination, missed polyps, and rare risk of colonic perforation. Good bowel preparation is paramount. High-definition

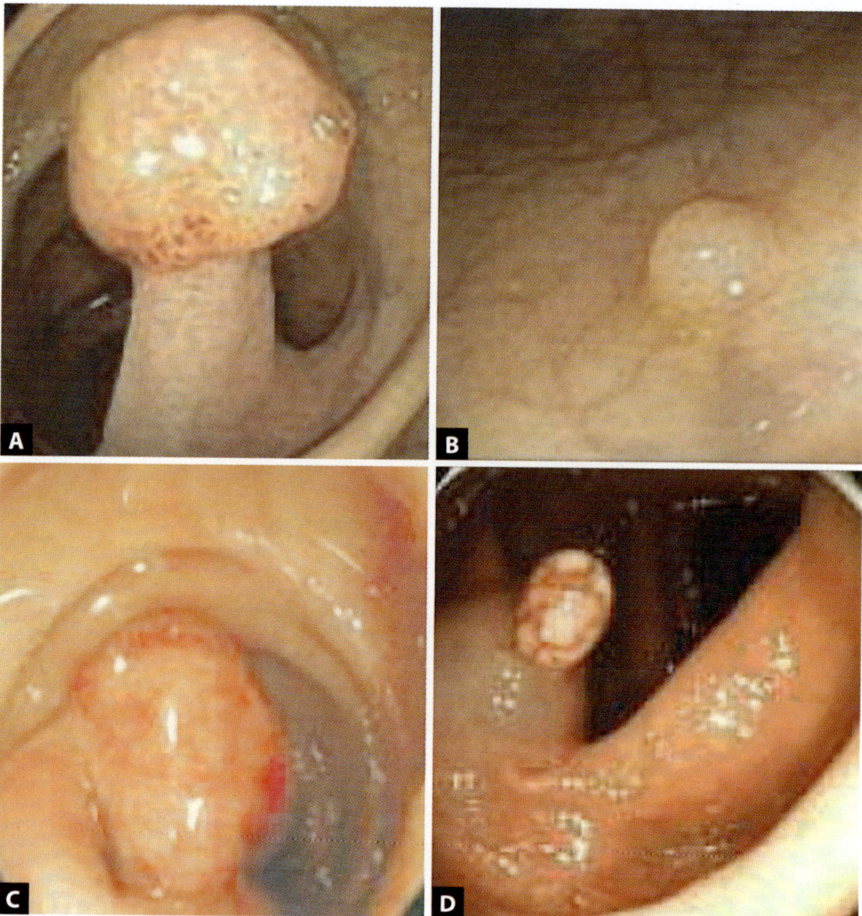

Figs. 4A to D: Histological types of polyps: (A) Adenomatous polyp; (B) Hyperplastic polyp; (C) Harmartomatous polyp; and (D) Inflammatory polyp.

(HD) colonoscopy and chromoendoscopy are very helpful. Careful withdrawal of colonoscope from cecum to anus taking >6 minutes, appropriate position change, periodic suction and water irrigation, and careful examination behind haustral folds will all ensure higher adenoma detection rate (ADR). Use of novel devices such as Endocuff and Third Eye Retroscope are also found to improve polyp detection rate.

- Virtual and capsule colonoscopies are attractive alternative modalities for screening high-risk groups. If pathology is noted, such patients could be referred for therapeutic colonoscopy.
- *Virtual colonoscopy **(Fig. 5)**:*
    - High-resolution CT scan along with "Fly through" software permits us to have CT colonography where in even polyps as

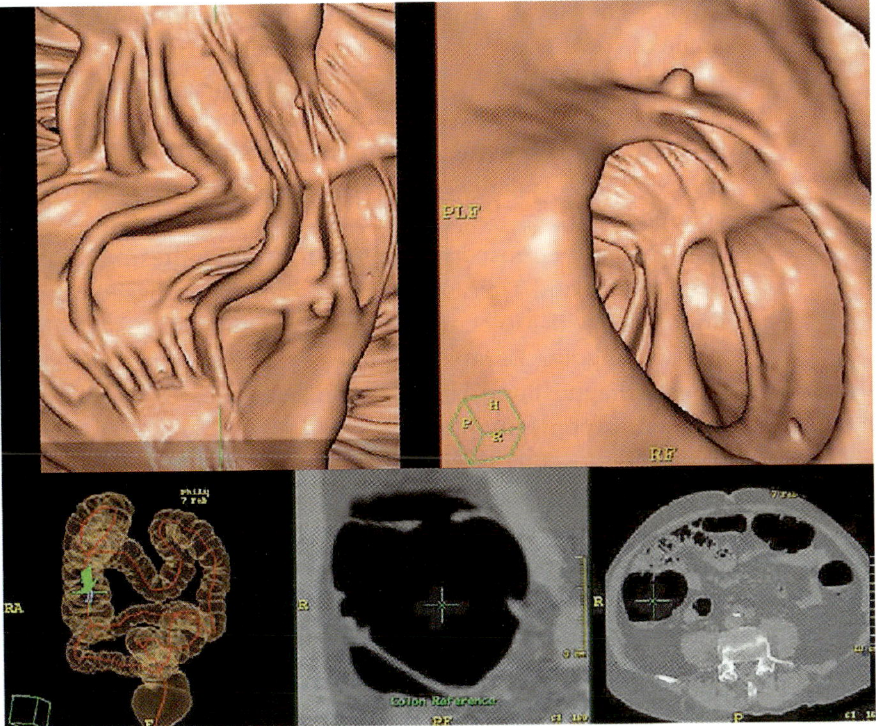

Fig. 5: Virtual colonoscopy.

small as 5 mm can be located. Fecal residue artifacts can be nullified.

- In case of incomplete colonoscopy or where colonoscopy is not feasible, consider this noninvasive modality for diagnosing any colonic pathology.

- *Capsule colonoscopy* ***(Fig. 6)****:*
  - Benefits of capsule enteroscopy are obvious, and hence, it has become an important tool in the algorithm of management of obscure GI bleeding.

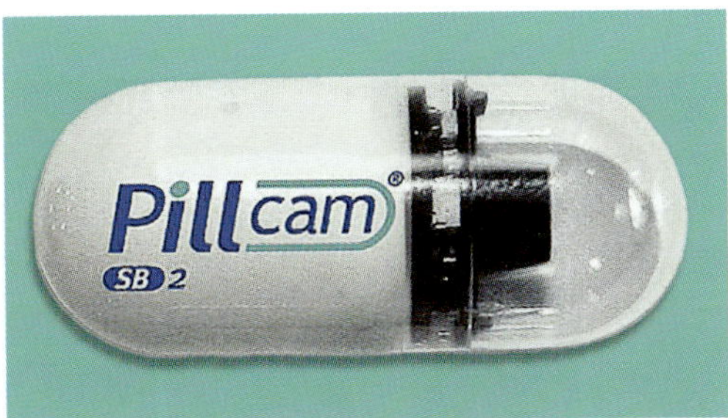

Fig. 6: Capsule endoscopy.

- Colonic capsules have cameras on either side with much wider angle of view. They feature 2-hour delay in activation and then transmit images at four frames per second.
- It can be considered for patient not fit or not willing for colonoscopy or after incomplete colonoscopy.
- It has 50–70% sensitivity and 70–90% specificity in detecting colonic polyps.
- The Versatile Endoscopic Capsule for Gastrointestinal Tumor Recognition and Therapy (VECTOR) and Nano-based capsule Endoscopy with Molecular imaging and Optical biopsy (NEMO) are two ongoing European studies evaluating more advanced types of diagnostic and interventional capsules.

6. **Advances in endoscopic imaging (Figs. 7A to C)**
   - White light endoscopy could easily miss small flat lesions in the bowel. But recent advances in endoscopic imaging could come to endoscopist's rescue.
   - Chromoendoscopy is a technique in which one sprays the colon with a contrast agent like indigo carmine to delineate the lesion clearly.
   - Electronic chromoendoscopy or image enhancement techniques along with magnification will improve the chances of lesion localization and lesion characterization.
   - Types of image enhancement:
     - Narrow-band imaging (NBI) (Olympus)
     - I-SCAN (Pentax)
     - FICE (Fujinon)
   - *Narrow-band imaging* is based on the presence of green and blue filters which helps to bring out greater mucosal details and vascular pattern.
     - NBI uses two discrete bands of light using blue filter at 415 nm and green filter at 540 nm. Blue light displays superficial capillary networks, while green light displays subepithelial vessels and when combined offer an extremely high-contrast image of the tissue surface.

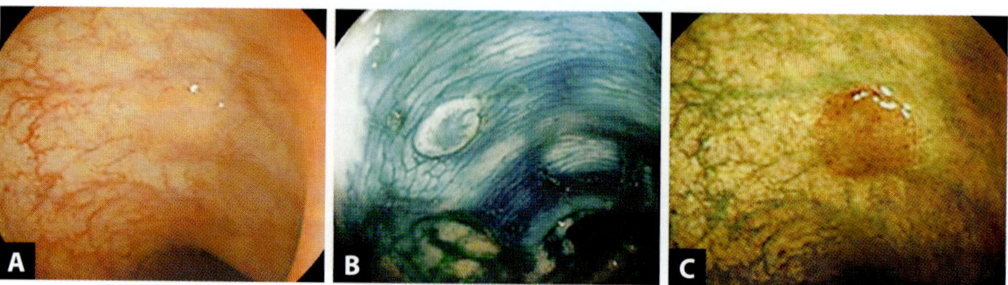

Figs. 7A to C: (A) White light; (B) Chromoendoscopy; and (C) Narrow-band imaging (NBI).

- *NBI image on the monitor:* Capillaries on the surface are displayed in brown and veins in the subsurface are displayed in cyan. It helps to detect subtle changes and flat lesions more easily. It also aids in more accurate in vivo diagnosis and precise target biopsy.
- All polyps can be classified as non-neoplastic and neoplastic based on Kudo's classification and NICE (NBI International Colorectal Endoscopic) classification.
- Sessile serrated adenoma can be distinguished from hyperplastic polyps in the presence of cloud like surface with indistinct border in white light colonoscopy while NBI would show presence of mucus cap, dark spots inside the crypts and varicose microvascular pattern along with type 2 Kudo's pit pattern **(Figs. 8A to F)**.
- Pentax I-SCAN technology is based on the postprocessing of reflected light.
    - I-SCAN can be switched on and off by simply pushing a button on the endoscope. It has three modes, namely, (1) surface enhancement (SE) mode, (2) contrast enhancement (CE), and (3) tone enhancement (TE) mode. SE highlights surface tissue architecture which may be used for the detection of circumscribed lesions or to highlight diffuse alteration (e.g., inflammation and atrophy). TE focuses on vascular and tissue architecture. These details are helpful to correctly characterize mucosal lesions. Neoplastic vessel and tissue patterns may be differentiated from non-neoplastic patterns. Three standardized I-SCAN settings are now readily available

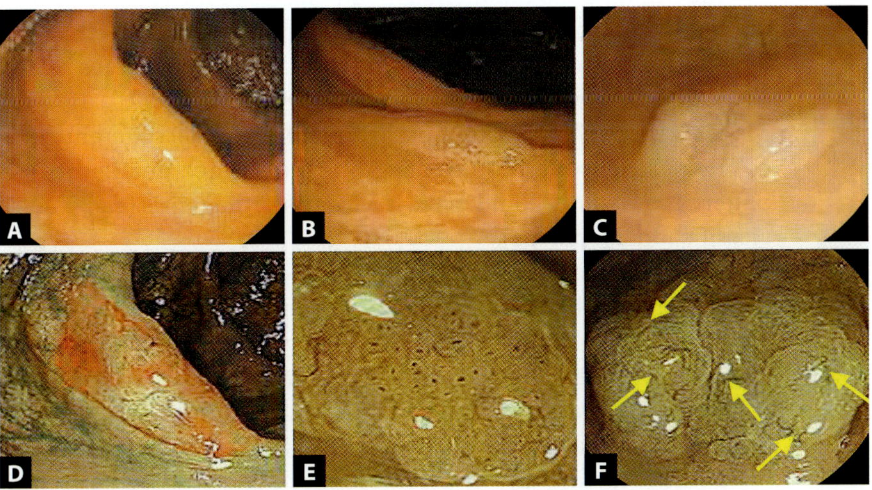

Figs. 8A to F: Sessile serrated polyp in white light and narrow-band imaging (NBI).

in the factory settings of the processor, including I-SCAN 1 (SE) recommended for detection, I-SCAN 2 (combination of SE and TE) recommended for lesion characterization, and I-SCAN 3 (combination of SE, TE, and CE) recommended for lesion demarcation, with I-SCAN 2 being probably the most widely used.

- FICE (Fujinon Intelligent Chromo Endoscopy, flexible spectral imaging color enhancement) is based on spectral estimation technology.
    - Spectral estimation technology takes an ordinary endoscopic image from the video processor and arithmetically processes, estimates, and produces an image of a given, and dedicated wavelength of light. More recent innovation is blue laser imaging (BLI) by Fujinon. BLI uses two monochromatic lasers (410 ± 10 nm and 450 ± 10 nm) instead of xenon light to obtain image-enhanced endoscopy. The BLI system utilizes three modes: (1) BLI mode, (2) BLI-bright mode, and (3) white light mode. Following steps of examination with BLI are recommended during colonoscopic evaluation of any lesion.
    - At the beginning, perform an overall observation of the lesion using the white light mode with normal magnification. White light mode may provide a clearer image than that using conventional xenon light. Next, the BLI-bright mode without magnification is applied. The extent of the lesion should be evaluated using this mode. Then, use the BLI-bright mode to identify the region with advanced histological atypia based on changes in color tone and superficial structure. Finally, apply the BLI mode to obtain magnified images of the surface pattern and vascular pattern by focusing on the region identified.
    - Compared to NBI, BLI gives brighter and clear images of any lesion
- Magnification by optical lens or digital method in all different types of HD colonoscopes could bring out the surface details like pit patterns so well, we could make in vivo tissue diagnosis (e.g., Kudo's classification of polyps).
- Artificial intelligence (AI) (EndoBrain) also could help us with making accurate optical diagnosis and guide us regarding plan to intervention. AI technology will highlight the sites of polyps so we could pay more attention to those sites and hence help to improve ADR.
- Endoscopic ultrasound will allow us to clearly recognize various layers of bowel wall and hence help to assess whether polyp is mucosal or submucosal and any invasion of muscularis mucosa as seen in malignant polyps (e.g., villous adenoma rectum) **(Figs. 9A and B)**.

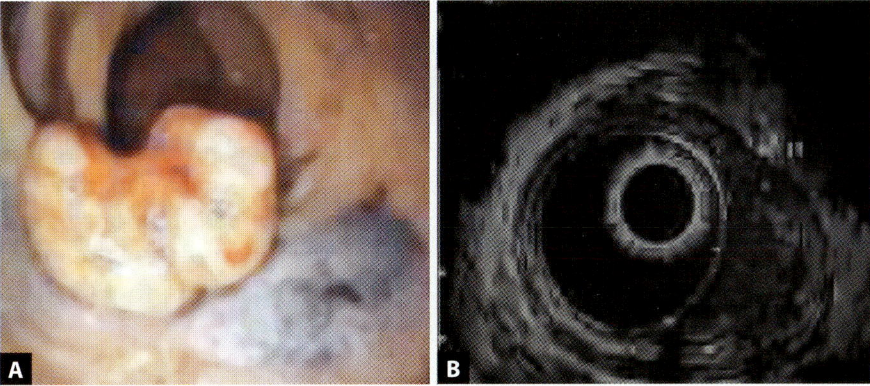

Figs. 9A and B: Endoscopic ultrasound.

7. **Treatment modalities: Endoscopic, laparoscopic, or open surgery**
   - Most of the polyps can be tackled endoscopically. Snare polypectomy is the technique wherein the pedunculated polyps are garlanded with a diathermy wire and strangled and cut using monopolar diathermy taking care to avoid bleeding and perforation. Submucosal saline elevation helps in removal of flat polyps **(Figs. 10A to C)**. Endoscopic submucosal dissection (ESD) is rapidly evolving technique wherein

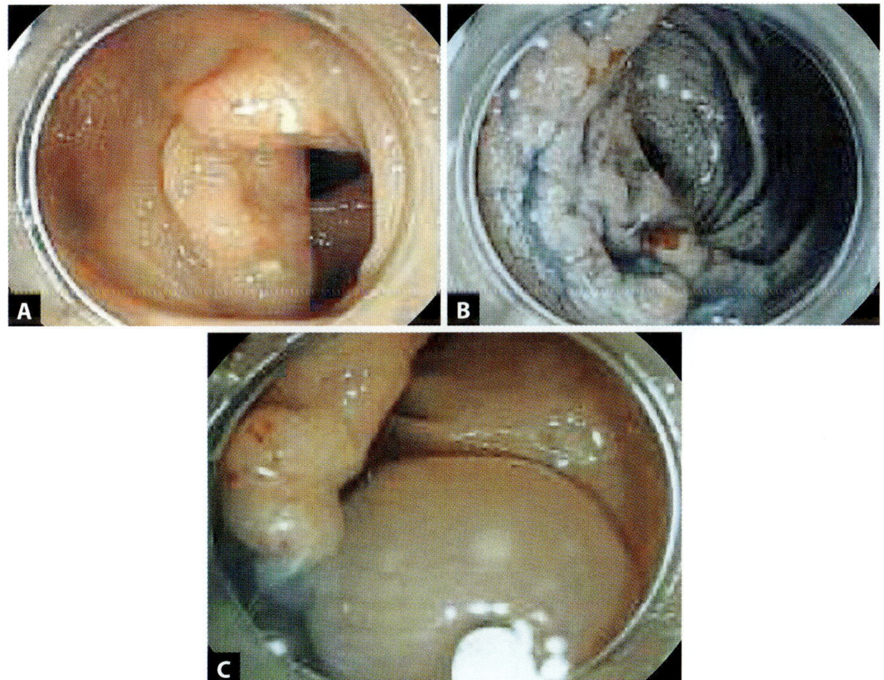

Figs. 10A to C: Endoscopic mucosal resection (EMR).

even very large flat lesions could be removed with the help of special accessories and expertise. Even lesion encroaching on superficial third of submucosa (SM1) would be amenable to ESD.

- If polyps are too large and difficult or dangerous to remove through colonoscopy, then it can be injected with India ink or indocyanine green and sent for surgical removal. This will enable laparoscopic surgeons to clearly visualize the portion of colon harboring the polyps during surgery. Laparoscopic endoscopic collaborative surgery is an evolving interesting field for surgeons **(Figs. 11A to C)**.

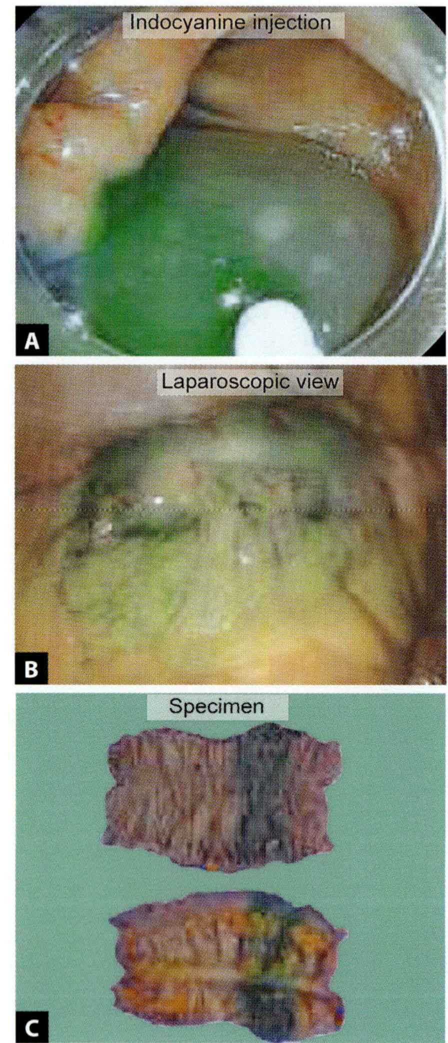

Figs. 11A to C: Laparoscopy-assisted colonoscopic polypectomy.

8. **Pathology report comes as malignant polyp: What is next?**
    - Malignant polyps can be suspected if large flat lesions are nongranular with areas of depression. Irregular surface vessel pattern and nonlifting sign on submucosal saline infusion are other signs to suggest invasive malignant lesions.
    - Polyps should be retrieved and send to pathologist after their removal. If the dysplastic changes breach muscularis mucosa then it is called malignant polyp.
    - Higgitt et al. described a classification system for pedunculated polyps with levels of invasion ranging from 0 to 4 **(Fig. 12)**.
        - *Level 0*: Indicates carcinoma in situ or intramucosal carcinoma
        - *Level 1:* Lesions have adenocarcinoma invading through the muscularis mucosa into the submucosa but are strictly limited to the head of polyp.
        - *Level 2:* Invading to neck of polyp
        - *Level 3:* Invading into stalk of polyp
        - *Level 4:* Invasion into bowel wall below the polyp stalk and is limited to submucosa.
    - Kikuchi classification is more relevant for describing the submucosal invasion in malignant sessile polyps **(Fig. 13)**.
        - Sessile polyps do not contain stalks and are considered equivalent to a level 4 pedunculated polyp with respect to their incidence of lymph node metastasis.
        - Submucosal invasion is classified into thirds with SM1 lesion exhibiting invasion into the upper third of the submucosa, SM2

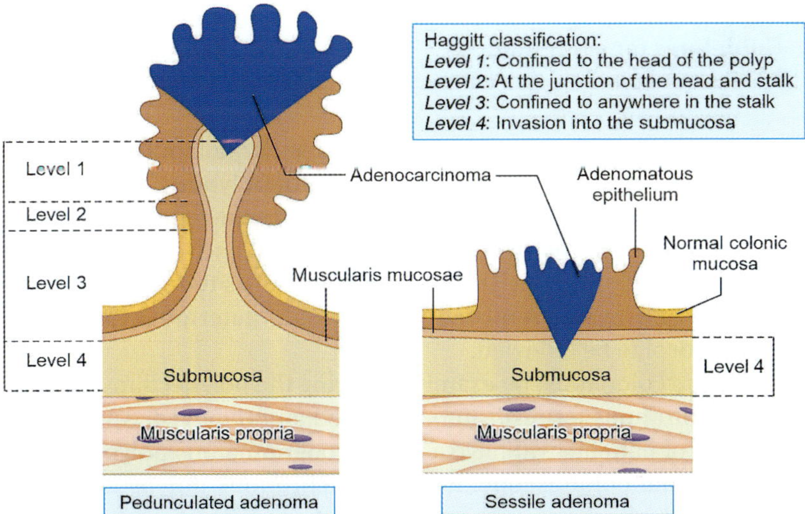

Fig. 12: The Haggitt classification of depth of invasion in malignant pedunculated and sessile polyps.

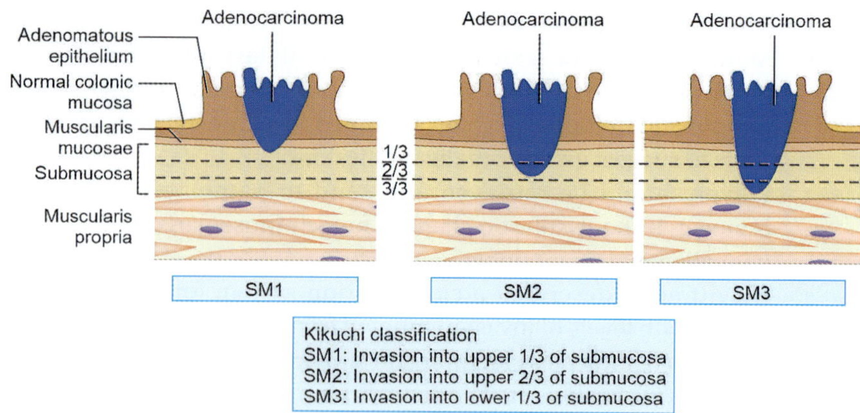

Fig. 13: The Kikuchi classification of depth of invasion into the submucosa of a malignant sessile polyp.

invasion into middle third of submucosa, and SM3 invasion into lower third of the submucosa.

- If histological report of the polyp shows any of the below mentioned findings. Then we should consider that colonoscopic polypectomy is inadequate and plan for further surgical excision of involved segment of bowel with nodal dissection for oncological clearance.
  - Haggitt level 4 lesion
  - Malignant polyp with margin of resection <2 mm
  - Evidence of vascular or lymphatic invasion
  - Sessile lesion with SM3 invasion (Kikuchi)
  - Incomplete resection or inability to assess margin (piecemeal technique)

9. **Guidelines for surveillance**
   - Risk of colonic cancer increases with age with >90% of cases occur beyond 50 years
   - Risk groups like people with family history of familial polyposis or family history of cancer (hereditary nonpolyposis colonic cancer) **(Fig. 14)** or Peutz–Jeghers syndrome need regular surveillance colonoscopy to pick up lesions early and advise treatment accordingly. These risk factors and as well as the size, number, and type of previous removed polyps would determine the screening protocol to be followed.
   - Entire colon must be examined during the polypectomy so that any synchronous lesions can be detected and removed. Approximately 50% of patients will have a second adenomatous polyp at the time of initial colonoscopy, while metachronous polyps are found in 20–50% of patients within 5 years of the initial polypectomy.
   - *Screening colonoscopy protocol* ***(Table 1)****:*
     - For people with average risk (in USA) start colonoscopy from age 50 years and repeat after 10 years

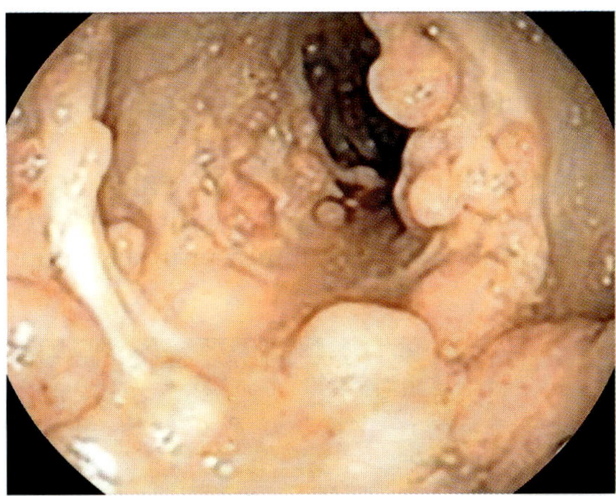

Fig. 14: Hereditary nonpolyposis colorectal cancer (HNPCC).

TABLE 1: Screening colonoscopy protocol.

Risk category	*When to start colonoscopy*	*Frequency of colonoscopy*
Average risk	50 years	Once in 10 years
Known colonic cancer, after surgery	1 year after surgery	3 yearly
F/H of colon cancer in first-degree relatives	40 years or 10 years less than age at diagnosis	1–2 yearly
F/H of HNPCC	25 years or 10 years less than age at diagnosis	1–2 yearly
F/H of FAP	10 years	Yearly up to 40 years and then 2–3 yearly
Inflammatory bowel disease	10 years after diagnosis	Yearly

(F/H: family history; FAP: familial adenomatous polyposis; HNPCC: hereditary nonpolyposis colorectal cancer)

- Patient with known colonic cancer and resection should undergo check colonoscopy 1 year after surgery and then repeat 3 yearly.
- People with family history of carcinoma colon (first-degree relatives) should undergo colonoscopy either at 40 years or 10 years less than the age at diagnosis in their relatives.
- Relatives of hereditary nonpolyposis colorectal cancer (HNPCC) syndrome should undergo colonoscopy 1–2 yearly from age 25 years or at least 10 years less than the age at diagnosis in the index patient.
- People with family history of familial adenomatous polyposis (FAP) should undergo annual colonoscopy from age 10 years till 40 years and then 2–3 yearly. Colectomy is performed if dysplastic polyps are noted.

10. Primary prevention of polyps (Fig. 15):
- Diet rich in fresh fruit and vegetables, low-fat diet
- Weight reduction
- Abstinence from alcohol and smoke

Though there is insufficient evidence to support, intake of following substances has shown to decrease the incidence of colonic polyps namely, calcium, folic acid, selenium, aspirin, and sulindac.

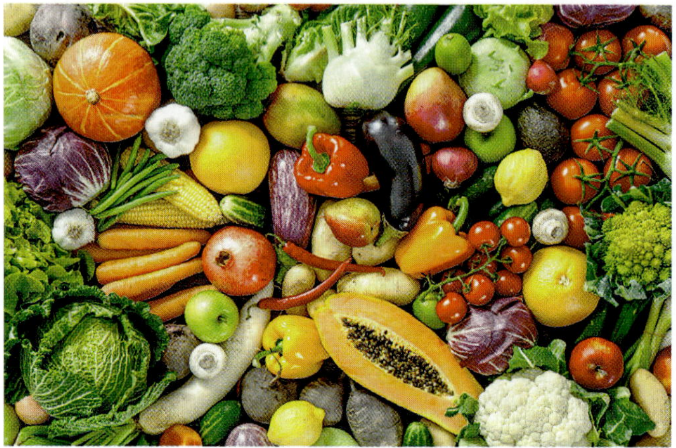

Fig. 15: Primary prevention of polyps.

SUGGESTED READING

1. Goh LY, Leow AH, Goh KL. Observations on the epidemiology of gastrointestinal and liver cancers in the Asia-Pacific region. J Dig Dis. 2014;15:463-8.
2. Kim NH, Jung YS, Park JH, Park DI, Sohn CI. Risk of developing metachronous advanced colorectal neoplasia after colonoscopic polypectomy in patients aged 30 to 39 and 40 to 49 years. Gastrointest Endosc. 2018;88(4):715-23.
3. Rex DK, Boland CR, Dominitz JA, Giardiello FM, Johnson DA, Kaltenbach T, et al. Colorectal cancer screening: recommendations for physicians and patients from the U.S. Multi-Society Task Force on Colorectal Cancer. Am J Gastroenterol. 2017;112(7):1016-30.
4. Rex DK, Lieberman DA. Feasibility of colonoscopy screening: discussion of issues and recommendations regarding implementation. Gastrointest Endosc. 2001;54:662-7.
5. Sung JJ, Ng SC, Chan FK, Chiu HM, Kim HS, Matsuda T, et al. An updated Asia Pacific Consensus Recommendations on colorectal cancer screening. Gut. 2015;64(1):121-32.
6. Triantafillidis JK, Vagianos C, Malgarinos G. Colonoscopy in colorectal cancer screening: current aspects. Indian J Surg Oncol. 2015;6(3):237-50.
7. Wilt TJ, Harris RP, Qaseem A. Screening for cancer: advice for high-value care from the American College of Physicians. Ann Intern Med. 2015;162:718-25.

Expert's Comment

Colonic polyps, although often asymptomatic, play a crucial role in preventing colorectal cancer. Their detection, classification, and management are essential components of effective screening strategies. In this chapter titled *"10 practical points about colonic polyps"*, the author highlights practical, evidence-based approaches that can enhance diagnostic accuracy and improve therapeutic decision-making in everyday clinical practice.

Polyp detection tips:

- Ensure optimal bowel preparation; split dosing improves mucosal visibility.
- Use retroflexion in the rectum to avoid missing flat lesions.

Classification insights:

- Differentiate between hyperplastic and adenomatous polyps by considering size, location, and histology.
- Recognize serrated polyps, especially in the proximal colon, as they are often under-recognized.

Management strategies:

- Discusses multiple treatment strategies and the need for complex polyp multidisciplinary team (MDT) in decision-making and management
- Follow-up intervals should align with updated national guidelines.

This chapter provides actionable insights for budding colonoscopists, particularly regarding polyp detection, classification, and treatment. It aligns with the current medical guidelines and accurately references pathology and surveillance protocols.

Additionally, it discusses advanced imaging methods (e.g., narrow-band imaging, flexible spectral imaging, color enhancement, and blue light imaging) as well as artificial intelligence (AI) tools like EndoBrain, demonstrating an awareness of cutting-edge diagnostics. The text is written in an accessible tone.

As our tools and techniques evolve, our clinical instincts must adapt as well. By staying attuned to the subtleties of polyp morphology and management, we can significantly impact patient outcomes. The practical points outlined here are more than just procedural; they represent preventive medicine in action.

Dr Chelliah Selvasekar
Manchester, UK

CHAPTER 13

Overview of Therapeutic Colonoscopy

Chapter Outline

Keywords: Hot snare polypectomy, hot biopsy, cold biopsy, EMR, ESD, colonoscopic hemostasis, colonoscopic decompression

INTRODUCTION

Colonoscopy has both diagnostic and therapeutic potentials. For efficient endo therapy, we should strive to acquire adequate training, appropriate accessories, and ample number of competent staff. As we start gaining more experience, we would be able to perform more complex therapeutic procedures with acceptable morbidity.

HOT BIOPSY (FIGS. 1A AND B)

Indication: Small sessile polyps <5 mm would be suitable.

Equipment: Hot biopsy forceps and diathermy with connecting wires.

Procedure:

- Grab the polyp with cusps of the hot biopsy forceps and lift it off the surface while applying brief spell of coagulation current and snap it and send the specimen for histology.

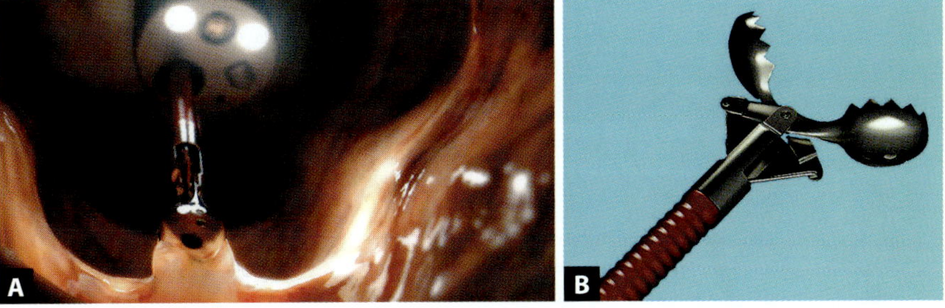

Figs. 1A and B: Hot biopsy forceps.

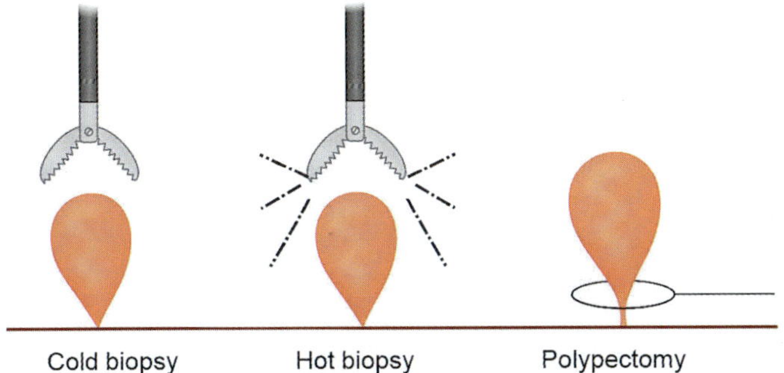

Fig. 2: Methods of biopsy.

- This should achieve hemostasis of base of polyp while the tissue bit within the cusps of the hot biopsy forceps is available for histology (though it often gets damaged due to diathermy).
- Cold snaring is a better alternative for such small polyps <5 mm with acceptable bleeding and availability of tissue for histology **(Fig. 2)**.

SNARE POLYPECTOMY

Indication: All polyps are >5 mm (both sessile and pedunculated). Consider endoscopic submucosal dissection (ESD) for larger sessile polyps.

Equipment ***(Fig. 3)****:*

- *Various sizes and shapes of polypectomy snares:*
  - Standard snare—2.5 cm diameter
  - Mini snare—1 cm diameter
- Diathermy unit and cables and returning pad
- 23F size and 210 cm long injection needle for dilute adrenaline in saline injection
- *Polyp retrieval forceps:* 3 or 5 Prong forceps, Roth Net, and Dormia basket
- Endoloops and hemoclips for hemostasis

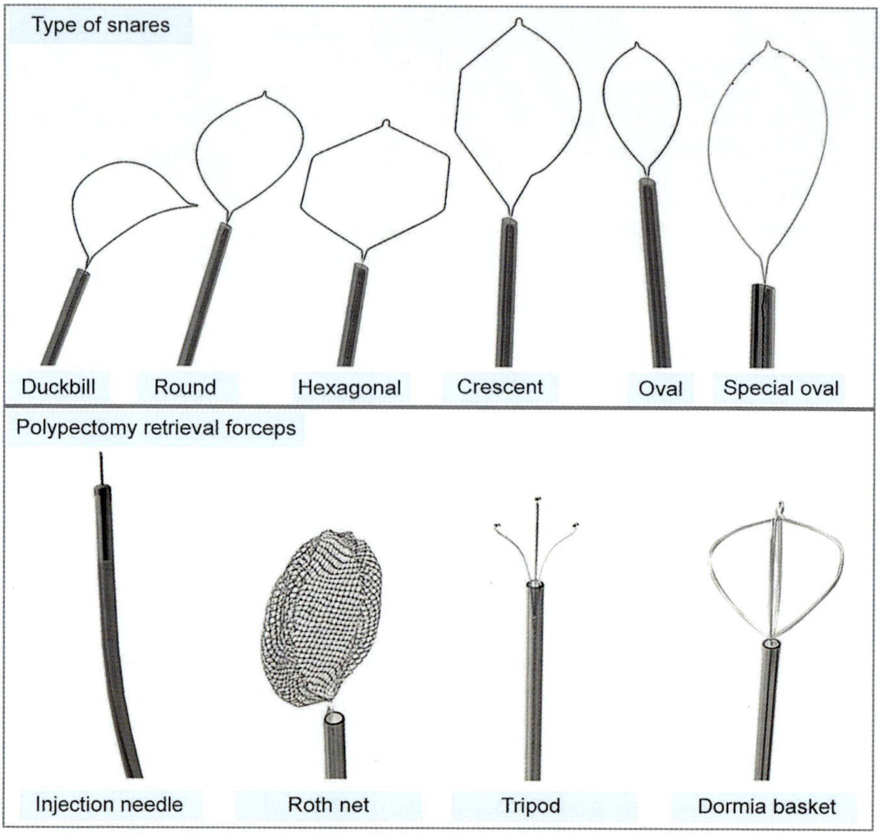

Type of snares

Duckbill Round Hexagonal Crescent Oval Special oval

Polypectomy retrieval forceps

Injection needle Roth net Tripod Dormia basket

Fig. 3: Snare polypectomy equipment.

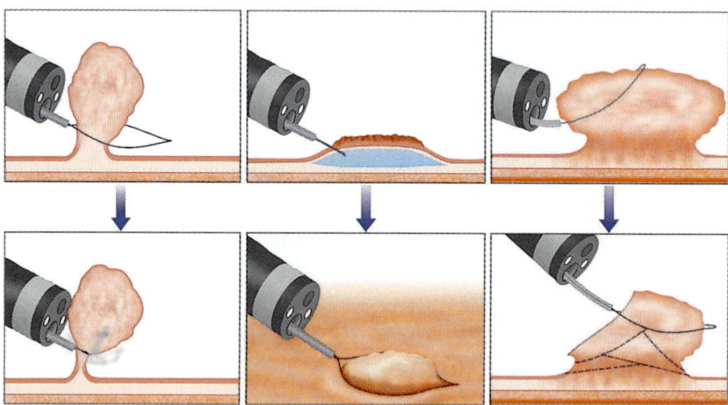

Fig. 4: Steps of polypectomy.

Steps of the procedure ***(Fig. 4)****:*

- Take appropriate size and shape of a snare. Start gently closing the snare and note the point when the wire completely disappears within the sheath. Mark that point in the snare handle using a marker pen. We should stop closing the handle any further while trying to garland a polyp or else there is a risk of guillotine or cold snaring by undue force.

- Perform colonoscopy to locate the polyp and dock the colonoscope to bring the polyp to the optimal position to garland using the snare (bring the polyp to the bottom half of the monitor and preferably in the bottom right quadrant).
- Pass the snare through the access channel and open it enough to encircle and garland the polyp. Keep the snare catheter tip close to the polyp while closing the snare to tightly encircle it.
- Close the handle *just up to previously marked point in the handle* and then apply diathermy ("Endocut" mode) to the stalk and cut the polyp by increasingly tightening the snare **(Figs. 5A and B)**
- Ensure that the polyp is not in contact with opposite bowel wall or else there is risk of direct coupling current injury **(Fig. 6)**
- Piecemeal polypectomy can also be tried for larger polyps
- Recover the polyp using any of the retrieval forceps and send for histopathological examination (HPE)

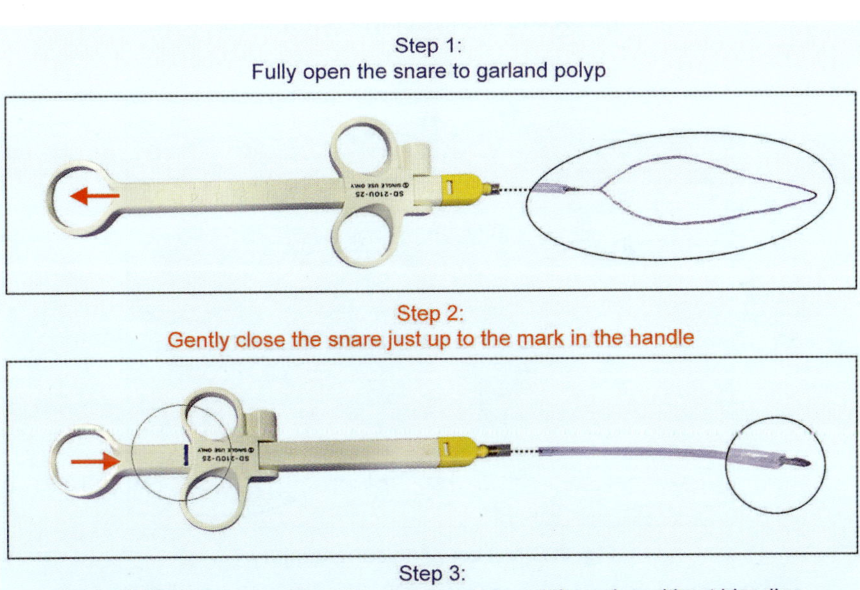

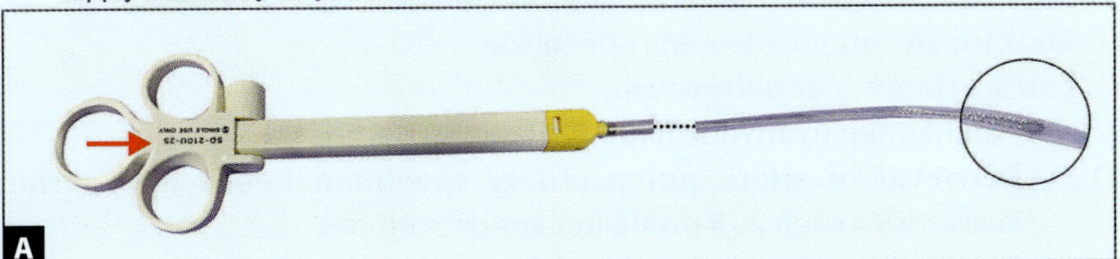

Fig. 5A

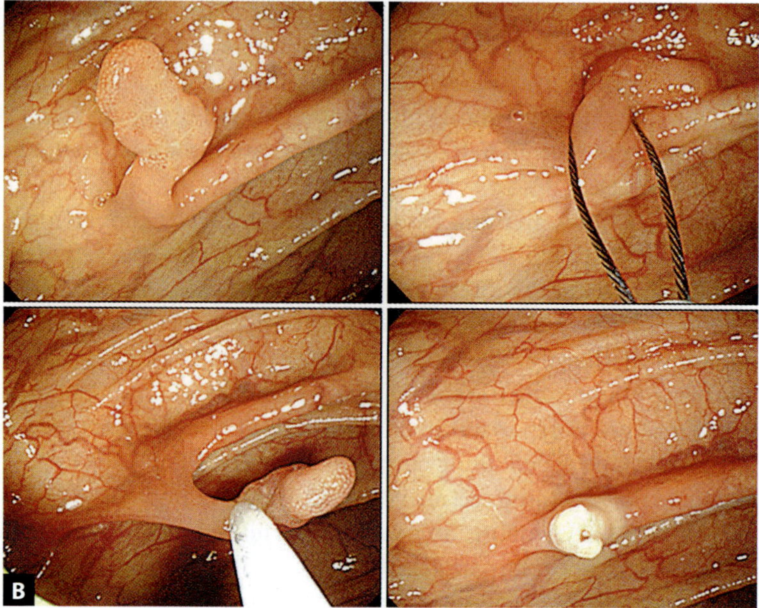

Figs. 5A and B: Snare polypectomy steps.

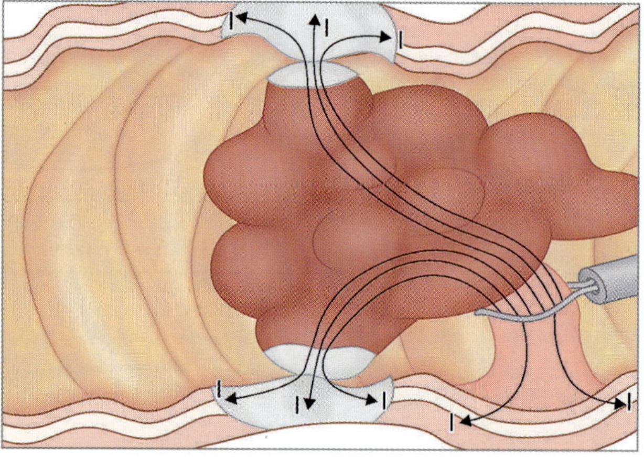

Fig. 6: Direct coupling current injury.

- Look for any undue bleeding and tackle
- *Lost specimen after polypectomy:*
  - Can happen to anyone if not vigilant
  - Retrieval of snare polypectomy specimen needs appropriate accessories such as 3 prong forceps or Roth Net
  - Small polyps can be found in the suction trap bottle or by sieving the stool specimen

SUBMUCOSAL SALINE CUSHION POLYPECTOMY

Indications:

- Useful in case of sessile or broad-based polyp to lift the polyp away from muscularis propria
- Failure to lift on submucosal injection is a sign of malignant infiltration and if so, we should abandon snare polypectomy.

Steps of the procedure **(*Fig. 7*)**:

- Take 23F 210 cm length sclerotherapy needle
- Prepare 20–100 mL of 1/100,000 adrenaline saline mixed with few drops of methylene blue
- Pass the needle through the access channel and once it exits the tip, ask the staff to push the handle to bring the bare needle out
- Tangentially enter the submucous plane and liberally infuse the prepared solution to raise a large submucosal wheal. It is advisable to start the injection at the farthest point of polyp, so the lesion starts lifting toward you rather than receding from your sight. Avoid injecting at multiple points unnecessarily to prevent leakage of fluid and quick disappearance of the wheal.
- Apply the appropriate-sized snare around the polyp and garland the lesion and gradually close the snare

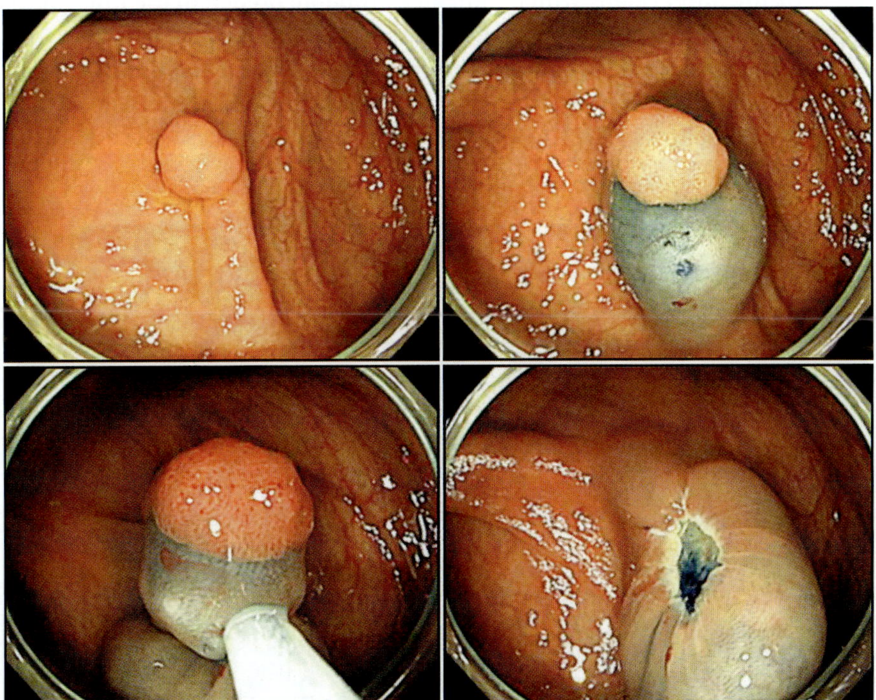

Fig. 7: Submucosal saline cushion polypectomy steps.

- Apply "Endocut" mode current while gradually squeezing the handle to snare the polyp
- Carefully see the floor of the polyp for any breach in the muscle layer or evidence of any residual lesion and manage accordingly

ENDOSCOPIC SUBMUCOSAL DISSECTION

Indication: In case of large sessile polyps like villous adenoma.

Steps of the procedure ***(Fig. 8)****:*

- Diathermy marking of the borders of the lesion
- Submucosal injection of a lifting agent (saline with dye) in the perimeter of the lesion
- Submucosal dissection with special insulated tip (IT) or hybrid knife with periodic further injection of lifting agent
- Complete resection of polyp. Snare may be useful at the end to garland and excise the lesion.
- Use of water jet and hemostatic forceps to locate and control the bleeders
- Retrieve the polyp, mount it on a board, fix it in 10% formalin and send for HPE
- Look for any bleeding spots and treat them using hemoclip or coagulation forceps
- Look for "target sign" which indicates probable breach in the muscularis propria layer. There will be a white center with surrounding stained area suggestive of breach in the muscle layer and likelihood of free perforation. Hence in such cases, we should consider immediate closure with hemoclips.

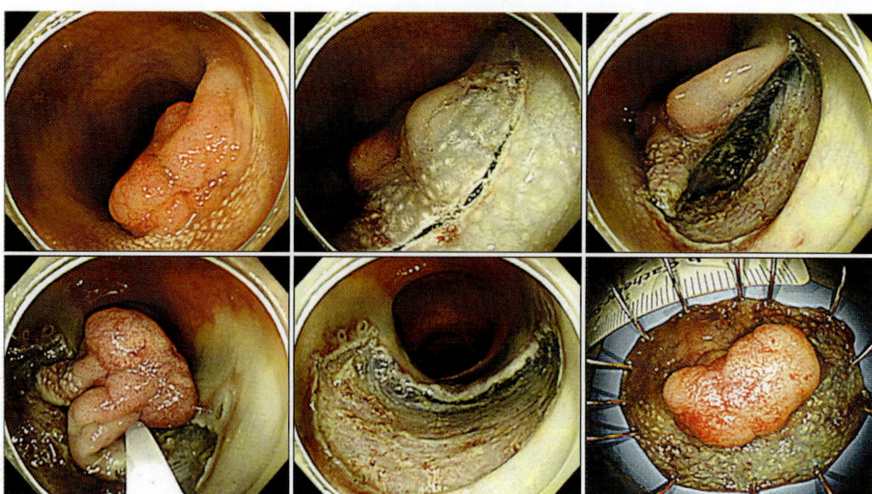

Fig. 8: Endoscopic submucosal dissection (ESD) steps.

COLONOSCOPIC HEMOSTASIS

Available modalities:

- Injecting the bleeding site with 1/10,000 dilute adrenaline
- Thermocoagulation
- Argon plasma coagulation (APC)
- Laser
- Hemoclip application
- Banding of piles

Injection with Dilute Adrenaline

Things required:

- 23G sclerotherapy resheathing retractable needle of 210 cm length
- Dilute 1 mL of 1/1,000 adrenaline to 10–20 mL by using saline to make it 1/10,000 to 1/20,000 dilution and take it in 10 mL syringes
- Water jet or irrigation system to flush the bleeding site
- Good suction unit

Trick of the trade:

- Reach and dock the colonoscope at the satisfactory position
- Pass the sclerotherapy needle through the biopsy channel and once seen at the distal end, instruct the assistant to push the "bare needle out" from the sheath for about 5 mm
- Pass it tangentially just outside the margin of the bleeding lesion
- Inject 1 cc of dilute adrenaline in each quadrant to achieve blanching by tamponade effect and initiate vasospasm and inflammatory reaction and thrombosis
- Subsequently one may choose to inject the base of the bleeding site with 1–2 injection of 1 mL each site
- If bleeding persists, one may choose combination of modalities like adding thermal method (e.g., bipolar diathermy using a gold probe) or even hemoclip application.

Thermal Method (Figs. 9A to C)

- Bipolar diathermy using the "gold probe"

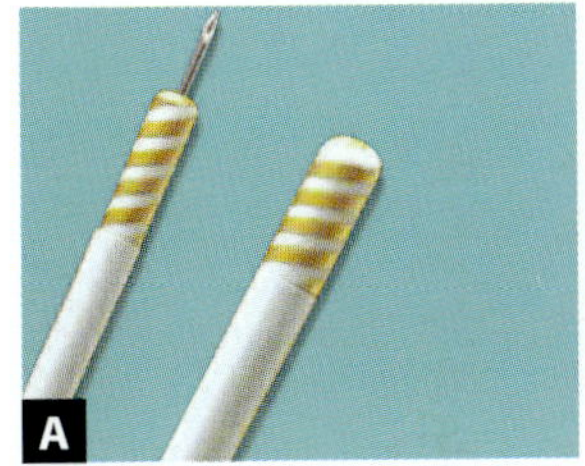

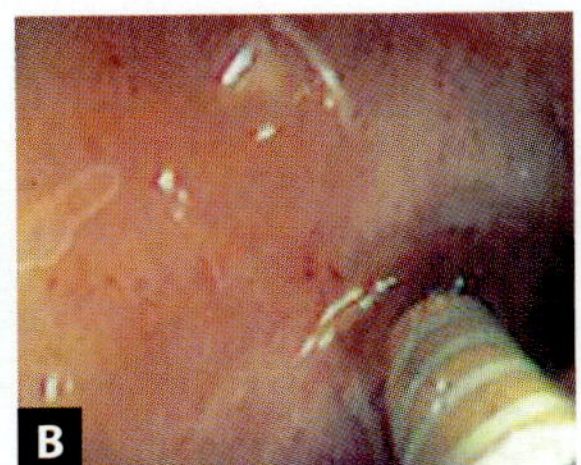

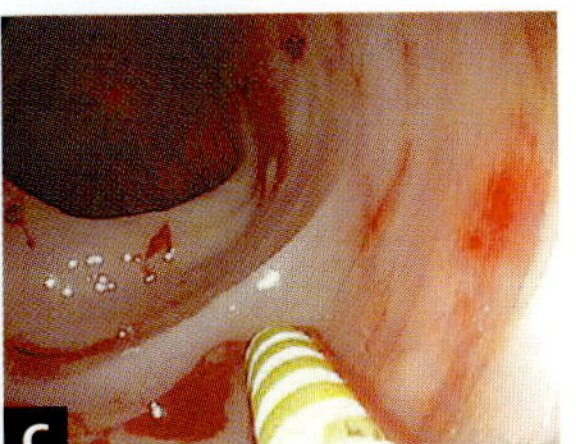

Figs. 9A to C: Gold probe.

- Usually as a combined method following the injection with dilute adrenaline
- Apply the gold probe over the bleeding spot, e.g., angiodysplasia colon, to achieve pressure effect and then activate the diathermy to achieve superficial coagulative thrombosis (coaptive coagulation).

Hemoclip Application (Fig. 10)

Indications:

- Base of bleeding polyp
- To close any defect following ESD

Types of hemoclip ***(Fig. 11)***:

- Disposable preloaded hemoclips
- Reusable hemoclip applicator with clips in separate cartridges
- Choose the one that can be rotatable and with adjustable width

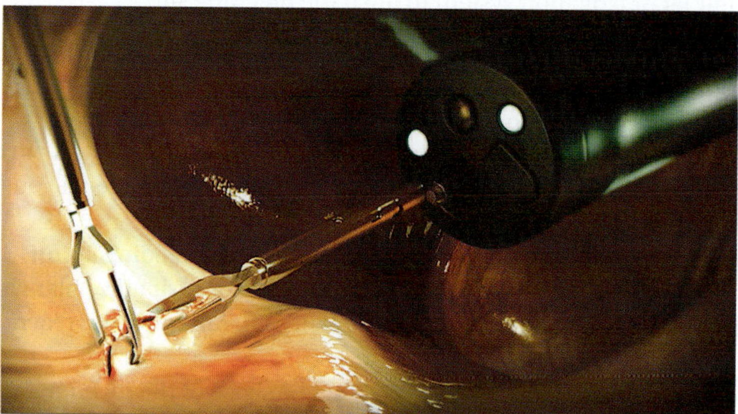

Fig. 10: Hemoclip application.

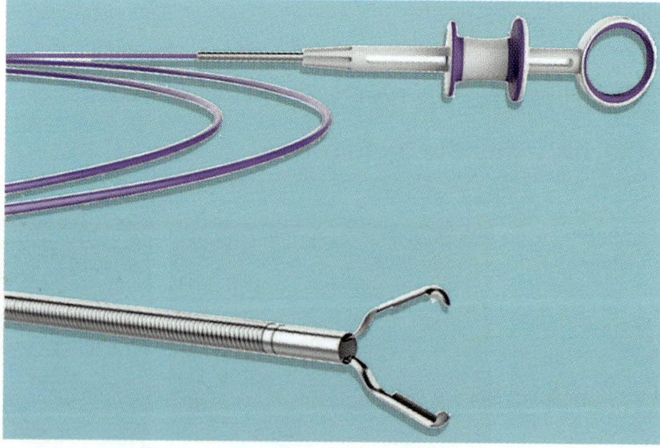

Fig. 11: Types of hemoclip.

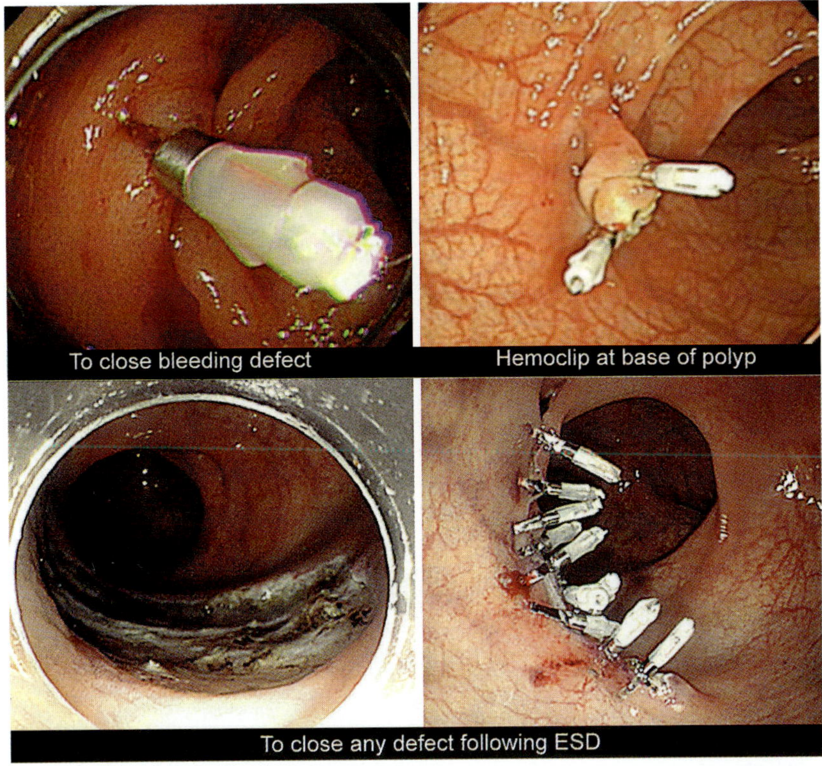

Fig. 12: Closing defect following endoscopic submucosal dissection (ESD).

Tricks of the trade ***(Fig. 12)***:

- Dock the endoscopy at the satisfactory position
- Load the clip from cartridge on to the applicator
- Pass the hemoclip applicator with clip hidden in the retractable sheath through the biopsy channel
- Bring out the clip and adjust the trajectory angle and its width
- Release clip by pushing the thumb grip handle once you have grabbed the tissue at the desired position.
- You may need few more clips depending on the situation.
- Avoid any thermal methods at the site following hemoclip

Argon Plasma Coagulation (Fig. 13)

Indications:

- Radiation proctocolitis
- Angiodysplasia
- Residual polyp after snare polypectomy

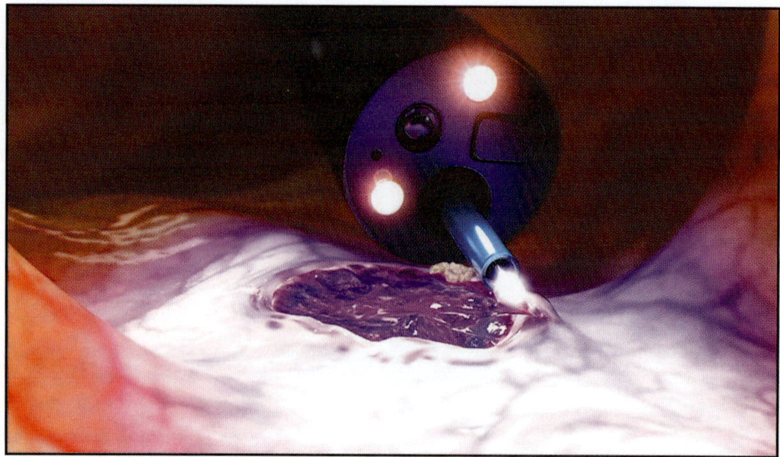

Fig. 13: Argon plasma coagulation.

Things required:
- Diathermy with APC provisions (ERBE or Valleylab)
- Argon plasma gas cylinder
- *Spray catheter:* Side and end firing types
- Good suction unit

Tricks of the trade: A case of radiation proctitis
- Check colonoscopy to verify site and extent of bleeding lesions
- Take the APC spray catheter (side firing or end firing) through the biopsy channel **(Fig. 14)**

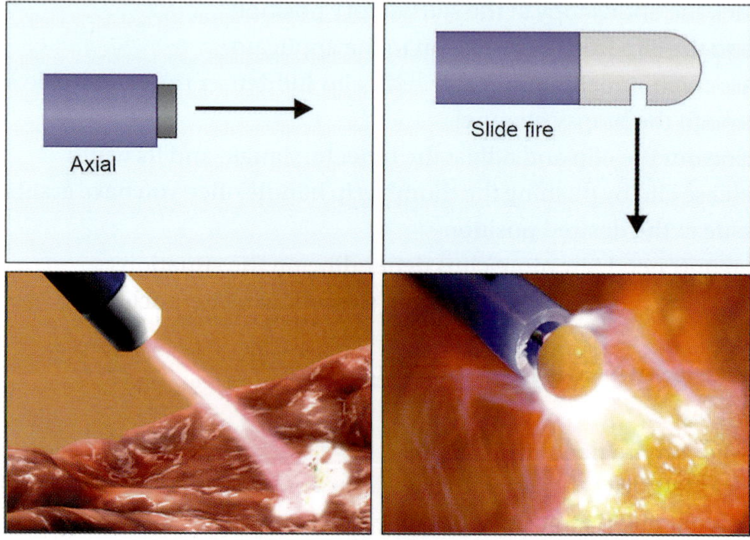

Fig. 14: Argon plasma coagulation (APC) probe opening.

- Ensure recommended diathermy and gas flow setting
- Activate the pedal to achieve superficial coagulative necrosis and hemostasis
- The catheter is close to but not touching the mucosa ("noncontact" mode).
- Keep the spray catheter unmoving but projecting 1 cm from distal end of colonoscope. Now manipulate the endoscopy and catheter as one unit to spray the area with APC (also called "paintbrush technique")

BALLOON DILATATION OF STRICTURE (FIG. 15)

Indications:

- Crohn's colonic stricture
- Anastomotic stricture
- Following nonsteroidal anti-inflammatory drug (NSAID) colitis or ischemic colitis

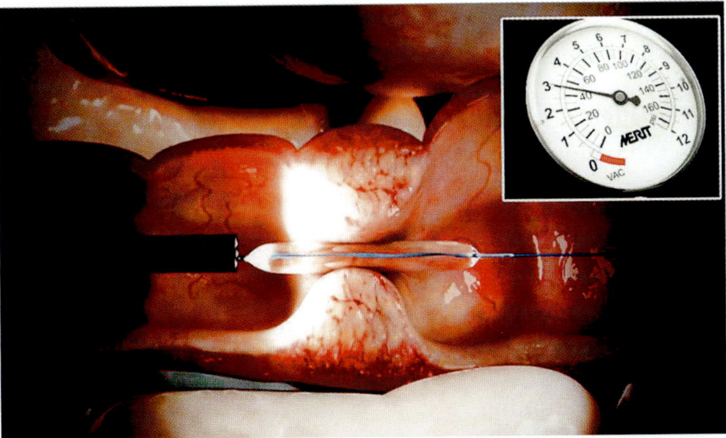

Fig. 15: Balloon dilatation of stricture.

Steps of the procedure:

- Use 10-12-15 mm 6 cm length controlled radial expansion (CRE) balloon with inflation device **(Fig. 16)**
- CRE balloon is a TTS device (through the scope) and hence could easily be passed through the biopsy channel of colonoscope.
- Apply some silicone gel in the access channel prior to passing the CRE balloon
- Pass the CRE balloon though the stricture with the help of guidewire if needed so that all but last 2 cm of balloon is inside the stricture area.
- Attach the Alliance gun or inflation device with saline to expand the balloon and carefully watch the pressure shown in the pressure gauge. The expansion diameter is according to the pressure reached (psi).

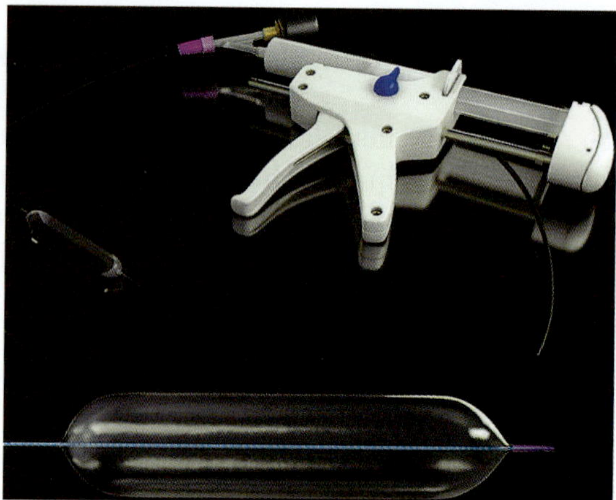

Fig. 16: Controlled radial expansion (CRE) ballon inflation device.

- There will be radial expansion of stricture area which could be visualized, thanks to the transparency of balloon.
- Partly deflate the balloon and try to pass the scope through the stricture gently
- This is ideally suited to dilate a tight, concentric ring-like structure.
- Deflate the balloon completely prior to taking it out through the access channel.

COLONOSCOPIC STENTING (FIG. 17)

Indication: Obstructive left-sided colonic tumor.

Methods of stent deployment:

- Radiological positioning
- Colonoscopic positioning

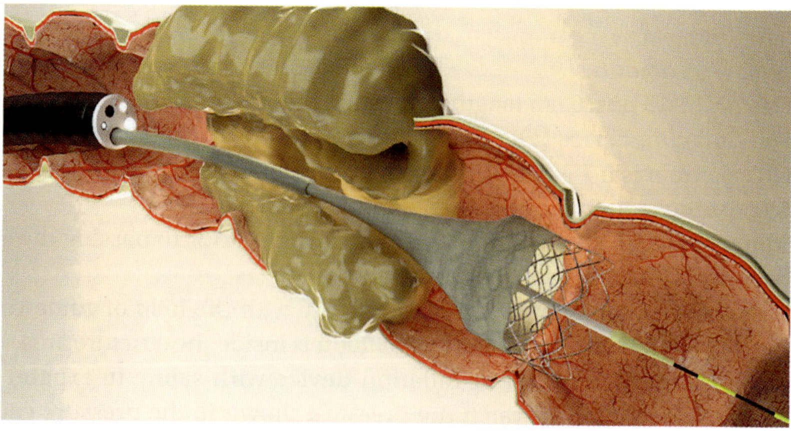

Fig. 17: Colonoscopic stenting.

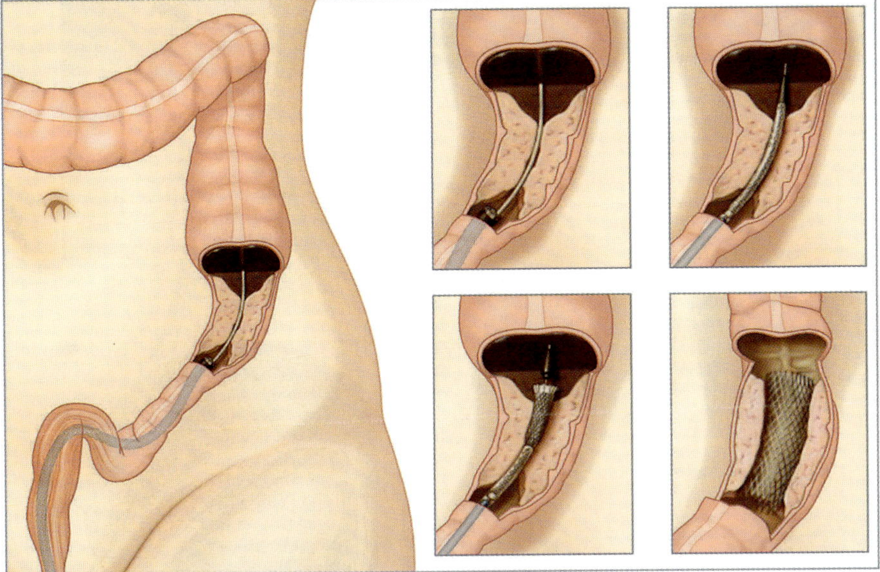

Fig. 18: Stent deployment.

Steps of deployment **(Fig. 18)**:

- Locate the obstructive lesion and pass stiff guidewire across
- Inject water-soluble contrast to identify the site, length, and extent of stricture
- Deploy the chosen stent

COLONOSCOPIC DECOMPRESSION

- *Pseudo-obstruction:*
  - Perform colonoscopy and exclude any mechanical cause and any evidence of ischemia
  - Decompress the bowel as you withdraw the colonoscopy and insert a rectal tube to be kept for some time
- *Sigmoid volvulus:*
  - Either rigid sigmoidoscopy in prone jackknife position or video colonoscopy in left lateral position
  - Indicated if patient is stable with no clinical signs of ischemia and no guarding or rigidity
  - Gently insert the scope with minimal insufflation
  - Volvulus is noticeable at the rectosigmoid junction **(Fig. 19)**.
  - If there are no obvious ischemic changes and scope can be gently pushed through the twisted part, sudden gush of air and fluid feces signals successful decompression and rectal tube can be kept if possible.

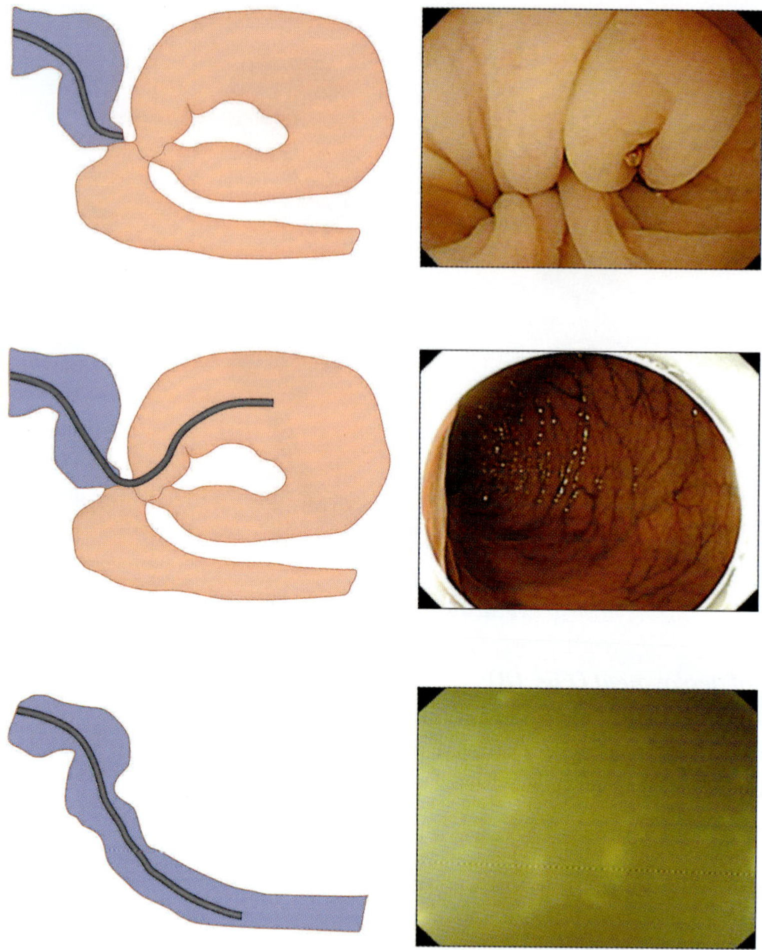

Fig. 19: Colonoscopic sigmoid volvulus decompression.

- Though detorsion and decompression is successful in most of the patients, elective sigmoid colectomy should be considered to prevent recurrence.

BANDING OF PILES

- *Direct banding:*
  - Use Baron's type of suction apparatus with rubber bands **(Figs. 20A and B)**
  - Apply the suction over the pile masses at 3, 7, and 11 o'clock position just above the dentate line and release the bands
- *Retroflex method* ***(Fig. 21)****:* In patient with short anal canal, bands can be loaded in flexible scope and retroflexed in the rectum and bands are applied from above.

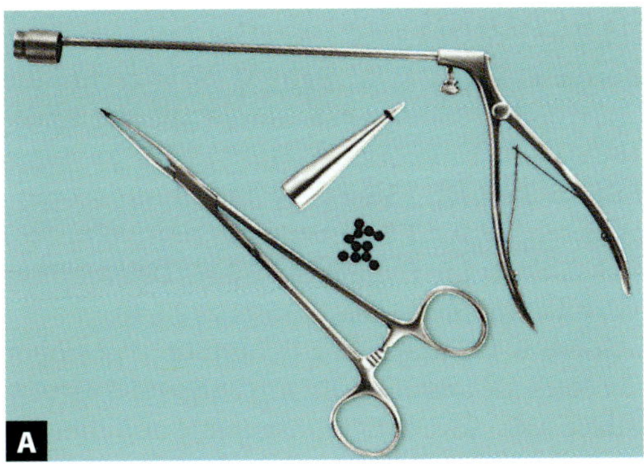

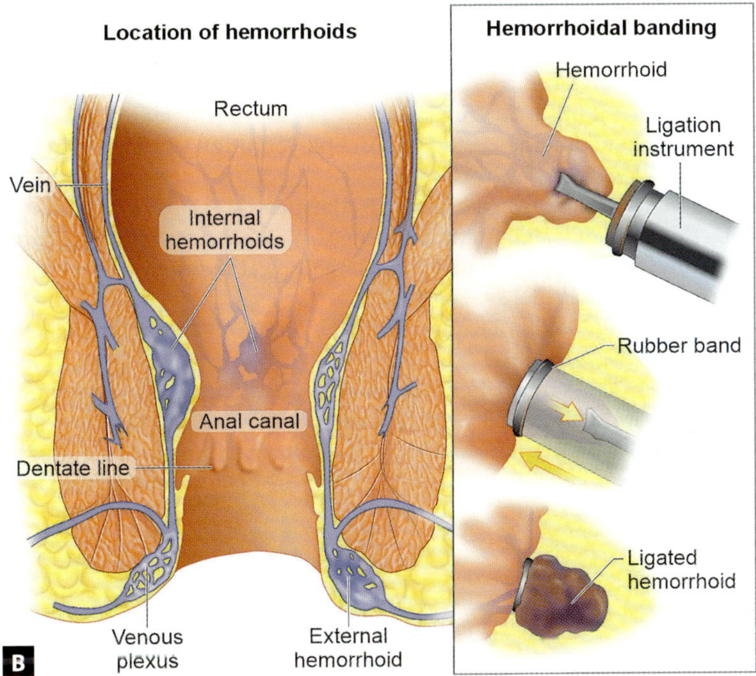

Figs. 20A and B: Banding of piles.

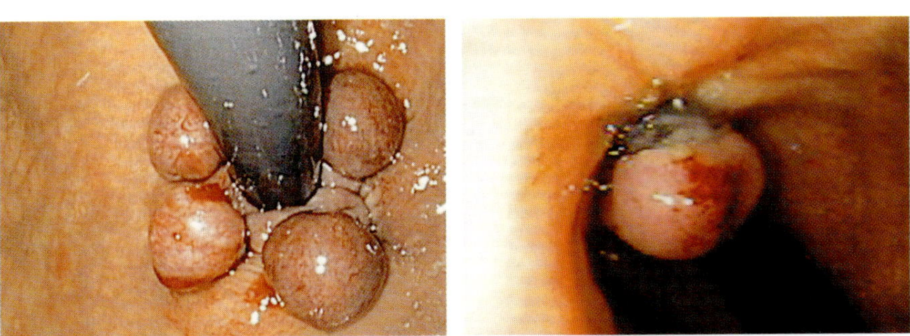

Fig. 21: Retroflex method of banding.

SUGGESTED READING

1. Aydin HN, Bertin P, Singh K, Arregui M. Safe techniques for endoscopic resection of gastrointestinal lipomas. Surg Laparosc Endosc Percutan Tech. 2011;21(4):218-22.
2. Bloomfeld RS, Rockey DC, Shetzline MA. Endoscopic therapy of acute diverticular hemorrhage. Am J Gastroenterol. 2001;96(8):2367-72.
3. Chen M, Shen B. Endoscopic Therapy in Crohn's Disease: Principle, Preparation, and Technique. Inflamm Bowel Dis. 2015;21:2222-40.
4. Cirocco WC, Golub RW. Endoscopic treatment of postoperative hemorrhage from a stapled colorectal anastomosis. Am Surg. 1995;61(5):460-3.
5. Gómez V, Wallace MB. Advances in diagnostic and therapeutic colonoscopy. Curr Opin Gastroenterol. 2014;30:63-8.
6. Holmes I, Friedland S. Endoscopic Mucosal Resection versus Endoscopic Submucosal Dissection for Large Polyps: A Western Colonoscopist's View. Clin Endosc. 2016;49:454-6.
7. Kaltenbach T, Milkes D, Friedland S, Soetikno R. Safe endoscopic treatment of large colonic lipomas using endoscopic looping technique. Dig Liver Dis. 2008;40(12):958-61.
8. Matsuda A, Miyashita M, Matsumoto S, Matsutani T, Sakurazawa N, Takahashi G, et al. Comparison of long-term outcomes of colonic stent as "bridge to surgery" and emergency surgery for malignant large-bowel obstruction: a meta-analysis. Ann Surg Oncol. 2015;22:497-504.
9. Raveenthiran V, Madiba TE, Atamanalp SS, De U. Volvulus of the sigmoid colon. Colorectal Dis. 2010;12:1-17.
10. Rogers BH. The safety of carbon dioxide insufflation during colonoscopic electrosurgical polypectomy. Gastrointest Endosc. 1974;20:115-7.
11. Uraoka T, Parra-Blanco A, Yahagi N. Colorectal endoscopic submucosal dissection: is it suitable in western countries? J Gastroenterol Hepatol. 2013;28:406-14.

Expert's Comment

Since the advent of flexible endoscopy almost 7 decades ago, we have seen exponential improvement in the endoscopic evolution and technologies. The advancements in microchips and high-resolution optics have transformed the way we perform endoscopy today. In this section on colonoscopy, I would like to highlight some key developments, though the author has very carefully covered all the salient aspects of therapeutic colonoscopy.

I would urge the aspiring endoscopists to spend enough time learning this procedure, as this is the most important diagnostic tool that will allow us to detect small adenomas and will, in turn, lead to a substantial drop in the need for elective colon cancer surgeries in the future. The Western data have already shown us the advantages of screening colonoscopy over the last decade, and we should learn from that. It is my humble request to all the readers of this chapter to keep in mind to screen high-risk groups of patients who have a family history of colon cancer and extend this screening tool to them.

Regarding the various advances of colonoscopic techniques, the author has described them in detail, so I would only add here the expanding horizons of endoscopic resections of established early colorectal cancers with techniques such as endoscopic mucosal resection (EMR), endoscopic submucosal dissection (ESD), submucosal tunneling endoscopic resection (STER), and endoscopic full-thickness resection (EFTR). I would also emphasize that those who want to venture on this path of colonoscopic diagnosis and treatments should consider investing in high-end equipment, which will enable you to detect subtle mucosal changes and therefore the minimum technology which you should have is high-resolution, magnification endoscopy with electronic chromoendoscopy features such as narrow-band imaging (NBI) and flexible spectral imaging color enhancement (FICE).

I hope that this chapter on colonoscopy will enhance your understanding of the intricacies of the procedure, and the effort that our author has made to bring it to all of us will be well utilized for patient safety and predictable outcomes. I wish you all the best in your endeavor to learn colonoscopy.

Dr Vipulroy Rathod
Mumbai

CHAPTER 14

Overview of Endoscopic Retrograde Cholangiopancreatography

Chapter Outline

- About the Hardware of Duodenoscope
- About the Fluoroscopy
- About the Commonly used Endoscopic Retrograde Cholangiopancreatography Accessories
- Preparation of Patient
- Steps of the Procedure
- Endoscopic Evaluation of Major Papilla
- Radiological Interpretation of the Bile and Pancreatic Ducts
  - Scout Film
  - Contrast Films
- Pancreatic Duct Imaging
- Bile Duct Imaging
- Understanding the Various Interventions Performed during ERCP
  - Selective Cannulation
  - Sphincterotomy
  - Sphincteroplasty
  - Biliary Balloon Sweep
  - Dormia Basketing
  - Mechanical Lithotripsy
  - Stenting
  - Nasobiliary Drainage Catheter Drainage
  - Needle-knife Sphincterotomy
  - Minor Papillotomy
- Complications of Endoscopic Retrograde Cholangiopancreatography

Keywords: Duodenoscope, sphincterotomy, sphincteroplasty, biliary fogarty balloon, mechanical lithotripsy, stenting

INTRODUCTION

Endoscopic retrograde cholangiopancreatography (ERCP) is the endoscopic visualization of the upper gastrointestinal (GI) tract and radiological evaluation of the pancreatic and biliary tract. It is an advanced endoscopic therapeutic procedure. ERCP relies on the cooperation and commitment of four teams, namely:

1. *E*xperienced endoscopist
2. *R*esponsible and agile assistants
3. *C*onsiderate and competent anesthetist
4. *P*roficient radiographer

ABOUT THE HARDWARE OF DUODENOSCOPE

Endoscopic retrograde cholangiopancreatography scope is a side-viewing duodenoscope. This allows us to see the side wall of second part of the duodenum.

It has the following special features, namely **(Figs. 1A and B)**:

- A side-viewing objective lens
- A side-positioned air/water nozzle
- Instrument channel 3.2 mm (standard scope) or 4.2 mm (therapeutic scope)
- A forceps elevator adjacent to the instrument channel outlet that allows fine linear instrument position changes. Its movement is controlled by a knob located adjacent to the big wheel in the control head.

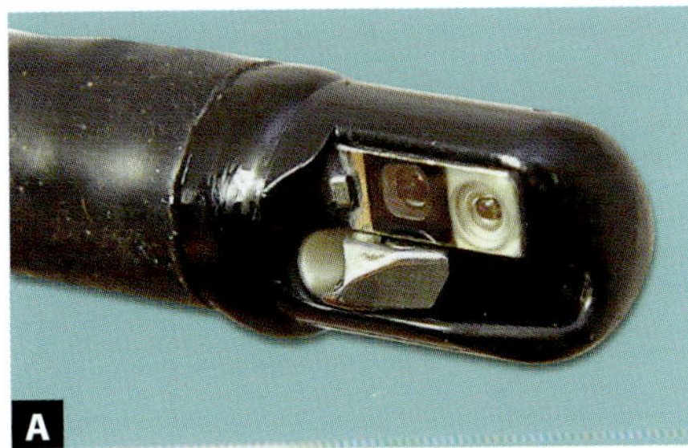

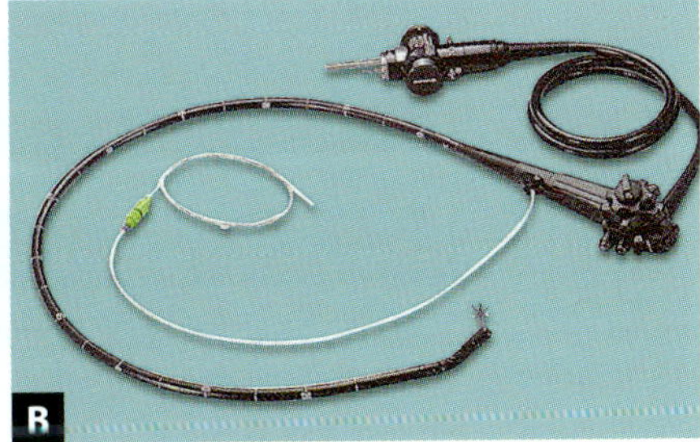

Figs. 1A and B: Side-viewing duodenoscope.

ABOUT THE FLUOROSCOPY

- Dedicated fluoroscopy unit with a table or portable C-arm unit with under table X-ray tube **(Fig. 2)**
- Ability to take spot pictures and also store the digital images and print them later
- The magnification factor of the images to be known before measuring the size of the duct or stone or length of the stricture
- Dual video monitors (for endoscopy and fluoroscopy images)
- Wear a lead apron and thyroid shield

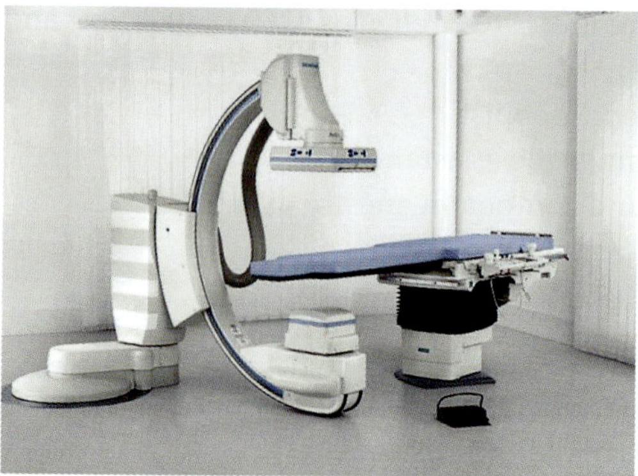

Fig. 2: Fluoroscopy unit.

ABOUT THE COMMONLY USED ENDOSCOPIC RETROGRADE CHOLANGIOPANCREATOGRAPHY ACCESSORIES

- *Sphincterotome* ***(Fig. 3)****:*
  - It aids us in selectively cannulating and cutting the desired duct with the help of the bow-like monopolar diathermy wire

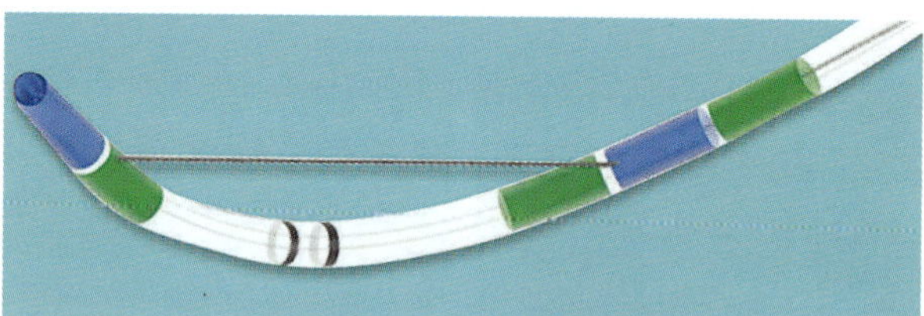

Fig. 3: Sphincterotome.

  - By controlling its handle, one could adjust the shape of the bow wire and its tension
  - Different designs are available to choose from various makers in the market.
  - In clevercut sphincterotomy, the bow wire is partly sheathed to avoid stray current and to achieve precise cut.
  - The tip of the sphincterotome could be short-nosed or long-nosed.
  - Usually, it has two separate ports for guidewire cannulation and contrast injection.
- *Guidewires* ***(Fig. 4)****:*
  - These flexible wires help us to navigate, negotiate, and reach various parts in the biliopancreatic tree and then we can railroad or exchange with various other accessories to perform different therapeutic procedures.

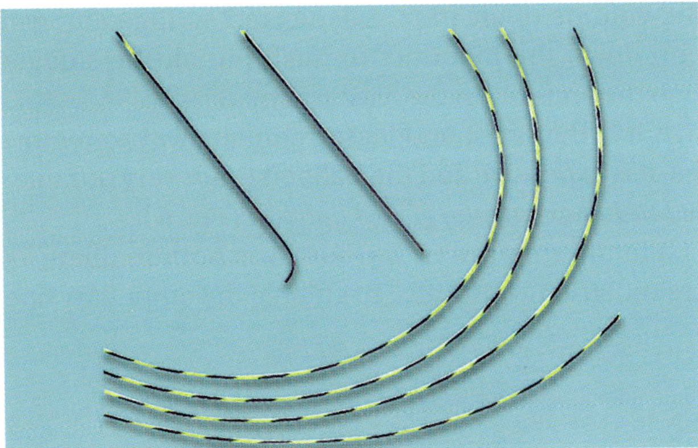

Fig. 4: Guidewires.

- There are vast numbers of guidewires in the market to choose from.
- Teflon-coated metal guidewires with flexible tips or nitinol wires with hydrophilic tips. Use the one you are comfortable with. Prefer the one with the hydrophilic steerable tip to aid easy cannulation of any stricture.
- Usually prefer 450 cm length and 0.035 inches guidewire (rarely 0.025)
- Radiopaque markers in the shaft of the wire aid its easy identification and measurement of the length of the stricture.
- Understand the characteristics, specifications, and capabilities of all different guidewires to improve our efficiency during the procedure.

▪ *Fogarty biliary balloon* ***(Fig. 5)****:*
  - This balloon works similar to an embolectomy balloon
  - This has a triple lumen for passing the guidewire, injecting the contrast, and also a separate port to inflate the balloon at its tip with air.
  - Once the balloon is inside the bile duct and inflated

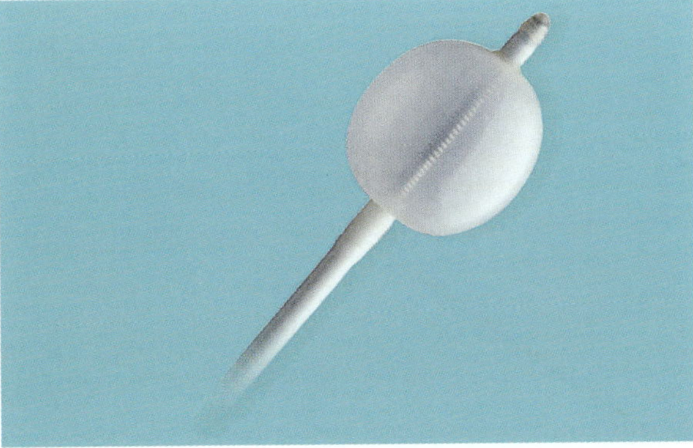

Fig. 5: Fogarty biliary balloon.

- Set the volume of air from a dedicated syringe and gently pull the balloon down the bile duct to flush out all the sludge and stones through the ampulla in the least traumatic way.
- Though it is the safest and least traumatic way to remove the biliary sludge, it is expensive and the balloon is not very durable.

▪ *Controlled radial expansion (CRE) balloon* ***(Fig. 6)****:*

- CRE balloons are used in various sizes both to dilate any biliary or pancreatic stricture and also to enlarge the ampullary opening.

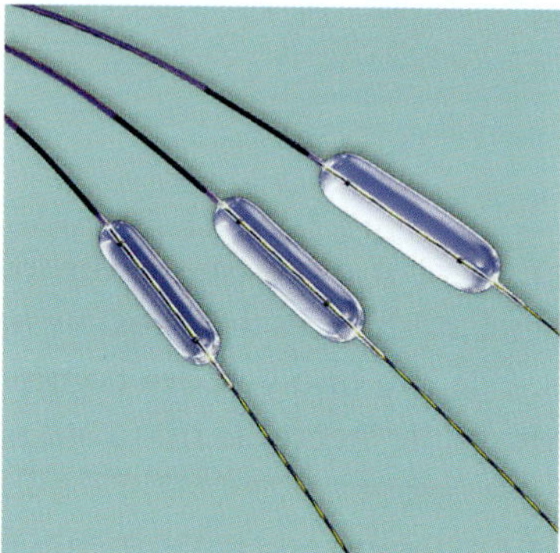

Fig. 6: Controlled radial expansion (CRE) balloon.

- Achieve the preset pressure with the help of a saline-filled inflation device to distend the balloon to the predetermined diameter
- Silicone gel is used to lubricate the balloon for easy passage through the channel.

▪ *Dormia basket* ***(Fig. 7)****:*

- These four- or six-wired baskets of different configurations and sizes to aid removal of biliary and pancreatic stones in the least expensive way.

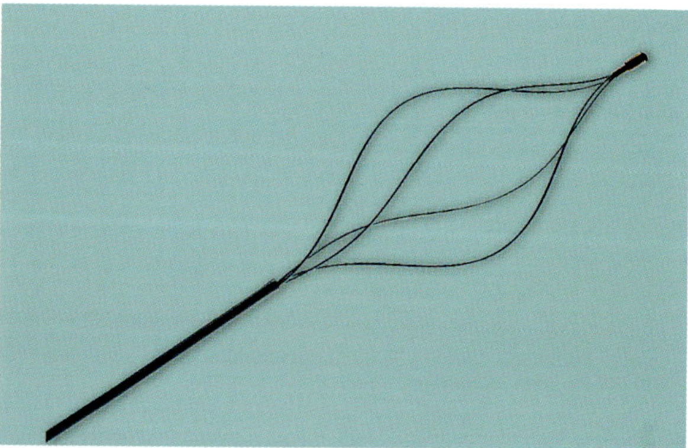

Fig. 7: Dormia basket.

- By plunging and pulling the handle, you could open and close the basket.
- There is usually a side port for flushing.

- *Precut sphincterotome* ***(Fig. 8)****:*
  - This needle knife sphincterotome helps to lance the ampulla like cutting a pear to expose the biliary and pancreatic opening
  - Useful in case of bulging ampulla with hidden or stenotic orifice

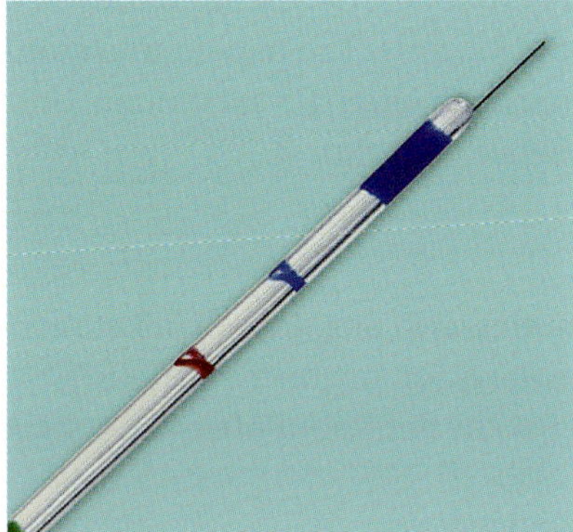

Fig. 8: Precut sphincterotome.

- *Cannula:* These are seldom used nowadays except for cannulating the minor papilla.
- *Mechanical lithotripsy basket with handle:* This tough-wired basket helps to grab and pulverize any hard and large stone with the help of a strong ratchet handle.

PREPARATION OF PATIENT

- Usually done as an inpatient procedure with overnight stay
- Ambulatory daycare ERCP is also commonly practiced in some centers
- Ensure overnight fasting or nil oral for at least 6 hours before the procedure
- Examine and document all the relevant history, clinical findings, investigation reports, any comorbidity, and list of drugs and drug allergies
- See liver function and international normalized ratio (INR) results
- Administer IV vitamin K 10 mg at least a day before [consider fresh frozen plasma (FFP) in needy patients with coagulopathy]

INVESTIGATIONS BEFORE ENDOSCOPIC RETROGRADE CHOLANGIOPANCREATOGRAPHY

- Liver function tests, amylase, renal parameters, and tumor markers such as α-fetoprotein (AFP), carbohydrate-associated antigen 19–9 (CA 19–9), and carcinoembryonic antigen (CEA)

- *Coagulation profile*: INR and activated partial thromboplastin time (APTT)
- ECG and X-ray chest
- Review all available imaging reports namely US abdomen, CT, MRI, or magnetic resonance cholangiopancreatography (MRCP) to ascertain the purpose of ERCP clearly.

INFORMED CONSENT

Endoscopic retrograde cholangiopancreatography is a complex procedure with significant potential hazards. The patient must understand the potential benefits, risks, limitations, and alternatives. Written, informed consent should be obtained in the presence of a witness.

ANTIBIOTICS

- Prophylactic antibiotics with one dose of injection cefotaxime 1 g/IV
- Endocarditis prophylaxis for any needy patient
- In patients with sepsis or persistent obstruction, continue antibiotics for 3–5 days

ANESTHESIA

- Conscious sedation using a combination of propofol and fentanyl or ketamine and midazolam
- General anesthesia in selected high-risk cases and children

POSITION OF THE PATIENT

- Prone position
- Left lateral position
- Supine (while doing ERCP during laparoscopic cholecystectomy or in a patient with hilar strictures)

ROOM LAYOUT AND REQUIRED INSTRUMENTS

- Dedicated ERCP room with fluoroscopy table or portable C-arm unit
- Endoscopy trolley with processor, light source, monitor, suction, and irrigation system
- Ergonomically placed twin monitors for endoscopy and fluoroscopy images side by side
- Monitoring assistant at the head end with nasal O_2, pulse oximeter, ECG, and BP monitoring
- Technical assistant standing next to the endoscopist with all the accessories
- Tissue responsive diathermy unit with “Endocut” provision (ERBE)

CONTRAST AGENTS

- Ionic contrast (iodine) like urografin (full strength for initial imaging to look for pancreatic duct and bile duct and half strength for subsequent filling of bile duct to look for stones or stricture)
- Nonionic contrast for patients with renal failure or a history of allergy
- Use 20 mL properly labeled syringes for injection of contrast and also for flushing the catheters with sterile water before guidewire insertion to prevent any stickiness.

STEPS OF THE PROCEDURE (FIGS. 9A TO E)

1. Place a mouth guard and intubate oropharynx blindly
2. Carefully traverse the esophagus and reach the body of the stomach
3. Torque the shaft of the scope to the right (clockwise) and pass along the greater curve to reach the pylorus
4. Ensure that the pylorus is at the 6 o'clock position of the monitor (sunset position of pylorus) **(Figs. 9A)**
5. Enter the duodenum and then turn the big wheel toward you (anticlockwise) and the small wheel away from you (clockwise) and gently pull out and shorten the scope to about 60 cm level while you turn your body clockwise from facing the patient to facing the monitor **(Fig. 10)**
6. You will now see the ampulla of Vater smiling at you as a pinkish protuberant structure
7. Major papilla is typically located at the top of the first longitudinal fold you encounter in the medial wall of second part of the duodenum and has distinct color and texture and appearance (neck and tie appearance).

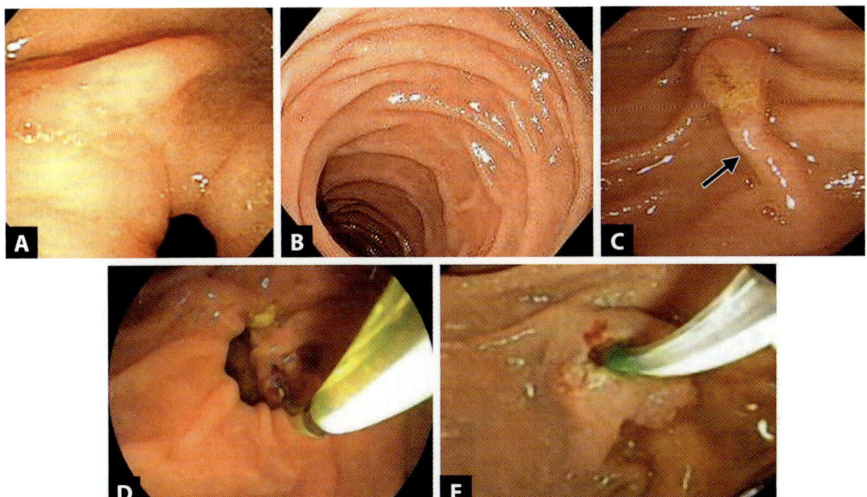

Figs. 9A to E: (A) Sunset sign; (B) D2; (C) Ampulla; (D) Periampullary diverticulum; and (E) Cannulation.

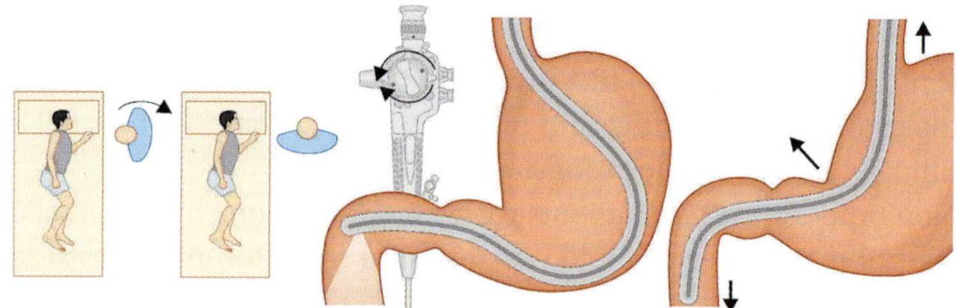

Fig. 10: Steps of endoscopic retrograde cholangiopancreatography (ERCP) procedure.

8. The minor papilla is like a tiny nipple seen 2 cm proximal to the major papilla in the second part of the duodenum between two horizontal folds.
9. Major papilla typically has four distinct parts **(Fig. 11)** namely (1) papillary orifice, (2) frenulum, (3) hood, and (4) infundibulum. The infundibulum may be large, small, or even absent giving varied looks to the major papilla. Sometimes, the papilla may be hidden by a large hood or situated in a periampullary diverticulum which could make the cannulation a challenging task.

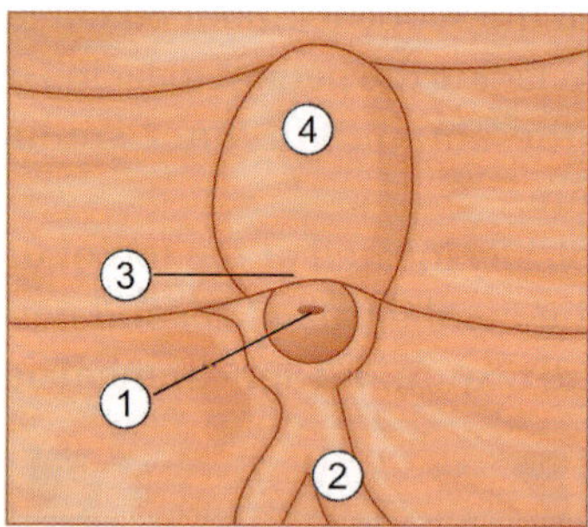

Fig. 11: Parts of ampulla. (1) Papillary orifice, (2) frenulum, (3) hood, and (4) infundibulum.

10. Fine adjustment for cannulation can be done by any of the following steps:
    - Namely turning big and small wheels, and the torque of the scope
    - Body movement of the endoscopist
    - Use of elevator
    - Pushing down or pulling up the scope or careful use of suction
11. Bring the scope below the papilla and see the major papilla in the center or the top left part of the monitor (10 o'clock). Cannulation is best done in the "en face" position.
12. Wire-guided sphincterotome is the best accessory useful for cannulation.
13. Approach the 10 o'clock position to cannulate the bile duct and between 1 and 3 o'clock to cannulate the pancreatic duct. This spatial orientation is vital for successful selective cannulation of the desired duct **(Figs. 12A and B)**.

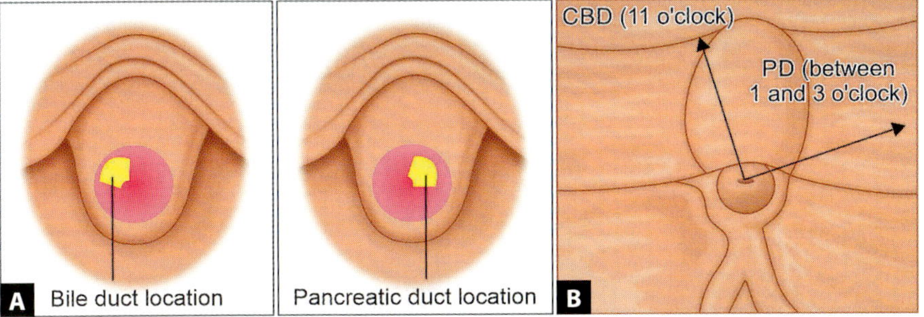

Figs. 12A and B: Direction of bile duct and pancreatic sphincterotomy. (CBD: common bile duct; PD: pancreatic duct)

14. Cannulation of the common bile duct (CBD) is usually achieved by approaching the papilla from below, in line with the axis of the CBD. It may be helpful to lift the roof of the papilla and to direct the cannula toward 10 o'clock.
15. Use fluoroscopy to aid wire-guided deep cannulation before injecting any contrast
16. Avoid unnecessary pancreatic duct cannulation or contrast injection to prevent pancreatitis
17. Full strength contrast should be used initially, and injected under fluoroscopic control. Consider switching over to dilute contrast when stones are visualized.
18. The left hepatic ducts usually fill before the right because they are more dependent on the patient lying prone. The gallbladder (GB) is usually filled except in cases with cystic duct obstruction.
19. Look at the biliary and pancreatic imaging carefully to make a clear diagnosis and plan for any therapeutic intervention accordingly
20. At the end of the procedure the endoscope is withdrawn and air suctioned from the stomach to minimize discomfort. The patient is then turned to a supine position and more radiographs may be taken in different projections.

ENDOSCOPIC EVALUATION OF MAJOR PAPILLA

- Recognize various appearances of the papilla and the presence of any periampullary diverticulum **(Fig. 13)**
- Ampullary stenosis or tumor
- Impacted stone at the major papilla
- Pus or infected bile pouring out
- Any choledochal duodenal fistula just above the papilla
- In the case of previous ERCP, recognize the location of biliary and pancreatic duct opening and the presence of any stent. The bile duct opening is usually found at the top end of the sphincterotomy.

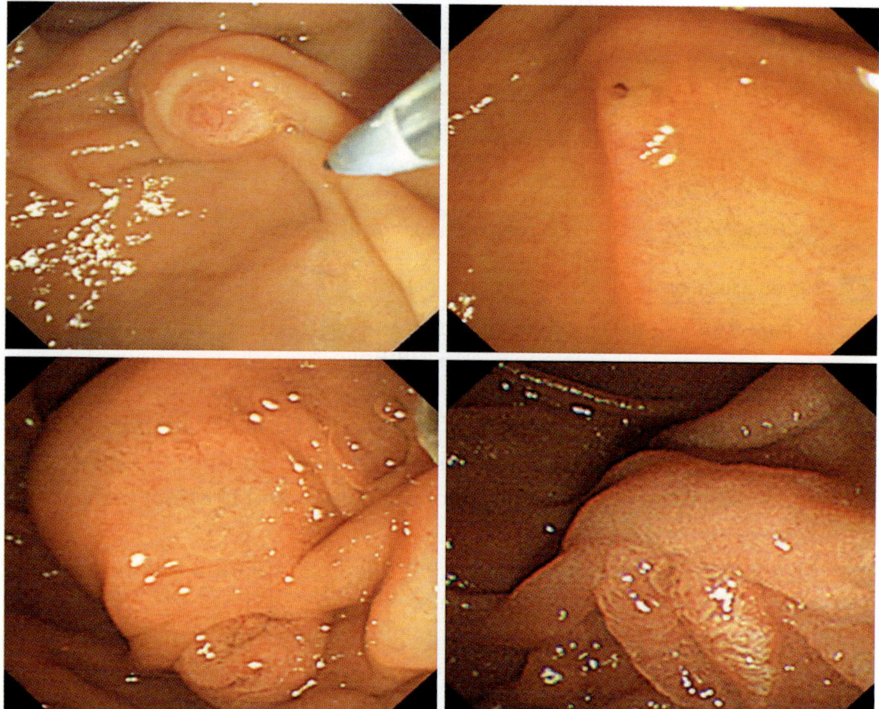

Fig. 13: Types of ampulla of Vater.

RADIOLOGICAL INTERPRETATION OF THE BILE AND PANCREATIC DUCTS

Scout Film (Figs. 14A to C)

A control film of the right upper abdomen should be taken with the scope in place before injection of contrast. With the patient lying prone and the scope in a short scope position, the calcified lesions above and to the right of the scope represent calcifications in the GB, liver parenchyma, or proximal bile ducts. Calcifications to the bottom left of the scope generally represent pancreatic calcification or, rarely, stones in the distal CBD. The presence of air within the bile ducts may be also seen as an air cholangiogram and suggests a patent communication between the bile duct and the gut such as a patent stent, a fistula, or a bilioenteric anastomosis.

Contrast Films

- Most diagnostic and therapeutic interventions are performed under fluoroscopic control; however, radiographs or stored images should be taken for documentation.
- Excess contrast injection may mask stones please beware.

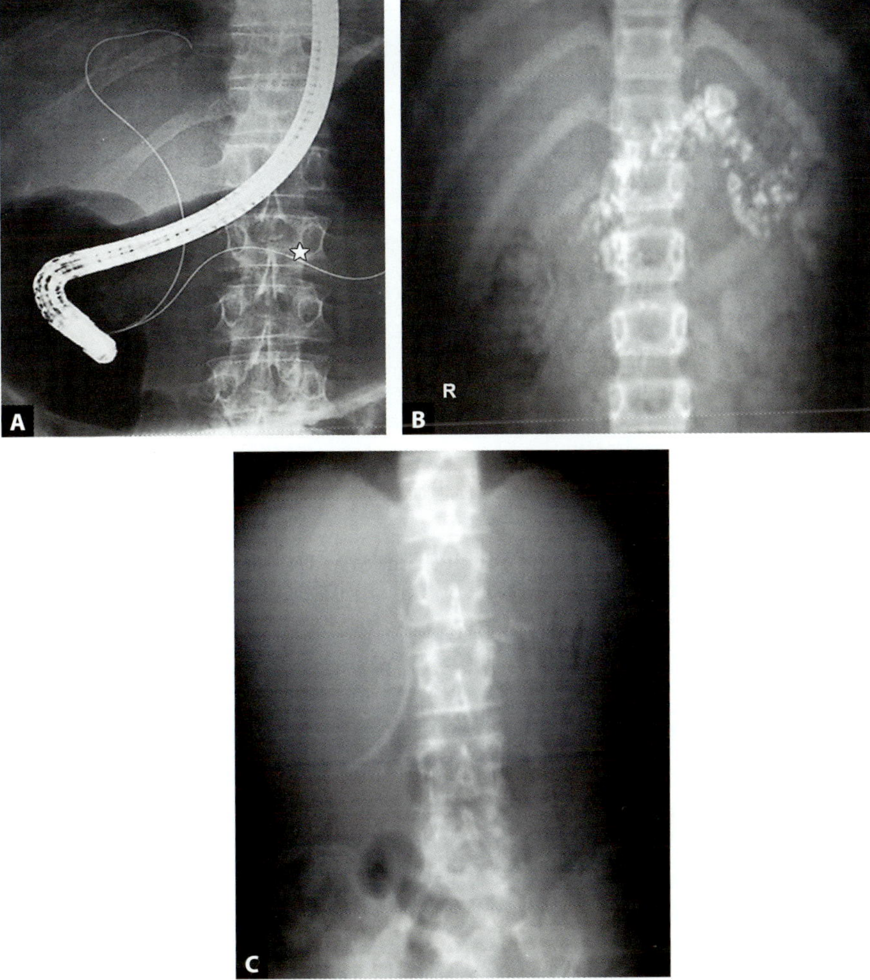

Figs. 14A to C: Scout film during endoscopic retrograde cholangiopancreatography (ERCP). (A) Guidewire position in bile duct and pancreatic duct (*) signifies pancreatic duct (PD); (B) Pancreatic calcification; and (C) Common bile duct (CBD) stent.

- In the prone position, contrast fills the left hepatic duct early, and hence head-down position to fill the right system may be needed.
- Be familiar with image orientation and get also focused magnified views when needed **(Fig. 15)**.

PANCREATIC DUCT IMAGING

Normal Pancreatic Duct

- Starts at the ampulla and has a smooth wavy course across the L1 vertebra with head, genu, body, and tail parts with gradual tapering

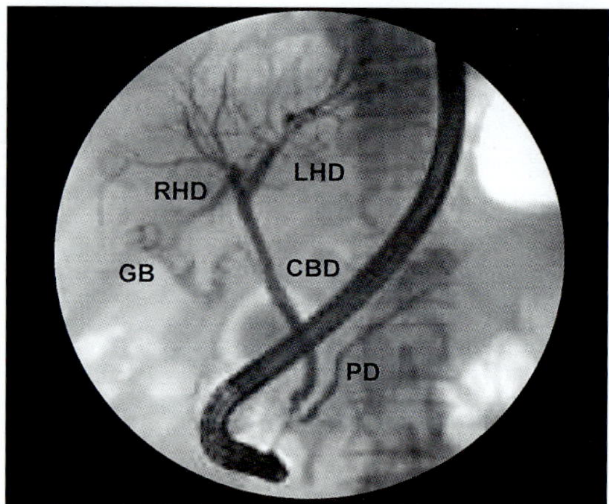

Fig. 15: Various parts of biliary and pancreatic ducts. (CBD: common bile duct; GB: gallbladder; LHD: left hepatic duct; PD: pancreatic duct; RHD: right hepatic duct)

- Branch ducts join the main duct at irregular levels at right angles
- The duct of Santorini is usually seen draining at the minor papilla
- Small ducts from the uncinate process may be seen
- Avoid acinarization or parenchymogram

Abnormal Pancreatogram (Figs. 16A and B)

- In patients with pancreas divisum, there is nonfusion of the dorsal and ventral ducts. The small isolated ventral pancreas drains through the main papilla. The dorsal (Santorini's) duct drains the bulk of the pancreas through the minor papilla.
- *Acute pancreatitis:* The pancreatic duct may appear slightly irregular with changes and irregularities of the side branches. The presence of a pseudocyst may cause complete obstruction of the pancreatic duct with or without communication with the duct.

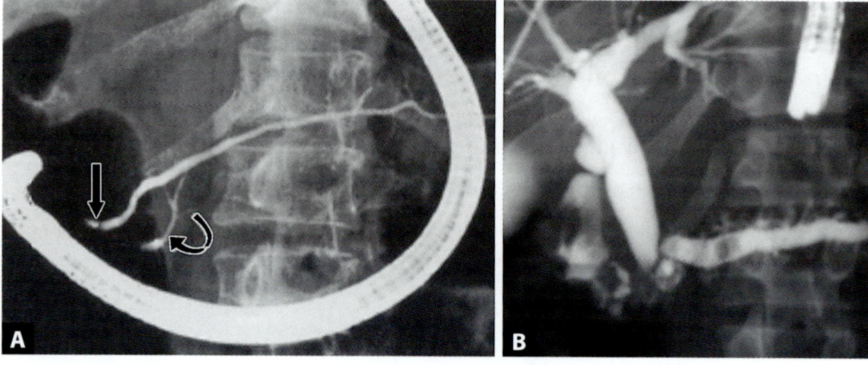

Figs. 16A and B: (A) Pancreatic divisum; and (B) Chronic pancreatitis.

- *Chronic pancreatitis (Cambridge classification):*
  - *Mild pancreatitis:* A normal main pancreatic duct with three or more abnormal side branches.
  - *Moderate pancreatitis:* An abnormal main duct with irregularities in three or more abnormal side branches.
  - *Severe pancreatitis:* Irregularity with strictures and dilatation of the main duct, with filling defects suggestive of stones or filling of cavities or cysts.
- *Traumatic pancreatitis:* Leakage of contrast from a transected pancreatic duct with nonfilling of the upstream duct.
- *Carcinoma head of the pancreas:* Double-duct sign with stricture of the head portion of duct with upstream dilatation of both pancreatic and bile ducts.

BILE DUCT IMAGING (FIG. 17)

Normal Cholangiogram

- With the filling of both extra- and intrahepatic ducts and cystic duct and possibly the GB
- The upper limit of bile duct diameter is about 7 mm (with 30% magnification)
- Beware of common anomalies like low insertion of the cystic duct and abnormal drainage of intrahepatic ducts, e.g., right posterior sectoral duct drainage
- Balloon occlusion cholangiogram may be needed in case of upstream strictures to fill the ducts under pressure.

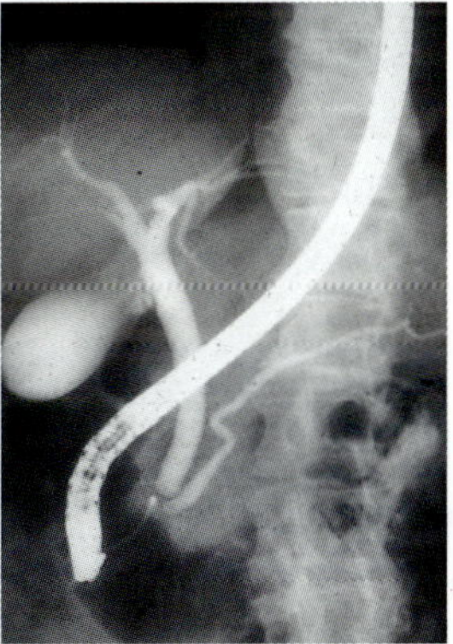

Fig. 17: Normal cholangiogram.

Abnormal Cholangiogram (Figs. 18A to C)

- *Bile duct stones:* Seen as meniscus sign or filling defects. See the size, shape, and number of the stones. Mid CBD stones may be hidden by the scope and hence change the scope to long route position to evaluate that area

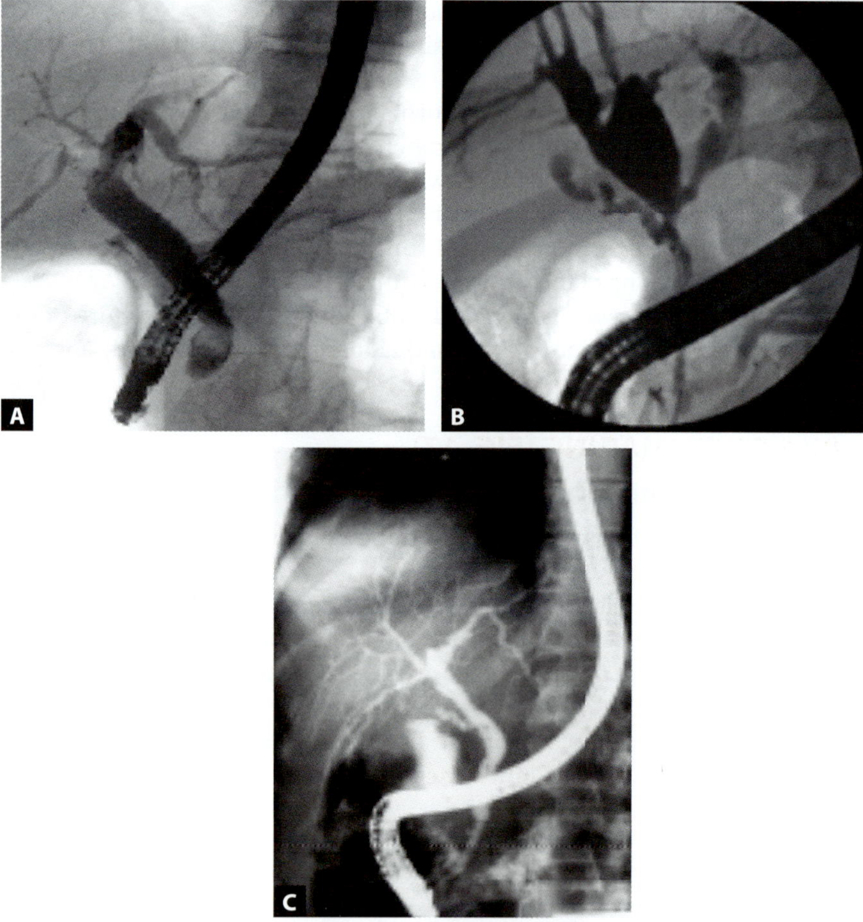

Figs. 18A to C: (A) Large stone common bile duct (CBD); (B) Hilar stricture; and (C) Cystic stump leak.

- *Bile duct strictures:*
    - *Benign postoperative strictures:* short and smooth
    - *Malignant stricture:* smooth or irregular stricture with upstream dilatation. This may be due to cancer of the bile duct, GB, pancreas, or nodes at the hilum
    - *Sclerosing cholangitis:* Multiple strictures and diffuse irregularity of the extra- and intrahepatic biliary system.
- *Parasites:* As linear filling defects
- *Liver parenchymal pathology:*
    - Crowded and tortuous intrahepatic ducts in cirrhosis
    - Irregular or displaced or splaying of ducts in space-occupying lesions
- *Bile leaks:* For example, postlaparoscopic cholecystectomy cystic duct stump leak
- Fistulous communications

UNDERSTANDING THE VARIOUS INTERVENTIONS PERFORMED DURING ERCP

Selective Cannulation (Fig. 19)

- Technique of cannulating the preferred duct for diagnosis and therapy
- Remember bile duct is at the 10 o'clock position and travels upward from right to left while the pancreatic duct is situated between the 1–3 o'clock position and courses horizontally and to the right
- There are two different approaches to achieve this feat, namely contrast-directed approach and guidewire-directed approach
- Guidewire approach is usually preferred.

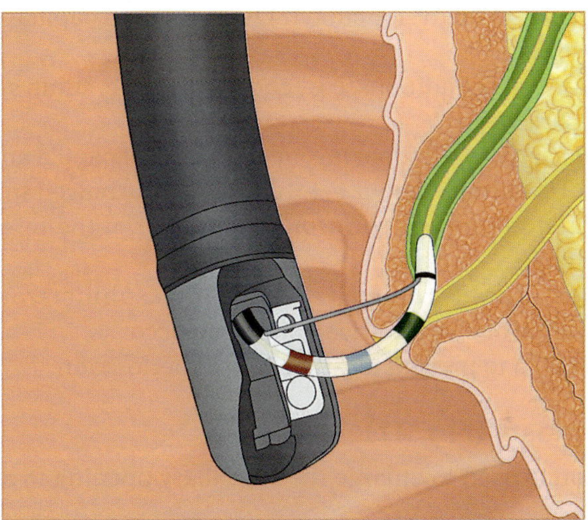

Fig. 19: Selective biliary cannulation.

Sphincterotomy (Fig. 20)

- Use the bow-like diathermy wire to cut and enlarge the ampullary opening at the desired place (10 o'clock for the bile duct and 2 o'clock for the pancreatic duct)
- Endocut mode is normally preferred wherein the cutting occurs with little pauses of coagulation thereby minimizing undue bleeding.
- Ensure the patient had INR checked before ERCP and received injection vitamin K 10 mg IV on the previous day (or frozen plasma in case of coagulopathy).
- Common indications for sphincterotomy are as follows:
  - Before removal of CBD stones
  - Facilitation of biliary stent placement for benign and malignant strictures

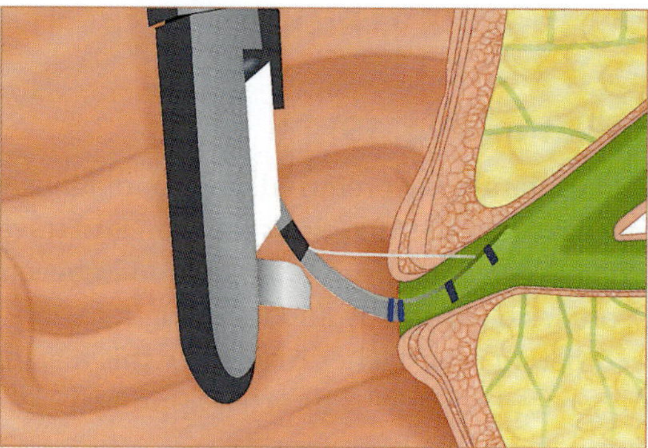

Fig. 20: Sphincterotomy.

  - Sphincter of Oddi dysfunction (SOD) or benign papillary stenosis
  - Biliary leaks
  - Miscellaneous conditions, e.g., choledochocele, sump syndrome, and biliary parasites
- *Size of sphincterotomy:* It depends on the shape of papilla and diameter of distal CBD. Usually, it is about 1–1.5 cm so that the bowed sphincterotome or an inflated biliary balloon would come out of the opening without much resistance.
- Use proper coated guidewire inside the sphincterotome during sphincterotomy or else electrical injury can occur.
- Care to be taken to prevent any bleeding or perforation.

Sphincteroplasty (Fig. 21)

- CRE balloon is used to enlarge the ampullary opening to aid removal of the stones.
- First do a small sphincterotomy and then insert the CRE balloon well inside the major papilla with one-third of the balloon projecting toward the duodenum.

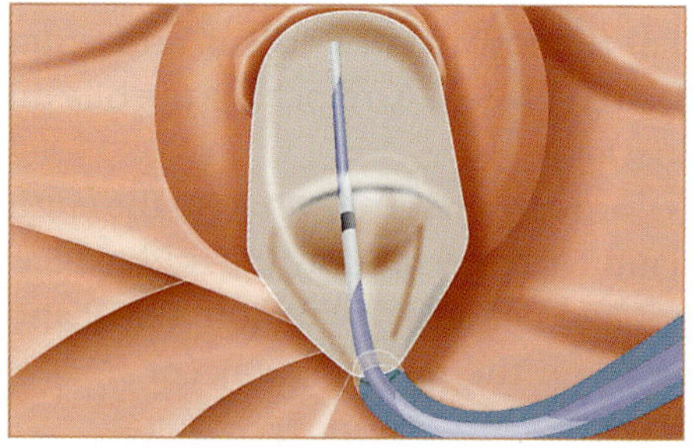

Fig. 21: Sphincteroplasty.

- Gently distend the balloon with the help of an inflation device to stretch the sphincter to the desired size dictated by the size of the proximal bile duct and the size of the stones.

Biliary Balloon Sweep (Fig. 22)

- Fogarty balloon is a simple safe and atraumatic way to remove biliary stones and sludge.
- Pass the guidewire-directed balloon deep inside the duct, inflate the balloon, and gently drag it out. All the sludge and stones below the distended balloon would be swept out to the duodenum.
- You could choose to perform a balloon occlusion cholangiogram to ascertain that all the debris has been cleared.

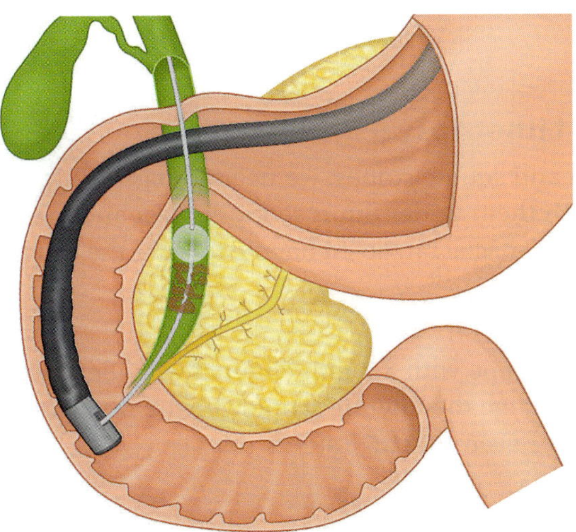

Fig. 22: Fogarty biliary balloon swipe.

Dormia Basketing (Fig. 23)

- The basket can be passed inside the duct and opened to grab the stones like a fish net and drag them out one by one starting from the lowest in the bile duct. Just jiggle the basket once it is inside the duct to trap the stone.
- Be patient and careful or else stone impaction may ensue and you will find it difficult to remove the basket out of the duct. Use a "Soehendra" lithotriptor when unexpected stone and basket impaction occurs during routine stone extraction and that is why it is often called the "lifesaver" to be kept in the ERCP room always.

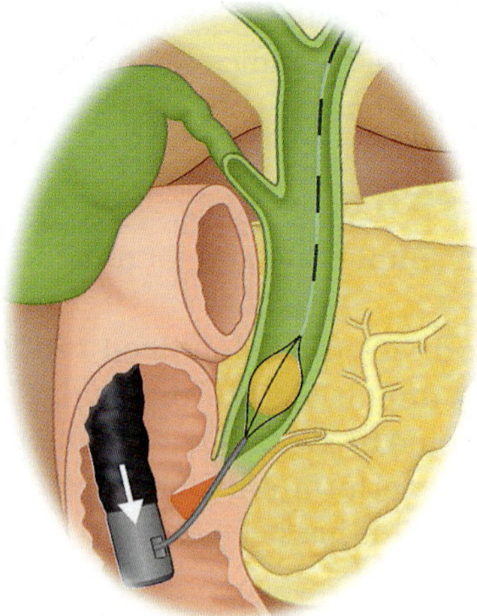

Fig. 23: Dormia basketing.

Mechanical Lithotripsy (Fig. 24)

For large hard and square stones, we need to pass the tough wired-guided baskets to catch them under fluoroscopy control and then pulverize them with the help of a special ratcheted handle to close the basket.

Stenting

Use of standard scope with 3.2 mm channel will allow placement of 5–7 F stent only while large therapeutic scope with 4.2 mm working channel will permit us to place even 10–11.5 F stents.

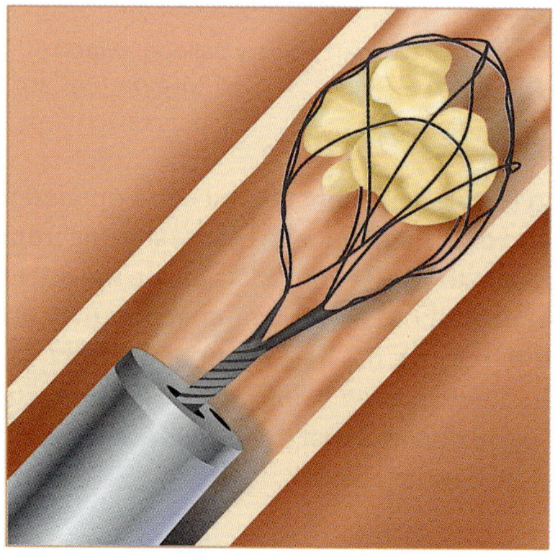

Fig. 24: Mechanical lithotripsy.

- *Plastic stents* **(Fig. 25)**:
  - Straight stents with flaps at the ends for anchorage or double or single pigtail catheters
  - Available in variable lengths from 6 to 15 cm
  - Be well versed with the stent release system composed of an inner guiding catheter and outer pushing tube passed over a 0.035 guidewires

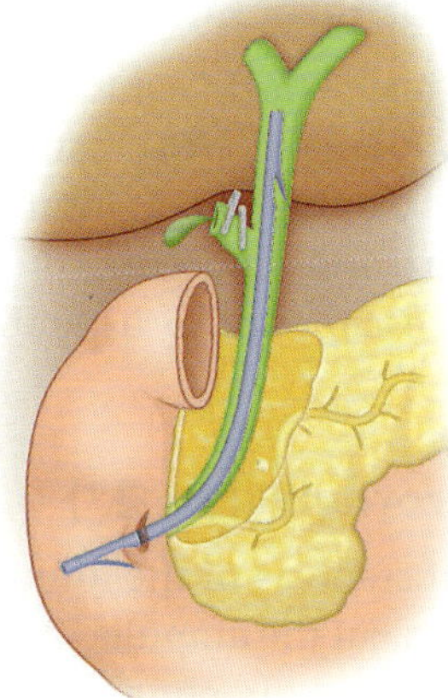

Fig. 25: Plastic stent.

- *Self-expandable metallic (SEM) stents* **(Fig. 26)**:
  - Covered versus uncovered
  - Sterile water or saline is initially injected to flush the system to minimize friction between the stent and the restraining sheath and

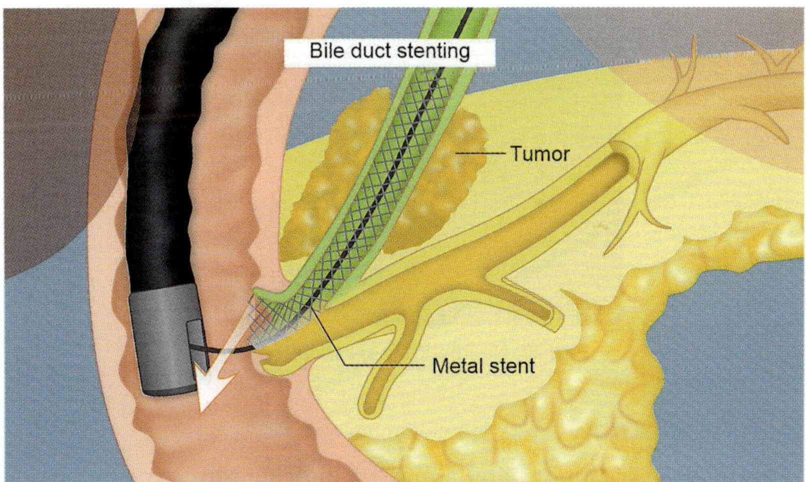

Fig. 26: Self-expandable metallic (SEM) stent.

to facilitate stent deployment. The whole system is placed over the guidewire and advanced through the obstruction. With the stent correctly positioned across the stricture, the overlying sheath is pulled back while the handle is held steadily to hold the guidewire in position. The stent is deployed slowly in a stepwise manner. Stent deployment can be monitored under fluoroscopic control using the radiopaque markers.

Nasobiliary Drainage Catheter Drainage

Pass a 0.035 guidewire deep inside the bile duct beyond any obstruction and then pass the 7 F nasobiliary drainage (NBD) catheter over it. Gently remove the scope and then pass a nasopharyngeal intubation tube and guide the NBD catheter to pass through it and come out of the nostril without any kinks. Check the position with fluoroscopy and by aspirating for bile. Then connect it to a drainage bag.

Needle-knife Sphincterotomy (Fig. 27)

It is indicated in the case of stenosis of the ampulla or impacted stone at ampulla. Use a needle knife to cut the ampulla like slicing a pear either from above downward in the presumed direction of the bile duct or from below upward. The risk of pancreatitis, bleeding, and perforation is higher with precut, so beware.

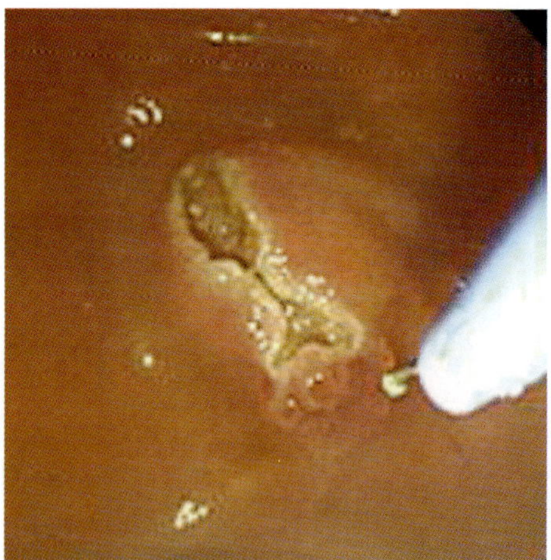

Fig. 27: Needle-knife sphincterotomy.

Minor Papillotomy

- Cannulation of minor papilla may be indicated in suspected cases of pancreas divisum causing recurrent attacks of pancreatitis

- Pancreas divisum is a congenital anatomic variant in which the ventral and dorsal pancreatic ducts fail to fuse. Minor papillotomy and stent insertion may be beneficial in preventing further attacks of pancreatitis.
- Minor papilla is usually cannulated in a long route position using a 3-mm fine metal tip cannula and then wire-guided sphincterotomy and stent insertion are done.

COMPLICATIONS OF ENDOSCOPIC RETROGRADE CHOLANGIOPANCREATOGRAPHY

Pancreatitis

- Transient post-ERCP hyperamylasemia can be of no clinical consequence.
- But serious pancreatitis could occur in cases such as difficult cannulation, precut papillotomy, overfilling of the pancreatic duct with contrast (parenchymogram), cases of the SOD, or in cases of pancreatic duct therapeutic interventions.

Cholangitis

- Due to an obstructed and undrained biliary system caused by stones or stricture, over injection of contrast, or using improperly disinfected scope and accessories
- Gram-negative bacilli such as *Escherichia coli, Klebsiella, Enterobacter, Proteus,* and *Pseudomonas*
- *Prevention:*
  - Always aspirate the biliary system before any contrast injection
  - Ensure wire-guided access to the proximal obstructed ducts before any injection of contrast
  - Avoid forceful or overfilling of proximal obstructed system
  - Prophylactic dose of antibiotic, e.g., IV cefotaxime

Bleeding

- In deviated or large cuts or in patients with coagulopathy
- Manage it by using an *occlusion balloon* for tamponade effect, injection of dilute adrenaline, *diathermy,* or even a hemoclip

Retroperitoneal Duodenal Perforation

- Due to deviated or excessive cuts at the papilla
- Retroperitoneal air better recognized by CT abdomen
- Mostly settle with conservative therapy

Stent Blockage

- Due to inspissated bile or infection and it is common when we use small caliber plastic stents.

- Consider stent exchange after 3–4 months in case of 10 F plastic stents used for palliation in case of malignant jaundice or else consider SEM stent.

Stent Migration

Inside the bile or pancreatic duct is a challenging complication to tackle use of rat-toothed forceps under fluoroscopy or SpyGlass system may be needed to retrieve such stents.

CONCLUSION

Endoscopic retrograde cholangiopancreatography is essentially a therapeutic modality for various pancreatic and biliary disorders. With proper training, one should be able to achieve a high cannulation rate and clinical success. Tools, teamwork, and temperament are paramount for success.

SUGGESTED READING

1. ASGE Standards of Practice Committee; Faulx AL, Lightdale JR, Acosta RD, Agrawal D, Bruining DH, et al. Guidelines for privileging, credentialing, and proctoring to perform GI endoscopy. Gastrointest Endosc. 2017;85(2):273-81. Erratum in: Gastrointest Endosc. 2017;85(5):1115.
2. ASGE Standards of Practice Committee; Maple JT, Ben-Menachem T, Anderson MA, Appalaneni V, Banerjee S, et al. The role of endoscopy in the evaluation of suspected choledocholithiasis. Gastrointest Endosc. 2010;71(1):1-9.
3. Elmunzer BJ, Scheiman JM, Lehman GA, Chak A, Mosler P, Higgins PD, et al. A randomized trial of rectal indomethacin to prevent post-ERCP pancreatitis. N Engl J Med. 2012;366(15):1414-22.
4. Freeman ML, Nelson DB, Sherman S, Haber GB, Herman ME, Dorsher PJ, et al. Complications of endoscopic biliary sphincterotomy. N Engl J Med. 1996;335(13):909-18.
5. Frossard JL, Morel PM. Detection and management of bile duct stones. Gastrointest Endosc. 2010;72:808-16.
6. Peery AF, Crockett SD, Barritt AS, Dellon ES, Eluri S, Gangarosa LM, et al. Burden of Gastrointestinal, Liver, and Pancreatic Diseases in the United States. Gastroenterology. 2015;149(7):1731-41.e3.
7. Rogers SJ, Cello JP, Horn JK, Siperstein AE, Schecter WP, Campbell AR, et al. Prospective randomized trial of LC+LCBDE vs ERCP/S+LC for common bile duct stone disease. Arch Surg. 2010;145(1):28-33.
8. Sun SX, Kulaylat AN, Hollenbeak CS, Soybel DI. Cost-effective Decisions in Detecting Silent Common Bile Duct Gallstones During Laparoscopic Cholecystectomy. Ann Surg. 2016;263(6):1164-72.
9. Teoh AYB, Cheung FKY, Hu B, Pan YM, Lai LH, Chiu PWY, et al. Randomized trial of endoscopic sphincterotomy with balloon dilation versus endoscopic sphincterotomy alone for removal of bile duct stones. Gastroenterology. 2013;144(2):341-45.e1.

Expert's Comment

Endoscopic retrograde cholangiopancreatography (ERCP) remains an essential tool in the surgical management of pancreatobiliary disorders. While initially developed as a diagnostic modality, ERCP has transitioned into a highly specialized therapeutic procedure, complementing—and often replacing—traditional surgical interventions in selected cases. It is a highly skilled procedure with a steep learning curve. A structured training program under expert guidance is essential before any endoscopist starts doing ERCP. For obvious reasons, surgeons have an advantage in learning the technique. The knowledge of anatomy and electrosurgical biophysics, adoptability, capacity to take quick decisions, and ability to handle a complication are some distinct advantages for surgeons to learn.

Endoscopic retrograde cholangiopancreatography offers minimally invasive access to the biliary and pancreatic ducts via a side-viewing duodenoscope, allowing real-time fluoroscopic visualization and therapeutic manipulation. Common surgical indications include choledocholithiasis, obstructive jaundice, biliary strictures (benign or malignant), bile leaks, and stent placement pre- or postoperatively. In the acute setting, ERCP can be life-saving in managing ascending cholangitis or postoperative biliary complications.

Understanding ERCP's capabilities and limitations is crucial for surgical planning, particularly when considering timing, coordination with endoscopists, or deciding between endoscopic, laparoscopic, or open approaches. Despite its minimally invasive nature, ERCP carries risks—including post-ERCP pancreatitis, bleeding, and perforation—necessitating careful patient selection and interdisciplinary collaboration.

As hepatopancreatobiliary care becomes increasingly multimodal, the surgeon's familiarity with ERCP enhances decision-making, facilitates timely intervention, and ultimately improves patient outcomes.

I congratulate Dr Easwaramoorthy, a champion among surgeon endoscopists for bringing out this valuable book. I am confidant that, like his earlier books, this will immensely help the readers to improve their understanding on various aspects of endoscopy, including therapeutic procedures.

Dr G Siddesh
Mysuru

CHAPTER 15

Top 10 Tips for Setting up an Endoscopy Unit

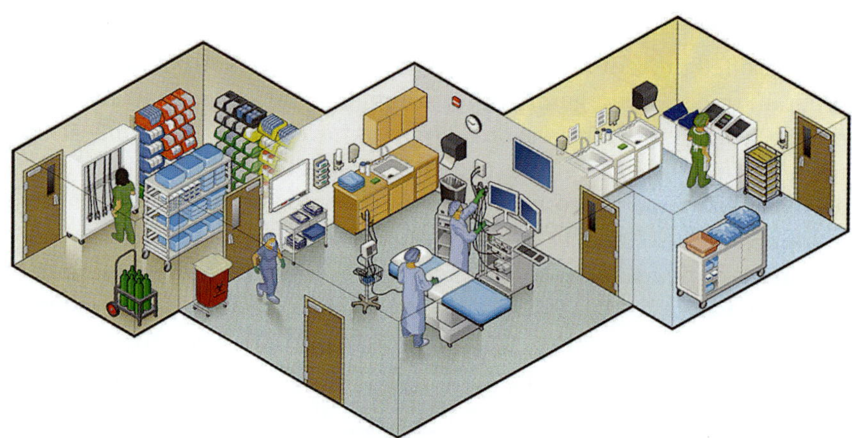

Chapter Outline

1. Ensure Sound Basics in Your Endoscopy Techniques
2. Improve Your Level of Endoscopy Training from Basic to Advanced
3. Acquire Good High-definition (HD) Endoscopes
4. Upgrade Your Endoscopy Suite
5. Identify and Train Your Staffs
6. Array of Accessories is Your Asset
7. Recording and Documentation
8. Focus Your Training and Accreditation
9. Obtain Appropriate Training Credentials
10. Importance of Associates and Association

Keywords: HD endoscopy, ergonomics in endoscopy, endoscopic accessories, template for endoscopy report

1. ENSURE SOUND BASICS IN YOUR ENDOSCOPY TECHNIQUES

- Ensure you always maintain a strict routine during your endoscopy procedures (preendoscopic rituals)
  - *Equipment checklist:* Check your endoscopic equipment to ensure they are in perfect condition and ready for use (*cockpit drill*)

- *Patient checklist*: Check your patient to know the indication for the endoscopic procedure, his/her comorbid conditions, drug history, previous bowel surgery, etc.
- Obtain *written informed consent* for the procedure after giving sufficient information regarding the procedure (provide well-written information leaflet in his/her language)
  - Remember the pneumonic "WHO" for obtaining consent:
    - *W*hy do we recommend endoscopy?
    - *H*ow do we perform?
    - *O*utcome: Benefits/risks/alternatives/what happens next, etc.
- *Systematic endoscopic examination:*
  - Be ambidextrous with the left hand holding the control head and the right hand holding the insertion section
  - Wheel movements, the torque of the scope, and your body movement determine the navigation of the endoscope tip
  - Ergonomics is essential for endoscopy. Ensure monitors are in the right place and at the right height.
- *Ensure safety during endoscopy procedure:*
  - Vigilance during the whole procedure
  - Administer nasal O_2
  - ECG/pulse oximeter
  - Have an anesthetist in selected cases
  - Access to defibrillator/resuscitation team
  - Proper disinfection of endoscopes and accessories
    - Manual or machine reprocessing of the endoscope
    - Enforce universal precaution by staff during endoscopy

2. IMPROVE YOUR LEVEL OF ENDOSCOPY TRAINING FROM BASIC TO ADVANCED

- Endoscopy training can be divided into levels 1, 2, and 3
- Level 1 training (basic) means the surgeon can perform diagnostic gastroscopy, colonoscopy, and simple therapeutic interventions such as foreign body (FB) removal and banding. The Endoscopy Fellowship of Indian Association of Gastrointestinal Endosurgeons (EFIAGES) by Indian Association of Gastrointestinal Endosurgeons (IAGES) and STEP 1 of Association of Surgeons of India (ASI) are classical examples.
- Level 2 training (advanced) means the surgeon is expected to perform more advanced therapeutic procedures such as dilatation, polypectomy, stent deployment, and percutaneous endoscopic gastrostomy (PEG) tube insertion. In addition, he/she could also perform basic endoscopic retrograde cholangiopancreatography (ERCP) procedures such as bile duct cannulation, sphincterotomy, and stenting. The Fellowship in

Advanced Gastrointestinal Endoscopy (FAGIE) colonoscopy course and FAGIE ERCP courses by IAGES and STEP 2 by ASI are seen as examples.

- Level 3 training means the surgeon is capable of performing more advanced procedures like advanced ERCP procedures like biliary self-expandable metal (SEM) stenting, pancreatic cannulation, and minor duct cannulation, and also procedures like endoscopic mucosal resection (EMR), endoscopic submucosal dissection (ESD), and peroral endoscopic myotomy (POEM). This level of training would require more time and dedication from the trainees and passionate trainers to guide them as well.

3. ACQUIRE GOOD HIGH-DEFINITION ENDOSCOPES (FIG. 1)

- High-definition (HD) endoscopes like Olympus CV 170, CV 190, CV 290/ Pentax i5000 and i7000/Fujinon EPK-4440 HD are essential for executing more advanced procedures with expertise.
- Unlike standard definition (SD) endoscopes, HD endoscope gives us sharper, more vivid, and colorful endoscopic images. Pristine pictures are due to more pixels in such HD endoscopes **(Fig. 2)**.

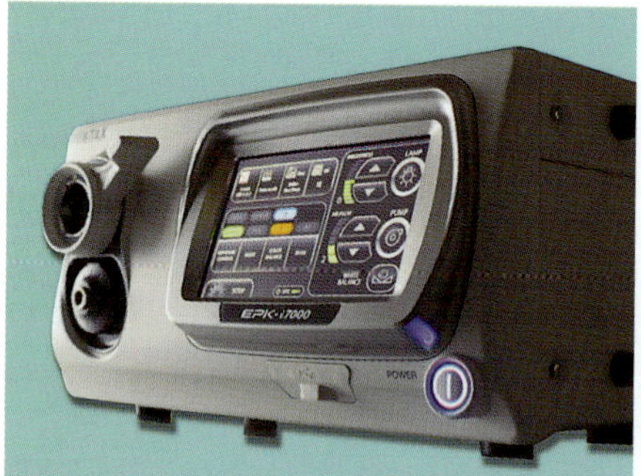

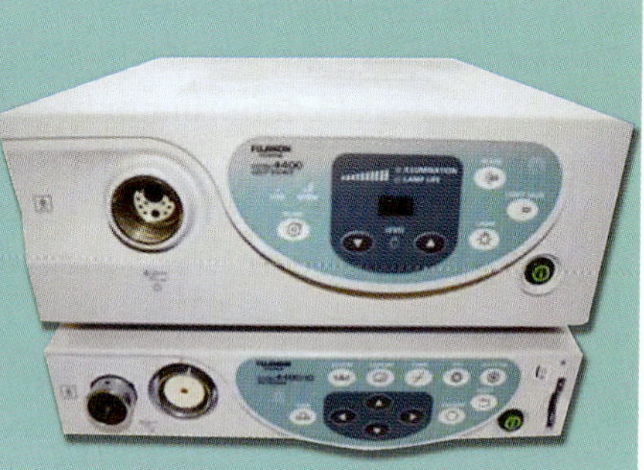

Fig. 1: High-definition (HD) endoscopes.

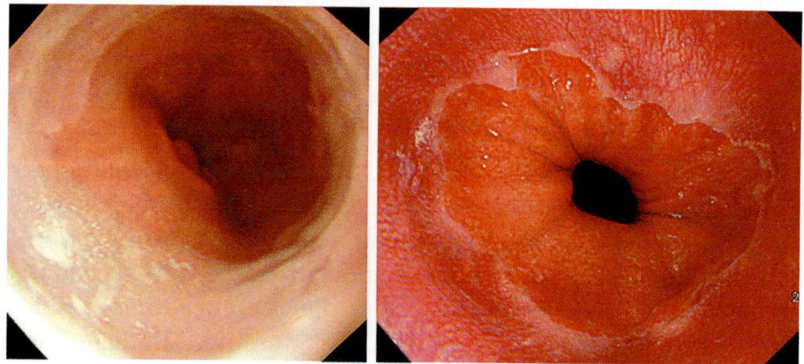

Fig. 2: Standard definition (SD) and high-definition (HD) endoscopes.

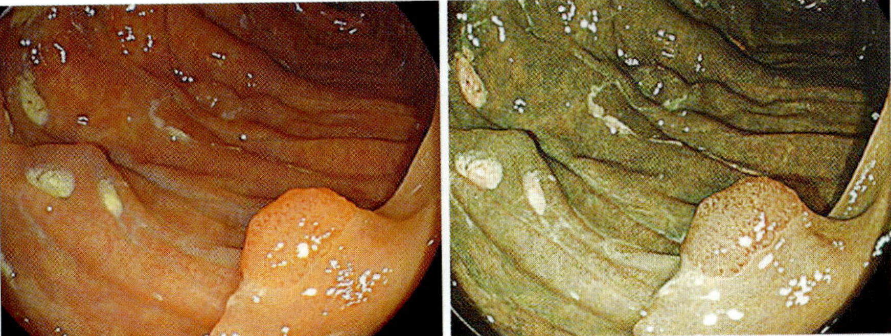

Fig. 3: Conventional and narrow-band imaging in colonic polyps.

- Ensure you also possess appropriate HD monitors and recording devices to enjoy the high-resolution output **(Fig. 3)**
- Magnification endoscopy and image contrast techniques are additional features that greatly improve your diagnostic and therapeutic capability and hence you are:
  - Able to detect "early" lesions/subtle changes
  - Able to make more "accurate" diagnosis
  - Able to perform a targeted biopsy of the suspected area

4. UPGRADE YOUR ENDOSCOPY SUITE

Features in an ideal colonoscopy suite:

- Size is at least 6 × 6 m or more
- Wide sliding doors for easy access and exit
- Centrally placed endoscope table with provision for C-arm imaging
- Compact tower trolley for endoscopes and its video processor with the light source
- Place for energy sources like diathermy/laser/argon plasma
- Monitors on ceiling-mounted pendants are preferable.
- C-arm facility or Scopeguide (preferable)
- Anesthesia workstation (optional)
- Central O_2 and suction and handwash
- Area for computer with recording and printing facility
- Storage cabinets for accessories
- Telephone and intercom facility
- Properly hidden cables and wires
- Ideal to have separate and dedicated endoscopy, colonoscopy, and ERCP rooms **(Figs. 4 to 6)**.

*Recovery area **(Fig. 7)**:*

- Located close to the endoscopy procedure room and also waiting area
- For immediate monitoring with pulse oximeter

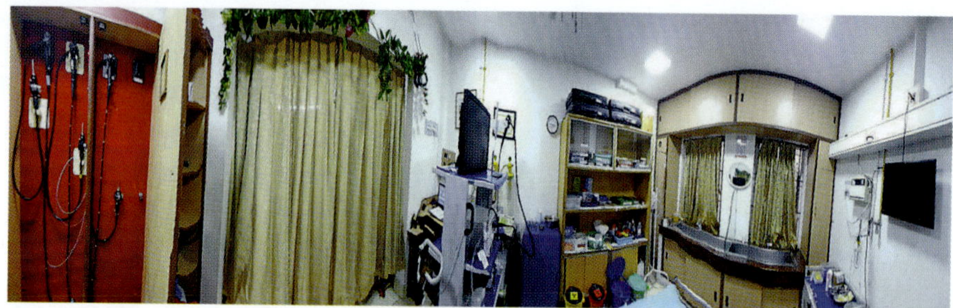

Fig. 4: Panoramic view of endoscopic room.

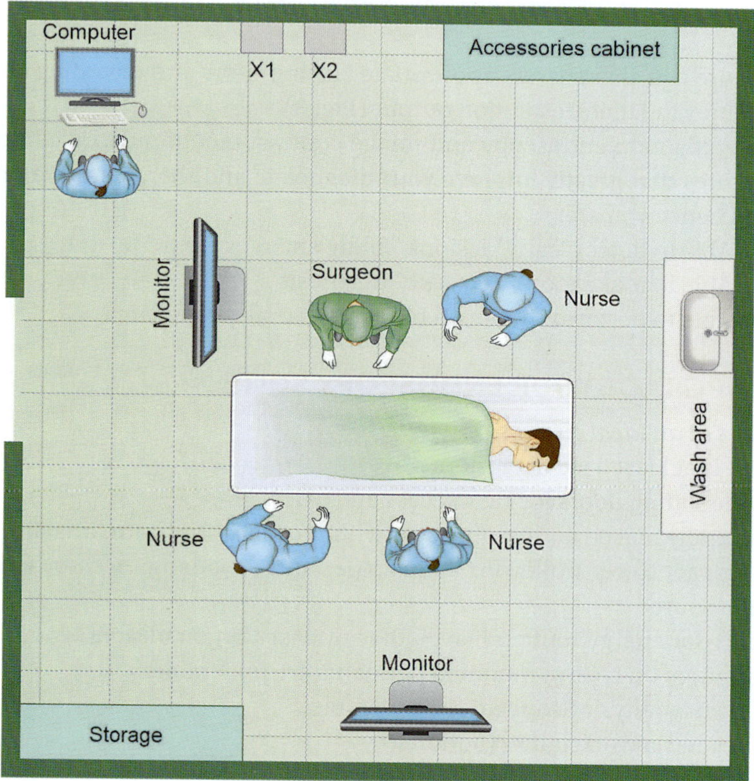

Fig. 5: Colonoscopy room layout.

- Provision of O_2 and suction
- Keep the movable crash cart with the defibrillator
- Facility to change dress
- Able to bring in relatives to discuss findings

Cleaning and disinfection area/storage area **(Fig. 8)**:

- Area for leak test and decontamination of scope
- Endoscope wash area with a sink

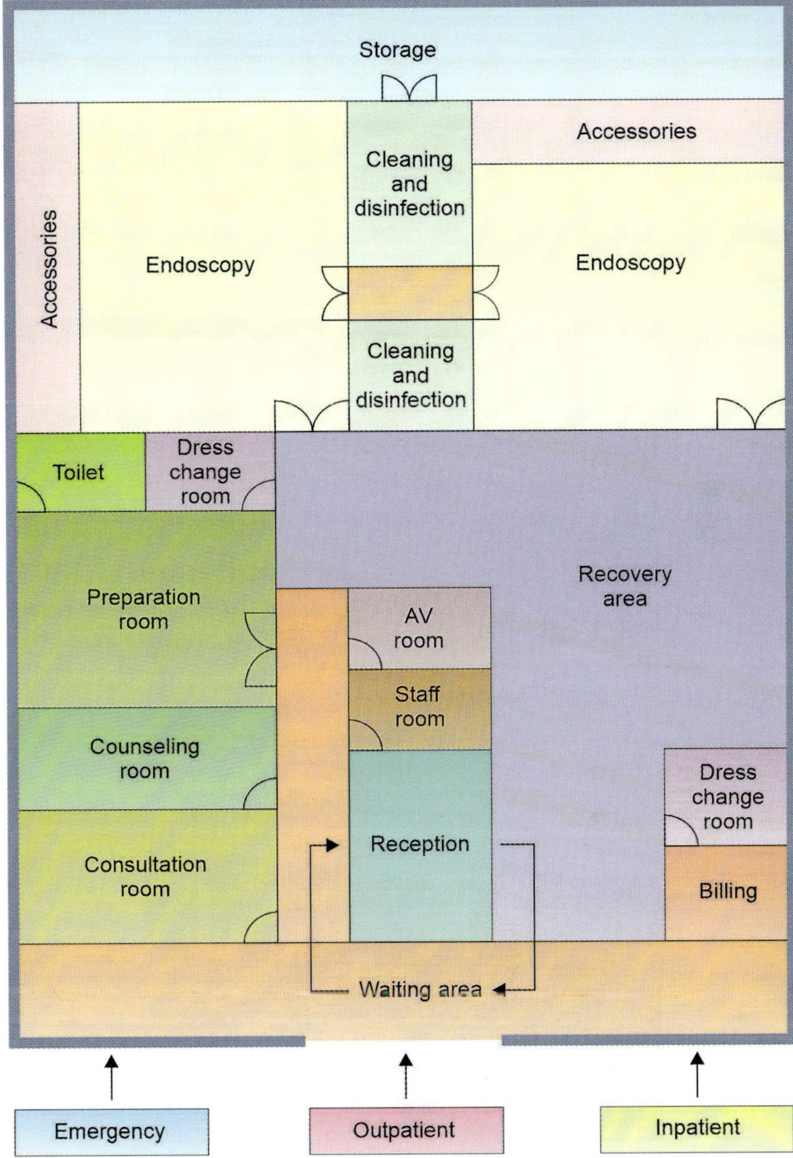

Fig. 6: Endoscopy suite layout.

- Sluice sink to drain all effluents
- *Disinfection:* Manual or machine (automatic endoscope reprocessor)
- Storage of scopes in well-ventilated and spacious cabinets
- *Accessories:* Properly labeled and stored in the cabinets under various categories
    - Biopsy forceps
    - Various sizes of snares

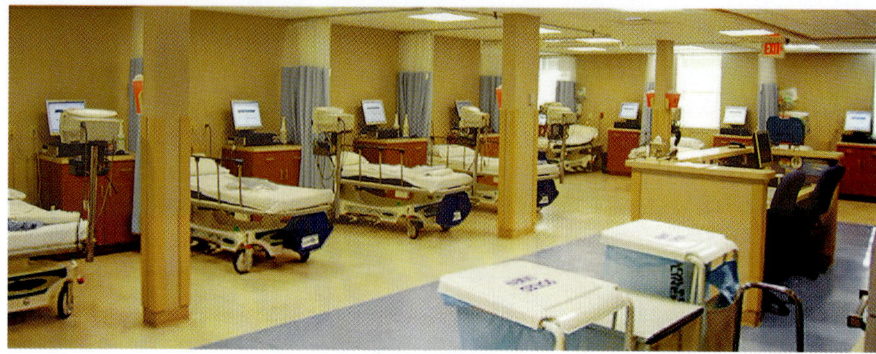

Fig. 7: Recovery area.

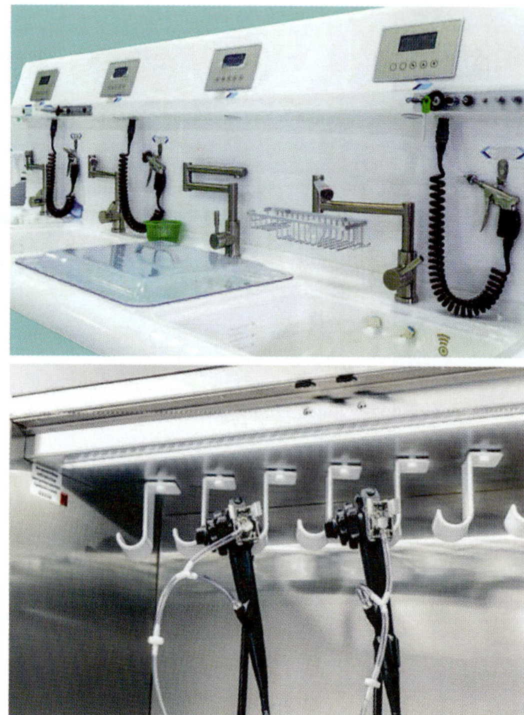

Fig. 8: Cleaning and disinfection and storage area.

- Hemostatic devices
- ESD devices
- FB removal devices
- Dilatation kits

- Either disposable or reprocessed using ethylene oxide (ETO) and ready for use **(Fig. 9)**

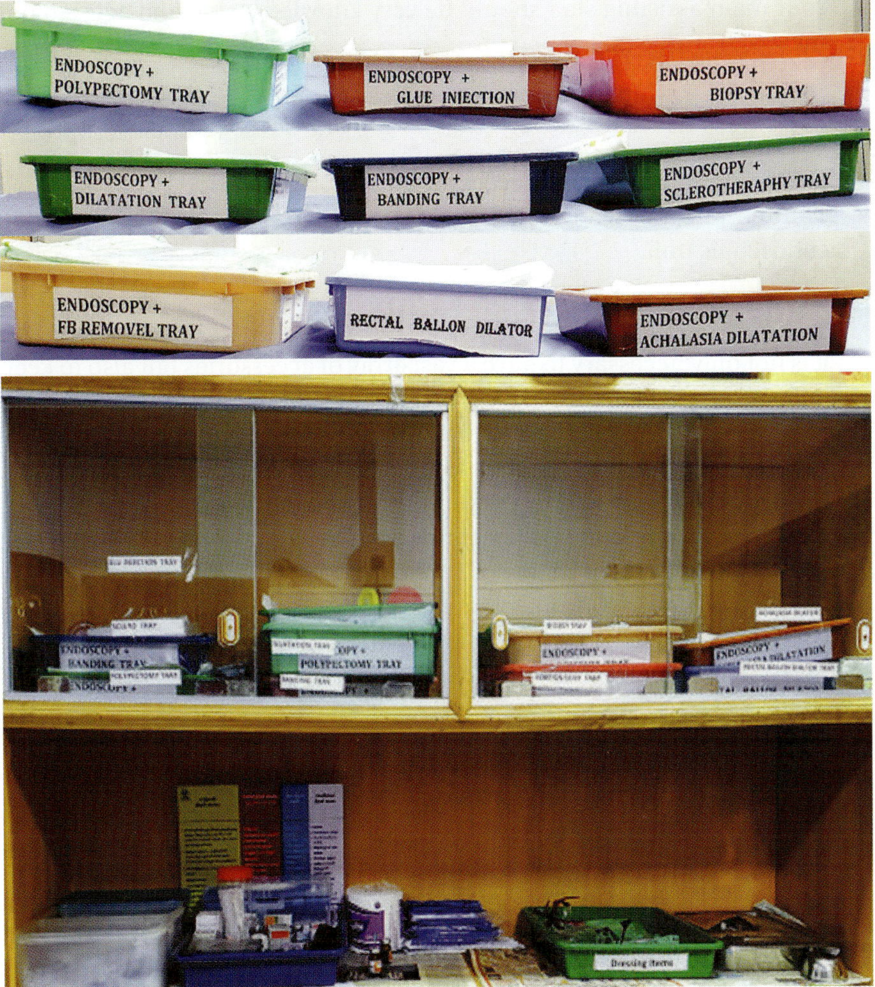

Fig. 9: Accessories in labeled trays.

5. IDENTIFY AND TRAIN YOUR STAFFS

- Ensure you have an adequate number of well-trained staff with clearly designated roles
- Even for simple diagnostic endoscopy, you would require 2–3 staffs for smooth conduct of the procedure
    - To monitor the vital signs and to restrain the patient and also to administer any drugs if needed
    - Assist you with appropriate accessories
    - Help to take pictures and report printouts

- Your main assisting staff should be very knowledgeable and agile so he/she:
  - Ably assists
  - Actively communicates
  - Anticipates
  - Arrange all the needed accessories
- Trained and dedicated staff are the biggest assets of any advanced endoscopic unit.

6. ARRAY OF ACCESSORIES IS YOUR ASSET

- It is not only necessary to have a vast array of accessories but also to keep them arranged in an orderly manner in individual properly labeled trays. This will ensure easy access to them in case of any emergency.
- Periodic checking of the accessories for their working conditions is important and it should be the routine for your endoscopy unit staff.
  - *Example:* The snare polypectomy tray should have **(Fig. 10)**
    - Various sizes of snares
    - 23 G 210 cm long injection needles
    - *Polyp retrieval forceps:* Roth Net and 3 or 5-prong forceps
    - Hemoclip application and clips

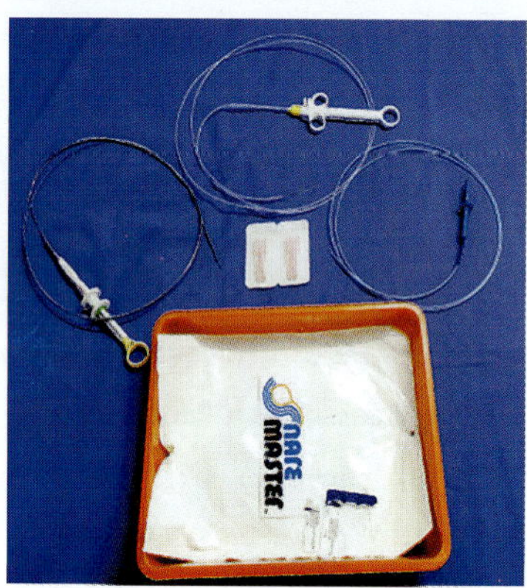

Fig. 10: Snare polypectomy tray.

7. RECORDING AND DOCUMENTATION (FIG. 11)

Endoscopic recording has come a long way since Rudolph Schindler employed an artist to paint watercolor pictures of the endoscopy images, he saw through his semiflexible gastroscope. One picture is equal to a thousand words. So, like radiologists, we should be also able to vividly describe what we see with the endoscope and be able to make the diagnosis and plan treatment. With the advent of video endoscopy, image capture software, and video recorders,

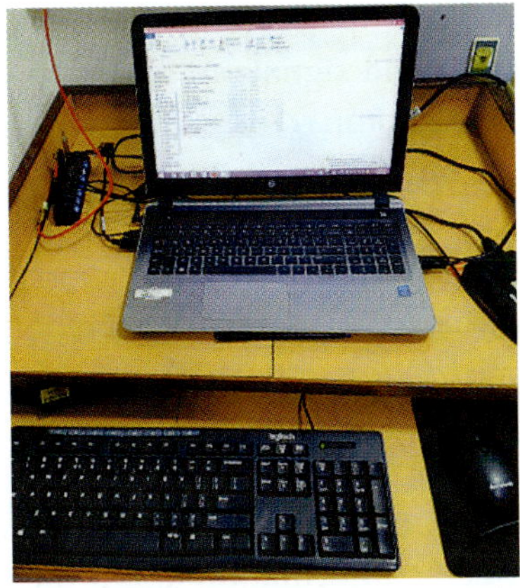

Fig. 11: Recording and documentation.

now endoscopic recording and documentation are becoming relatively easy and very essential aspects in everyday endoscopic practice.

We should understand the purpose and real benefits of endoscopic recording and documentation. We can collect the image data, analyze, annotate, validate, and then store the image and video files for the following reasons:

Benefits of recording and documentation:

- It facilitates continuity of patient care
- To communicate with colleagues, junior staff, and nurses
- It helps to teach the trainees with image atlas and master videos
- It becomes an important piece of document in the following situations:
    - Medicolegal proceedings
    - Insurance claims
    - As a marker of quality assurance [National Accreditation Board for Hospitals (NABH)]

Requirements for ideal endoscopy recording and documentation:

- Invest in a user-friendly image capture software
- Use standardized image terminology
- Custom-designed and well-structured template for the report

Image capture software:

- Key 10 steps of image capturing process
    1. Illumination by xenon/halogen light transmission
    2. Surface reflectance and magnification
    3. Reflected light is focused by the objective lens onto the charge-coupled device (CCD)
    4. CCD conversion of the reflected light to an electrical signal (photons to electrons)

5. Transfer of electrical signal through image guide cables
6. Reconstruction of the signals to an image in the processor unit (electrons back to photons)
7. Projection of the image onto an HD/SD monitor
8. Transfer of image data to the computer software
9. Image capturing, manipulation, annotation, and storage
10. Retrieval of the image data for writing a report on a template

- *Basic aspects of image capture software:*
  - There are plenty of endoscopy reporting software available in the market. Most of them use Digital Imaging and Communications in Medicine (DICOM) technology. DICOM is a standard for imaging that contains very specific information about the images, as well as the images themselves.
  - Image formats include bitmap (BMP), Joint Photographic Experts Group (JPEG)
  - Video formats include Moving Picture Experts Group (MPEG) MPEG1, MPEG2, MPEG4, Audio Video Interleave (AVI), and Windows Media Video (WMV)
  - Image and video storage sites include computer hard drives, universal serial bus (USB) storage devices ("memory stick"), conventional digital video disk, external hard drives, or offsite servers ("cloud")
  - If possible, link the Image and video data to the hospital patient management system software
  - Choose software that can store in HD format, has faster data transfer capacity, and provisions for compression of data.
- *Additional benefits of image capture software:*
  - Store both static image data and video files for future reference
  - Ability to do editing of video and image files, annotation, and voice addition
  - To make a hard copy on a CD for the patient and e-mail the data
  - Easy retrieval of patient clinical data for any future research
  - Options to overlay the patient data on images and videos allow you to brand yourself
  - Images can be simultaneously captured while the videos are getting recorded with the help of a foot switch and the captured images can be pushed to PowerPoint presentations.
  - Image and video editing tools to add annotations help the user to export the edited data to a DVD/Pen drive **(Fig. 12)**.

Standardized image terminology:

- Across the world, the same lesion should be described in the same way and should carry the same meaning.

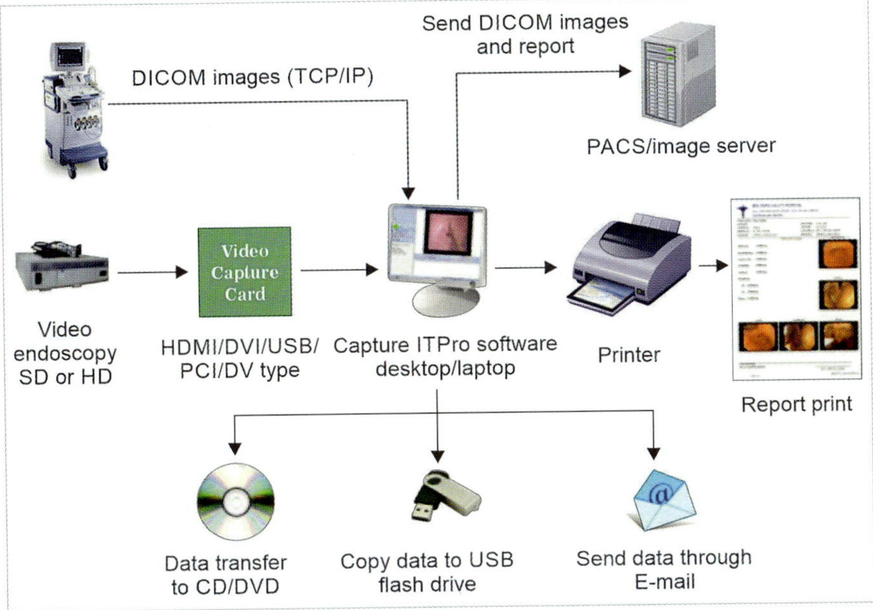

Fig. 12: Report processing.

- The World Organization of Digestive Endoscopy (OMED) initiated efforts to standardize endoscopic image reporting
- Minimal standard terminology (MST) has been endorsed by US and European endoscopic societies.
- Software developers should utilize these universally acceptable descriptive terminologies while designing a report.
- Also, we should not hesitate to write in the natural language in the text blocks rather than pointing and clicking some improper or confusing terminology from the menu.

Custom-made structured report format:

- It should be clear, concise, and easy to comprehend
- We should design separate templates for upper gastrointestinal (GI) endoscopy, colonoscopy, ERCP, and so on.
- Easy to use, fully customizable PDF/word base reports with prefilled fields and respective libraries help the end user generate quick reports
- Hospital logo, name, and address details along with surgeon's digital signature integration possibilities
- *It should contain the following data and images:*
    - *Pre-endoscopy documentation by nurses:*
        - Patient demographics
        - Vital signs
        - Antibiotics and sedation dosage and timing

    - Clinical diagnosis
    - Type of procedure
    - Name of endoscopist and assistants
    - Anesthesia
    - Indication for the procedure
    - Model of the instrument and accessories used
    - Extent of examination
  - *Details about the procedure:*
    - Time in and time out from the endoscopy suite, etc.
    - Template of various endoscopy procedure stations and findings
  - Postprocedure dietary and drug advice
  - Ample number of images
  - Diagnosis
  - *Any intervention done:* Biopsy/dilatation, etc.
  - *Advice:*
    - Regarding any further investigation
    - Timing and need for any surgical intervention
    - Postprocedure dietary and drug advice

Aim for a structured image documentation:

- Include a patient photo for authenticity
- Incorporate the picture showing the pathology
- Annotate the lesion if possible
- Include important images with negative findings
  - *To document the completion of the procedure:*
    - Ileocecal valve in colonoscopy
    - Ampulla of Vater in upper GI endoscopy
  - To reassure about remission of disease
  - Anastomotic areas to show the absence of any recurrent tumor

Sample endoscopy report ***(Fig. 13)****:*

Future developments in image capture and documentation:

- *Tele endoscopy:*
  - Real-time streaming by the distant observer or
  - Record the procedure and then upload it later for expert opinion
- Automated analysis and reporting by the computer (like blood and ECG reports)
- Endoscopy can recognize lesions and even initiate therapy automatically.

To conclude, image management systems are becoming an integral part of endoscopy units. Choose software that is user-friendly for entering patient data, recording and transferring image and video files, and preparing patient reports in a standardized format in quick time.

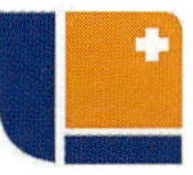

Lotus Hospital and Research Centre Limited
Poondurai Main Road, Erode-638 002, Ph: +91 9750028328
Dept. of Gastro Enterology-Dr. S. Easwaramoorthy MS FRCS (LON) FRCS (Gas) FRCS (Edin)

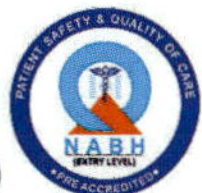

Patient Name: XYZ	
Contact #:	**Age/Gender:** 76 Yrs, Male
Hospital ID: 472011	**Visit Date:** 03/03/2025
Referred Dr:	**Consulted Dr:** Dr. S. Easwaramoorthy
Procedure: Endoscopy	**Medication:** Local 10% Xylocaine Spray

Under Xylocaine Spray

Diagnostic Images

Medication : 10% Xylocaine Spray
Esophagus : Normal
OG Junction at : Lax OG Junction Hill type 2
Hiatus hernia : Absent
Stomach : Distal erosive Gastritis, 1 cm polypoidal lesion @ cardia
Cardia : 1 cm polypoidal lesion
Fundus : Normal
Body : Normal
Pylorus : Erosive gastritis
D1 : Normal
D2 : Normal
Ampulla : Normal

Final Impression : GERD-Lax OG Junction Hill type 2
Distal erosive Gastritis
1 cm polypoidal lesion @ cardia

Additional Procedure Done : RUT-Negative

Advice : Snare polypectomy

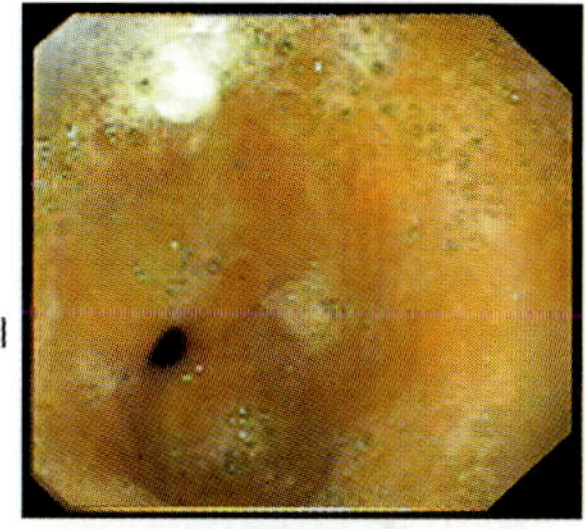

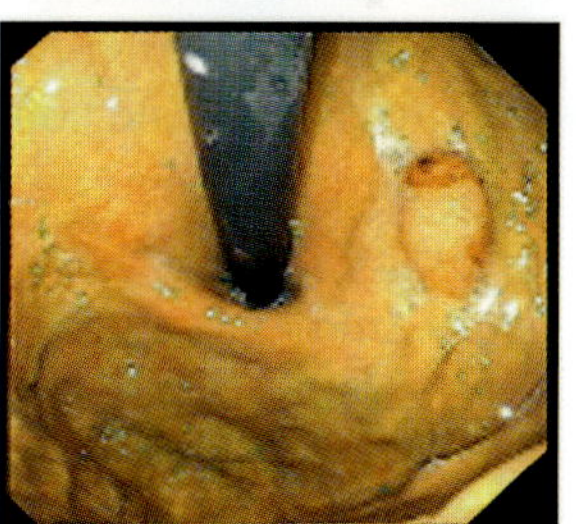

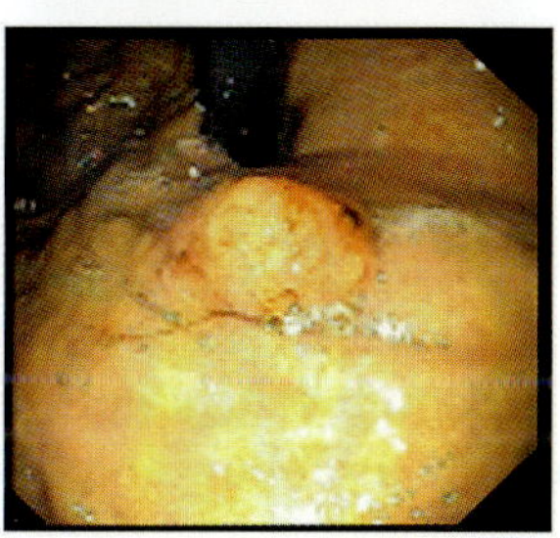

Fig. 13: Report format.

8. FOCUS YOUR TRAINING AND ACCREDITATION

- No incision. Endoscopic interventions would impress the patient group
- Even during laparoscopic surgery, endoscopy skills are essential in certain situations like:
    - Preoperative tattooing of polyp site or intraoperative colonoscopy in case of colectomy for colonic polyps

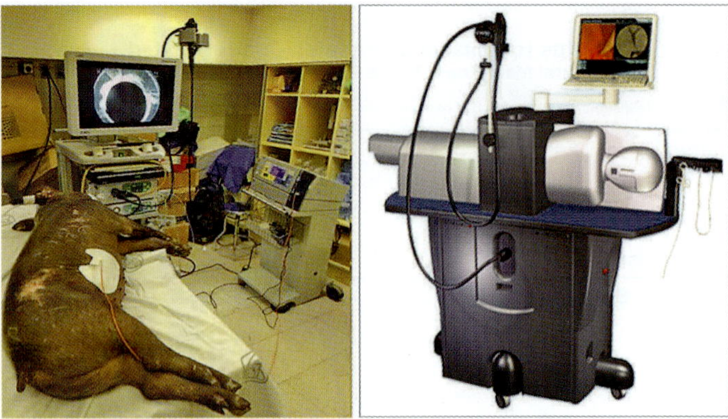

Fig. 14: Virtual and live simulators.

- Intraoperative endoscopy for obscure GI bleeding, etc. and cases of laparoscopic Heller's myotomy

- Akin to laparoscopy, endoscopy is also a rapidly expanding and exciting field with the potential for various therapeutic interventional procedures.
- Hence, we should concentrate our energy and spend time in certain areas of therapeutic endoscopy.
- ESD and endoscopic ultrasound (EUS) need specialized training provided you anticipate that you have enough volume to acquire the skill and able to pass through the learning curve swiftly and safely.
- Long-duration fellowship training is ideal but may not be feasible for all.
- Virtual simulation with GI mentor (Simbionix), live animal training, animal tissue training, and cadaveric training could shorten your learning curve and also would help us in skill assessment **(Fig. 14)**.

9. OBTAIN APPROPRIATE TRAINING CREDENTIALS

- We need not have negative thoughts and doubt whether we are legally permitted to perform endoscopy or colonoscopy.
- Let us follow the undermentioned points to successfully face any medicolegal battle
- The surgical postgraduate curriculum contains a syllabus of endoscopy and colonoscopy
- Following your postgraduation in surgery, attend hands-on certified courses to improve your knowledge and skills. We should obtain appropriate certification for all the training. Before performing any advanced procedure, ensure that you are competent to perform the procedure safely and effectively. You should have the manpower and materials to help you to accomplish the feat efficiently.

- Keep all the proof of your training credentials
- Document all the endoscopy procedures and outcomes for regular audit and self-improvement. Mention how many cases are done alone/under the supervision of a mentor/or assisting your senior. Also, keep a record of morbidity and mortality.
- Video record all the endoscopy procedures and save interesting and rare cases for future reference and presentations
- Always keep a copy of any journal article on endoscopy or colonoscopy topic written by you for future reference.
- We should never hesitate to seek senior help in case of any difficult case or complication following any procedure.

10. IMPORTANCE OF ASSOCIATES AND ASSOCIATION

- It always helps to be a member of various academic associations for endoscopic training. We should also be in constant touch with our mentors to seek their advice regarding any problem cases and before acquiring expensive equipment.
- IAGES is a large laparoscopic and endoscopic association with close to 12,000 members and is currently having several endoscopy fellowship programs for the benefit of its members, namely:
  - *EFIAGES:* Endoscopy fellowship of IAGES (basic endoscopy)
  - *FAGIE:* Fellowship in advanced gastrointestinal endoscopy
    - FAGIE ERCP course
    - FAGIE colonoscopy course
- Society of Gastrointestinal Endoscopy of India (SGEI)
- Indian Society of Gastroenterology (ISG)
- *Association of Surgeons of India (ASI):* STEP 1, 2, and 3 endoscopy training courses
- *Overseas affiliation:* ASGE/ESGE/SAGES, etc.
- Also join various discussion forums by these academic bodies to share and improve our knowledge and expertise.

CONCLUSION

Endoscopy training is not just optional but essential for every practicing surgeon. The diagnostic and therapeutic potentials of endoscopy are well-known and associated with very minimal morbidity. It is our moral and ethical obligation to train ourselves in all three modalities, namely open surgery, laparoscopy, and endoscopy so that we will enable us to make appropriate treatment choices for our patients.

There is no scope without a scope.

SUGGESTED READING

1. Adler DG, Hilden K, Wills JC, Quinney E, Fang JC. What drives US gastroenterology fellows to pursue academic vs. non-academic careers?: Results of a national survey. Am J Gastroenterol. 2010;105(6):1220-3.
2. American College of Gastroenterology Executive and Practice Management Committee. Ensuring competence in Endoscopy. [online] Available from https://www.asge.org/docs/default-source/education/practice_guidelines/doc-competence.pdf?sfvrsn=6 [Last accessed April, 2025].
3. ASGE Technology Committee. High-definition and high-magnification endoscopes. Gastrointest Endosc. 2014;80(6):919-27.
4. Atkinson M, Schmulewitz N. Downstream hospital charges generated from endoscopic ultrasound procedures are greater than those from colonoscopies. Clin Gastroenterol Hepatol. 2009;7:862-7.
5. Block B, Schachschal G, Schmidt HHJ. Endoscopy of the Upper GI Tract: A Training Manual. Stuttgart: Thieme; 2004.
6. Cotton PB, Eisen G, Romagnuolo J, Vargo J, Baron T, Tarnasky P, et al. Grading the complexity of endoscopic procedures: results of an ASGE working party. Gastrointest Endosc. 2011;73(5):868-74.
7. Cotton PB, Eisen GM, Aabakken L, Baron TH, Hutter MM, Jacobson BC, et al. A lexicon for endoscopic adverse events: report of an ASGE workshop. Gastrointest Endosc. 2010;71(3):446-54.
8. Faigel DO. Economic realities of EUS in academic practice. Gastrointest Endosc. 2007;65:287-9.
9. Haycock A, Cohen J, Saunders BP, Cotton PB, Williams CB. Cotton and Williams' Practical Gastrointestinal Endoscopy: The Fundamentals. UK: Wiley Blackwell; 2008.
10. Kroh M, Reavis KM (Eds). (2016). The SAGES Manual: Operating Through the Endoscope. Springer.
11. Ross AS, Roth J, Waxman I. Resource-intensive endoscopic procedures: do the dollars make sense? Gastrointest Endosc. 2008;68:62-6.
12. Waschke KA, Anderson J, Valori RM, MacIntosh DG, Kolars JC, DiSario JA, et al. Chair of 2017-18 ASGE Training Committee. ASGE principles of endoscopic training. Gastrointest Endosc. 2019;90(1):27-34.

Expert's Comment

This chapter gives an insight into the minute details of setting up an endoscopy unit. The safe performance of advanced endoscopy requires not only an expert endoscopic surgeon but also the presence of a competent team and the availability of appropriate tools and a state-of-the-art endoscopic theater.

A modern endoscopy theater is designed for safe and efficient performance of all endotherapy procedures. Adequate space is essential for keeping the image intensifier, energy sources, anesthetic machines, imaging devices, and several cabinets to store endoscopic accessories.

Ergonomics is essential for endoscopic surgeons, too. The height of the endoscopic trolley and the location of the endoscopic monitors should be appropriate for ease and comfort.

Laparoscopy–endoscopy cooperative surgery is the future. This requires additional gadgets for the coordinated performance of two surgical teams, as in the excision of gastric gastrointestinal stromal tumor (GIST) near the esophagogastric junction or the resection of a flat polyp in the base of the cecum.

Third-space endoscopy warrants a sterile operating environment with adequate monitoring devices.

We need to have a dedicated cleaning, disinfection, and storage area for a vast array of endoscopic equipment. There should be a clear mechanism for the reprocessing of several endoscopic disposable accessories.

Artificial intelligence and augmented reality have also come to the endoscopy suite with potential benefits. A good network communication facility allows for the prospect of telementoring and telesurgery. Documentation and archiving of data would help us in the efficient exchange of patient-related information and facilitate teaching budding endoscopic surgeons.

Dr M Kanagavel
Chennai

CHAPTER 16

ABC of Energy Sources for Endotherapy

Chapter Outline

- Classification of Energy Sources for Endoscopy
- Basic Aspects of Electrosurgery
- Thermal Effects of Diathermy on the Bowel Wall
- Importance of Understanding Your Diathermy Machine
- Explaining the Essentials of "Endocut"
- Classification of Electrosurgical Endotherapy Accessories
- Clinical Application of Endotherapy Accessories
- Diathermy in a Patient with Implantable Cardiac Electronic Device
- Use of Argon Plasma Coagulation
- Radiofrequency Ablation
- Use of Laser for Endotherapy

Keywords: Electrosurgery, argon plasma coagulation, radiofrequency ablation, laser

INTRODUCTION

Since the landmark invention of diathermy by Harvey Cushing and William Bovie **(Figs. 1A and B)** in 1926, we have come a long way in using various energy sources. Endoscopic surgeons should understand the functional and safety aspects of all different energy devices before performing any endotherapy.

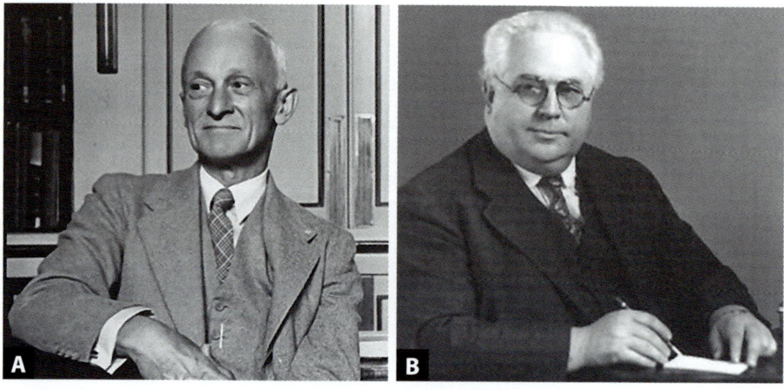

Figs. 1A and B: Harvey Cushing and William Bovie.

Even the most advanced Boeing 747 depends upon the knowledge and skill of a pilot for a safe flight! So, what matters most is not the machine but the man behind the machine to ensure the safe and effective use of any device!

CLASSIFICATION OF ENERGY SOURCES FOR ENDOSCOPY

- *Electrosurgery:*
  - Monopolar diathermy
  - Bipolar diathermy
- Argon plasma coagulation (APC)
- Radiofrequency (RF) ablation
- Laser

BASIC ASPECTS OF ELECTROSURGERY

- Electrosurgery and electrocautery are two different entities. Electrocautery works on the principles of passive transfer of heat generated by the passage of direct current through a resistance wire, e.g., a heater probe **(Fig. 2)**.
- But in electrosurgery, there is the active generation of heat because of the passage of alternate current through the tissue, e.g., insulated tip (IT) knife and bipolar gold probe **(Fig. 3)**

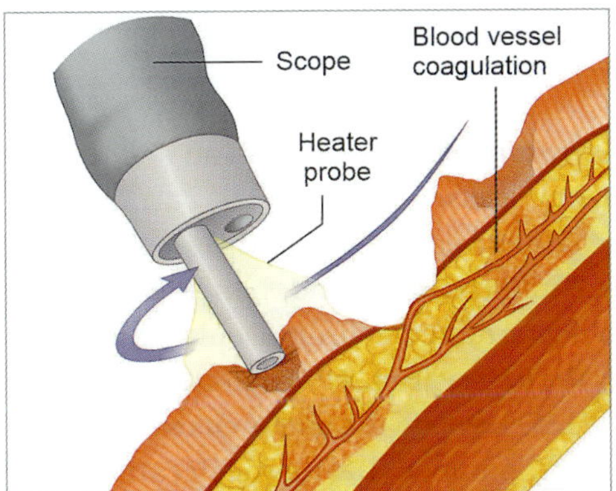

Fig. 2: Heater probe.

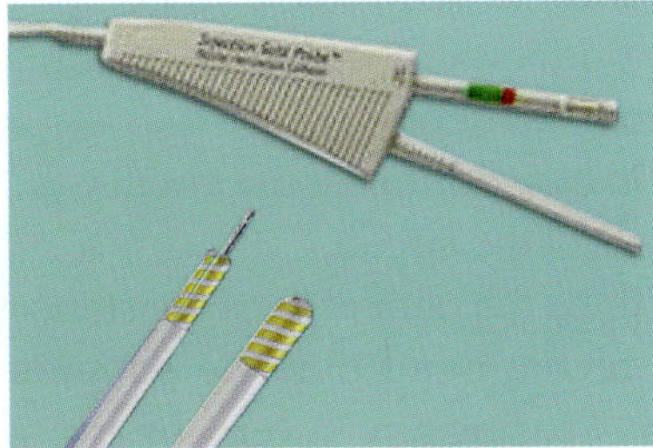

Fig. 3: Bipolar gold probe.

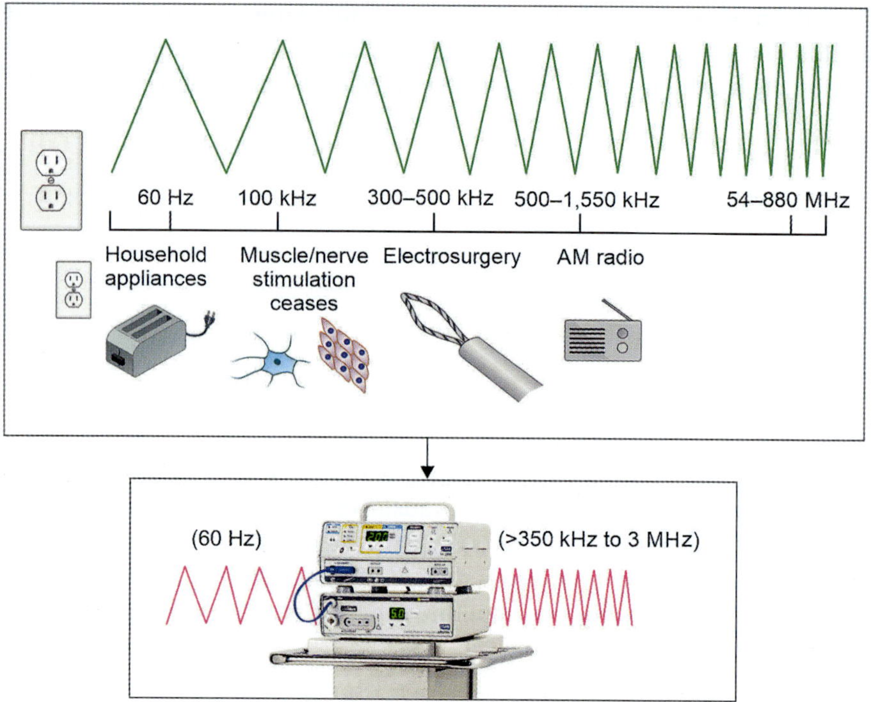

Fig. 4: Electromagnetic spectrum.

- *Function of electrosurgical unit (ESU):* The diathermy machine converts the low-frequency household alternate current (60 Hz) to very high-frequency alternate current (from >350 kHz to 3 MHz), thereby preventing the dangerous Faradic current and, hence, avoiding the risk of cardiac arrest and also unwarranted neuromuscular stimulation **(Fig. 4)**
- *Monopolar electrosurgery* ***(Fig. 5):*** When we activate the ESU, the current passes from the ESU through the active electrode to the tissue and causes the desired effect, namely cutting, desiccation, etc. Then, the same quantum of current passes through the patient's body and reaches the indifferent electrode or return pad, which is kept under the thigh. From there, the current returns to the ESU to complete the circuit. Hence, we should clearly understand these three fundamental principles of monopolar diathermy, namely:
  1. Current always likes to complete the circuit.
  2. The patient is part of the circuit.
  3. Current always finds the path of least resistance.

  That is why we recommend that the patients should not come to the endoscopy unit wearing any jewelry or earrings, which may cause alternate-site burns. Also, the patient has the risk of developing burns

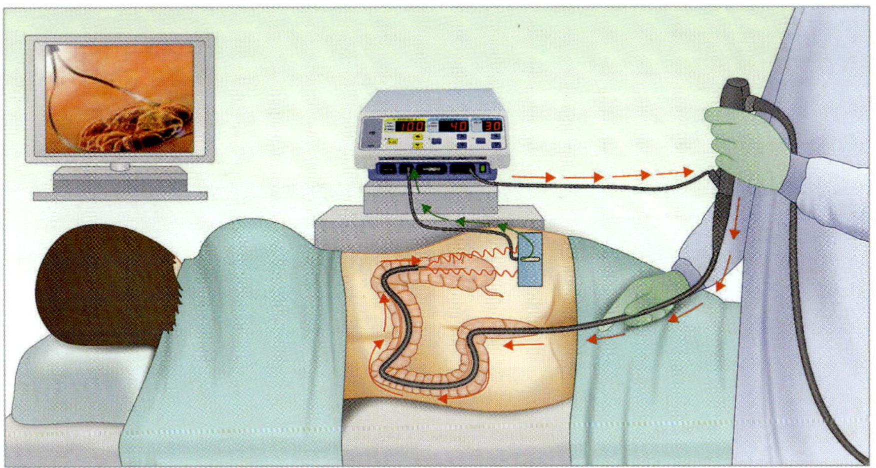

Fig. 5: Monopolar diathermy mechanism.

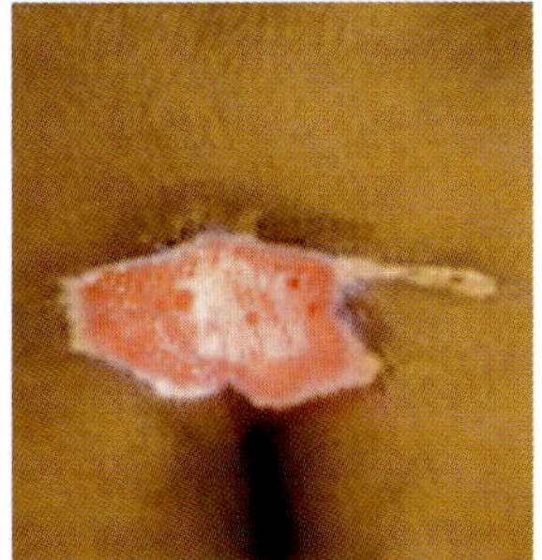

Fig. 6: Diathermy pad site burn.

at electrocardiogram (ECG) lead sites and wherever he/she has contact with metal objects, such as a drip stand and operation table (OT) **(Fig. 6)**. Fortunately, such alternate site burns are very rare now, as the present-day diathermy machines are isolated units and not ground-referenced units as it was before the 1970s. Also, we should always have the habit of using the lowest wattage of current to minimize any risk to the patient.

- *Bipolar electrosurgery* ***(Fig. 7)****:* Here, the current passes between the two jaws of the electrodes kept close to each other and causes the desired effect only to the tissue held by the device tip.
  - Here, the patient is not in the circuit. Hence, bipolar has a better safety profile.
  - But the bipolar current is not versatile and has less clinical applications
- *Electrophysiology of diathermy:*
  - When the alternating current passes through tissue, it causes movement of ions within the cells and hence produces heat.

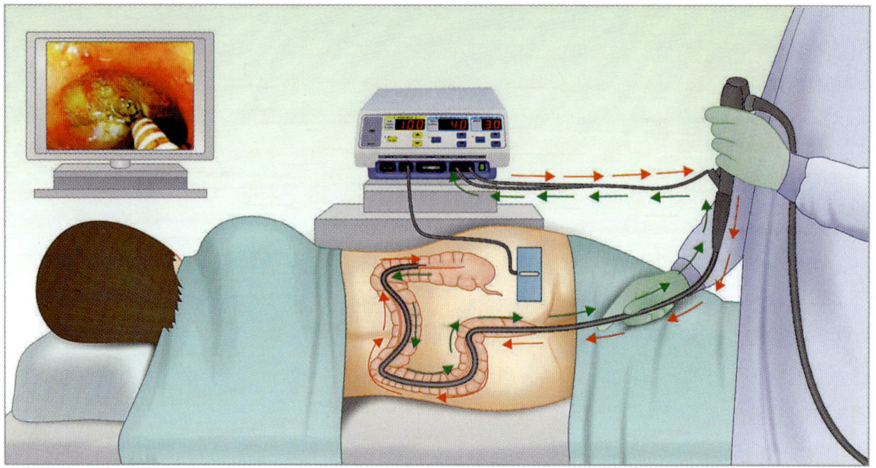

Fig. 7: Bipolar diathermy mechanism.

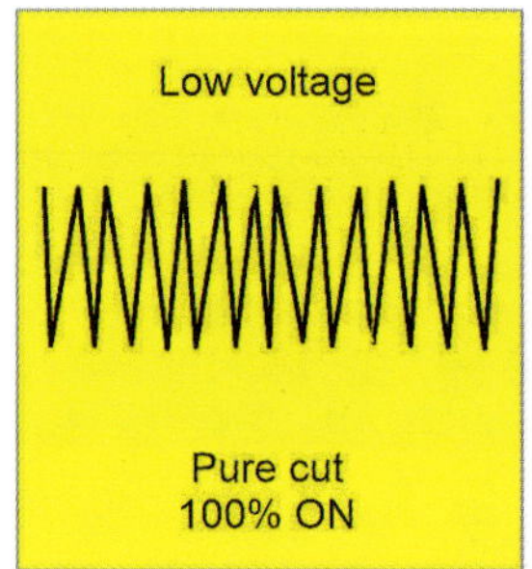

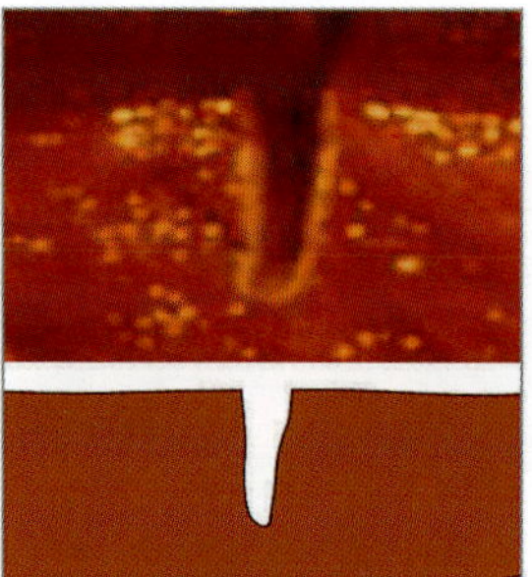

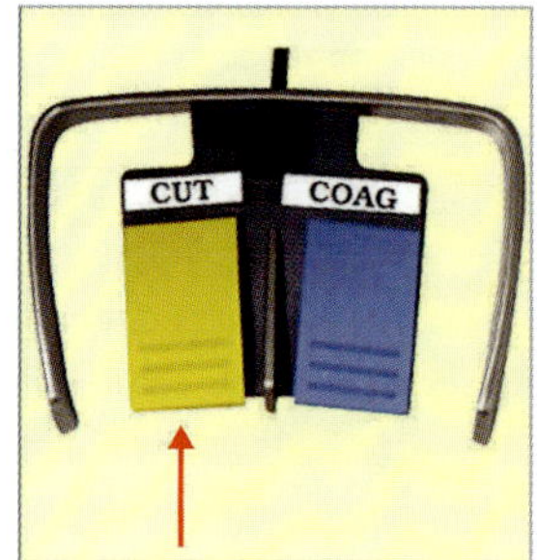

Fig. 8: Cutting mode.

- Cut mode **(Fig. 8)** (code: yellow) is a low-voltage, continuous waveform current that causes a rapid rise in heat within cells. Hence, there is the generation of steam and the explosion of cells. It is akin to microscopic flashes of lightning. Hence, we can achieve a cutting effect with minimal lateral thermal damage.
  - Example, precut sphincterotomy during endoscopic retrograde cholangiopancreatography (ERCP).
- Coagulation mode **(Fig. 9)** (code: blue) is high peak-to-peak voltage, and intermittent waveform current. Current passes only during 5% of the duty cycle. Hence, there is only a slow, gradual rise of temperature within cells. Hence, there is evaporation of water and shrinkage of cells, causing gradual tissue desiccation.
  - For example, using coagulation forceps to control bleeding during peroral endoscopic myotomy (POEM) **(Figs. 10A and B)**
- Cut mode causes cell explosion while coagulation mode causes cell dehydration! **(Fig. 11)**

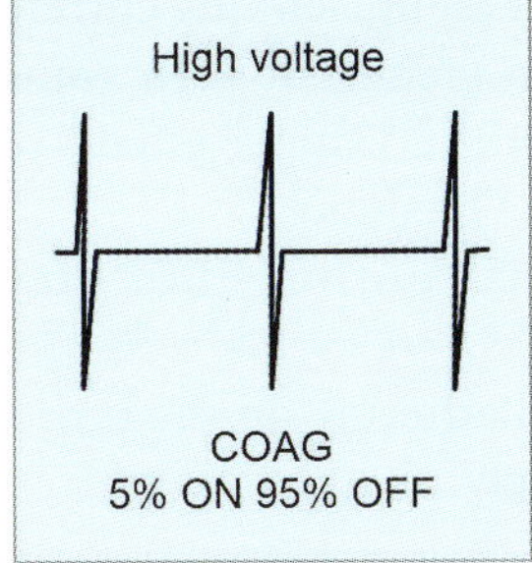

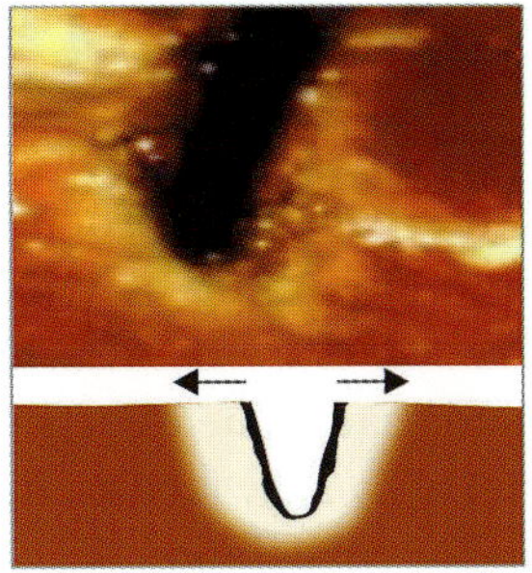

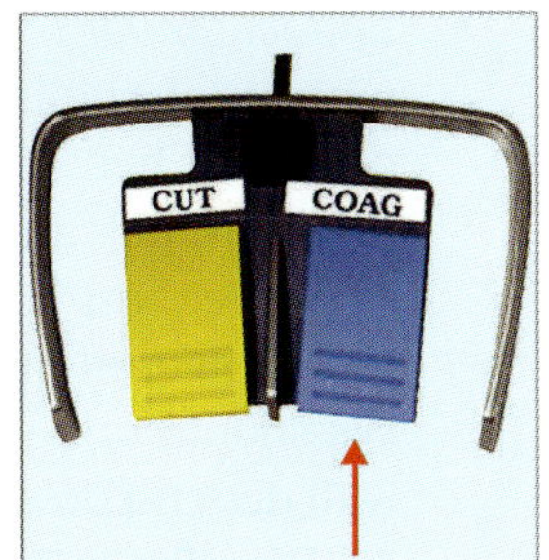

Fig. 9: Coagulation mode.

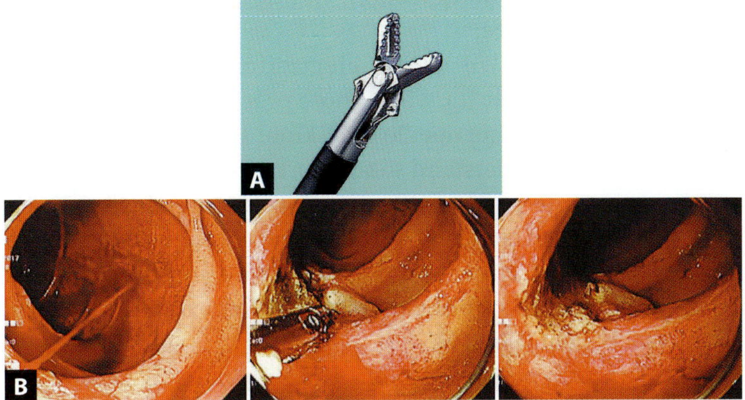

Figs. 10A and B: (A) Coagulation forceps; and (B) Endocopic hemostasis.

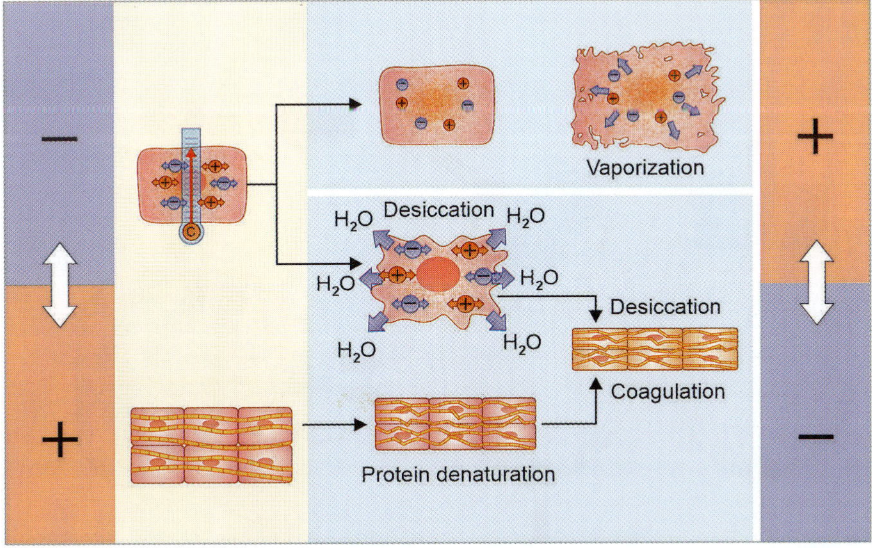

Fig. 11: Cutting versus coagulation mode.

- *Endocut mode (code: yellow)* is defined as incremental cutting current with brief spells of coagulation to ensure a clean cut with some degree of hemostasis. Hence, we can prevent the "Zipper effect" or uncontrolled fast cutting with the risk of undue bleeding.
  - For example, endocut mode is essential during ERCP and sphincterotomy.
- We should understand that tissue effects of diathermy on the bowel wall depend on a total of five key factors, namely:
  1. *Waveform:* Cutting or coagulation
  2. *Power setting:* Wattage level
  3. Size of the electrode
  4. Duration of current exposure
  5. Tissue impedance
- The smaller the size of the electrode, the higher the current concentration or density, with a more precise tissue effect.
  - For example, precut needle or IT knife
- We should also understand the importance of a "properly kept large return electrode pad" to ensure safety during electrosurgery. The same quantum of current that causes the cutting or coagulation effect has to return safely back to the diathermy unit through the return pad (indifferent electrode), thanks to its large surface area with easy dispersal of heat **(Fig. 12)**.
- *Units of measurement of current*:
  - *Voltage:* Volts
  - *Output power:* Watts
  - *Tissue impedance:* Ohm's

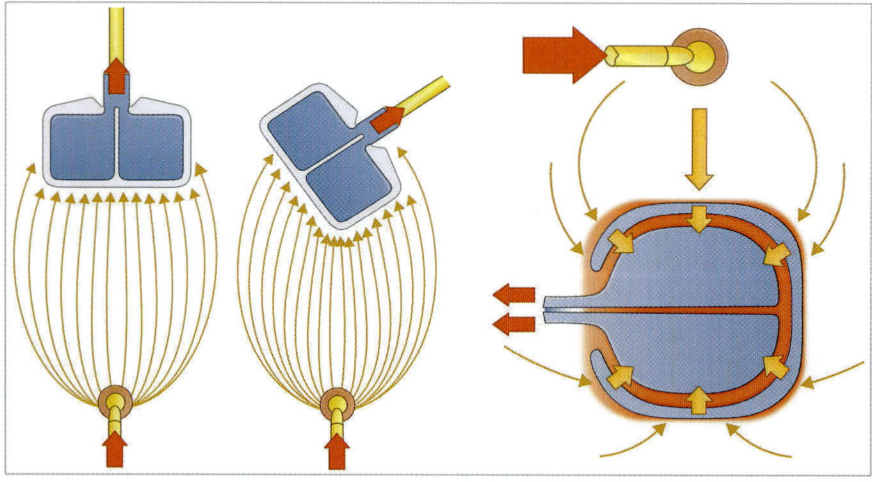

Fig. 12: Electrode pad.

- Importance of return electrode monitoring **(Fig. 13)**.
  - We should ideally use a split return electrode pad to ensure good contact with large vascular areas.
  - Newer diathermy machines have a contact quality monitoring system (CQMS). For this to work, we should use a split return pad. In modern diathermy units, there is an additional interrogation circuit between the machine and the two parts of the split pad. If there is no proper quality of contact, then the interrogation circuit is broken, which would automatically shut down the diathermy machine!

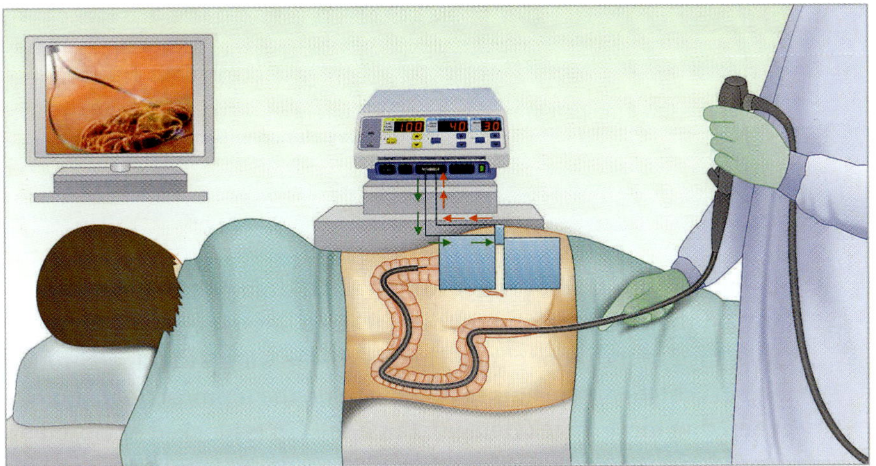

Fig. 13: Interrogation circuit.

  - Hence, by proper use of a return pad, preferably a split pad, we should prevent any contact burns at the site of the return pad **(Figs. 14A to C)**.
- *Importance of tissue-responsive generators* ***(Fig. 15)***:
  - Understanding Ohm's law or knowing the importance of terms such as voltage, tissue impedance, and wattage are made easy by using the

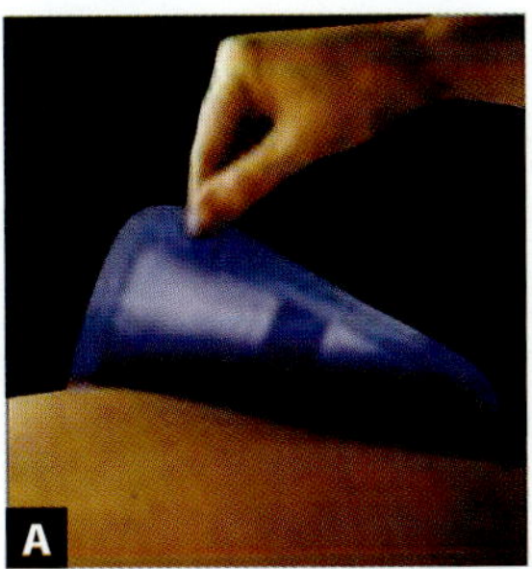

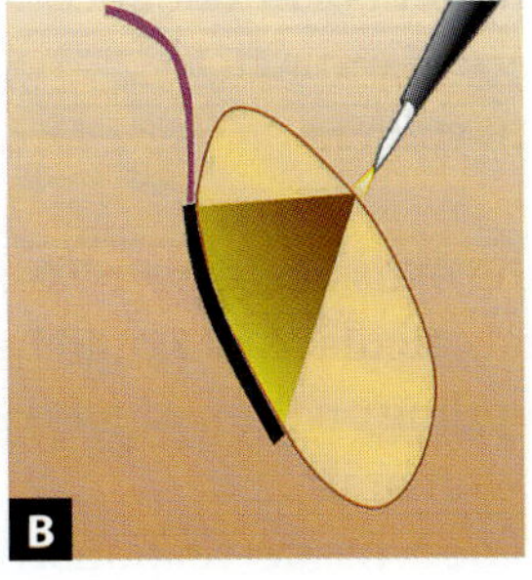

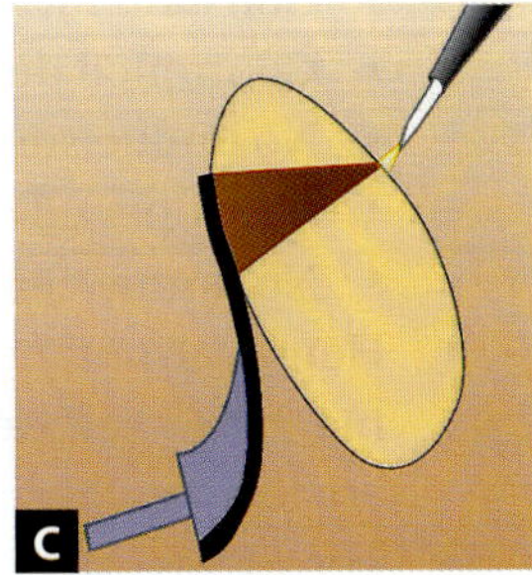

Figs. 14A to C: Split pad.

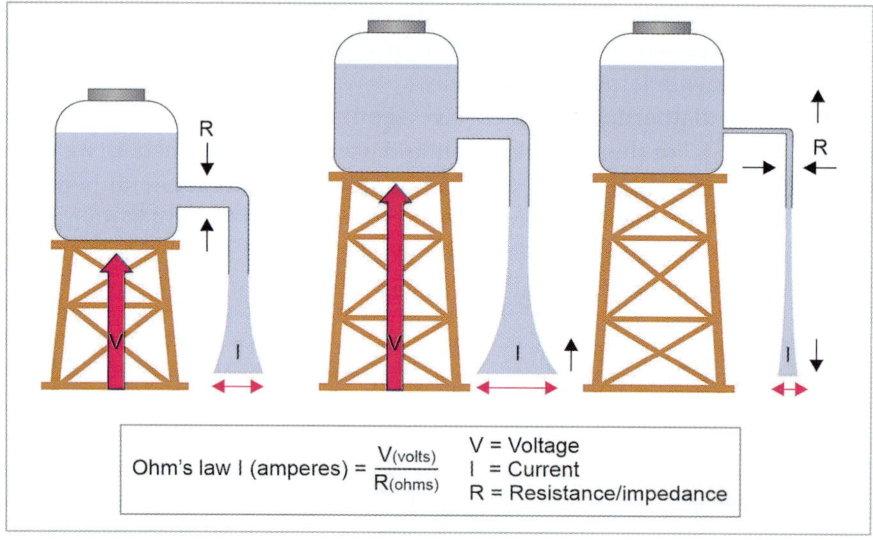

Fig. 15: Ohm's law.

analogy of the "flow of water from a tank." Imagine there is a water tank on the top floor of the hospital. Also, imagine there is a water tap in the ground-floor clinic. The flow of the water (wattage) through the tap is higher if the tank is very big or on the topmost floor, thereby generating more force (voltage). But if the tap is blocked or closed on the ground floor (tissue impedance), then there is no flow of water (wattage), whatever the force (voltage). If the tissue impedance is high as in less vascular tissue (e.g., charred tissue), current will not flow, and simply raising the voltage would invariably lead to the risk of serious complications. What forces current to travel is voltage, and what prevents current from passing through tissue is its tissue impedance!

- Tissue-responsive generators are microprocessor-controlled units with the following unique properties, namely:
  - Constant measurement of impedance
  - Controlled delivery of wattage
  - No undue surge in voltage
  - No zipper effect
  - No undue charring of tissue
- Hence, all our mental calculations would be automatically done by the machine itself, depending on the assigned job. Hence, these machines are like "diathermy with brain!"
- Let us invest in a good tissue-responsive diathermy unit for safe endotherapy!

THERMAL EFFECTS OF DIATHERMY ON THE BOWEL WALL

- There are five different types of thermal effects seen on applying diathermy to the bowel wall, namely:
  1. Thermal devitalization
  2. Thermal coagulation
  3. Thermal desiccation
  4. Thermal carbonization
  5. Thermal vaporization
- Thermal devitalization or cell death occurs when the temperature rises above 40°C.
- Thermal coagulation occurs when the temperature reaches above 60°C. It is akin to boiling an egg. It causes some contraction of collagen and blanching of the bowel.
- Thermal desiccation happens once the temperature reaches 100°C. There is a shrinkage of cells and contraction of collagen, hence aiding hemostasis. Also, there will be some stickiness of the electrode to the bowel wall.
- Thermal carbonization: This happens when the desiccated bowel tissue at a temperature nearing 200°C is exposed to the presence of oxygen! Smoke is generated, and hence visibility is affected, and there is also the risk of explosion. Hence, it is advisable to use CO_2 during endotherapy to avoid the risk of tissue carbonization.
- Thermal Vaporization happens when there is a rapid rise of temperature above 500°C, as in laser tissue ablation.
- Let us also understand the anatomical basis of electro-surgery during colonoscopy:
  - Colon is only 0.5–3 mm thick, and after insufflation, the wall can even be much thinner. Moreover, any damage beyond the submucosa would cause thermal injury to the muscularis propria, with the risk of delayed perforation **(Fig. 16)**. Hence, every surgeon should have sufficient knowledge of energy sources and the availability of good quality energy devices.

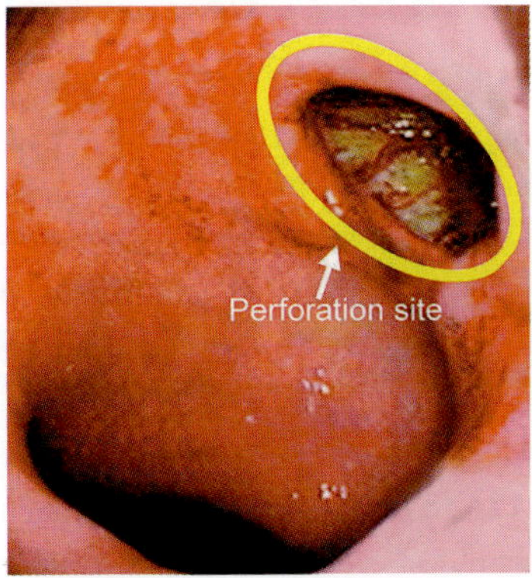

Fig. 16: Perforation site in colonoscopy.

- The following are the four common types of tissue effects achieved by diathermy, along with some classical examples:
  1. *Pure cut:* Noncontact mode cutting/dissection
     - *Needle knife Sphincterotomy, endoscopic submucosal dissection (ESD) using IT knife*
  2. *Blend/endo cut:* Contact mode cutting with pause.
     - *Snare polypectomy, bow wire sphincterotomy*
  3. *Desiccation:* Contact mode coagulation
     - *Swift or forced coagulation with the use of coagulation grasping forceps*
  4. *Fulguration:* Noncontact mode coagulation
     - *APC spray coagulation*

IMPORTANCE OF UNDERSTANDING YOUR DIATHERMY MACHINE (FIGS. 17A TO D)

- Different diathermy machines produce different types of tissue effects by different mechanisms.
- ERBE, KLS Martin, Valley laboratory, or Olympus diathermy machine could all achieve the desired tissue effects, provided we understand each one of them.
- Endocut in ERBE is what blends current in the Valley laboratory. Soft coagulation in ERBE is what contact coagulation is in KLS Martin.

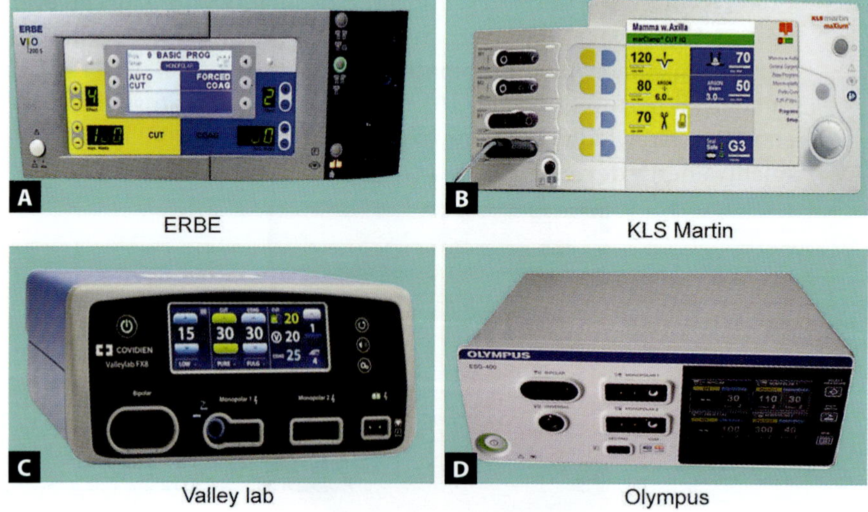

Figs. 17A to D: Various diathermy machines.

- Each machine can create a vast array of tissue effects.
  - ERBE is capable of following tissue effects
    - *Cut mode*:
      - Endocut, precise cut, and auto cut
    - *Coagulation mode*:
      - Swift coagulation, soft coagulation, spray coagulation, forced coagulation, etc.
- *Remember this*: We are working on a narrow therapeutic window. It is like walking on a tightrope! Hence, it is advisable to fully understand the potential and safety profile of any machine prior to use. Let us say this again, what matters most is the man behind the machine.

EXPLAINING THE ESSENTIALS OF "ENDOCUT"

- It is characterized by intermittent or installment cutting current with brief spells of coagulation, thus ensuring a clean cut with some degree of hemostasis.
- It is activated by continuously pressing the yellow pedal, but the cutting action is intermittent with typical beep-beep sounds during the whole duration of the endocut action.
- Endocut prevents the risk of the "Zipper" effect or rapid, uncontrolled cut.
- Specific programs for "Endocut mode" are chosen after taking three aspects into consideration, namely cut duration, cut interval, and effect **(Figs. 18A and B)**.
  - Cut duration (1–4) determines the length of the cut. A cut duration of four achieves a longer cut with each beep compared to a cut duration of one or two.
  - Cut interval (1–10) determines the speed of the cut. A cut interval of one means a faster beep with a faster speed of cut, but resulting in

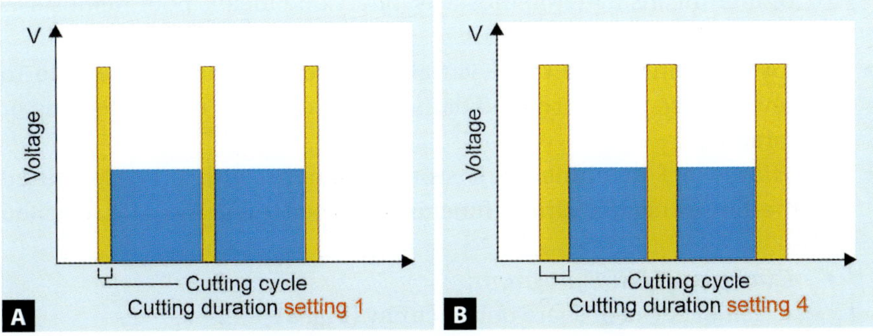

Figs. 18A and B: Cutting duration.

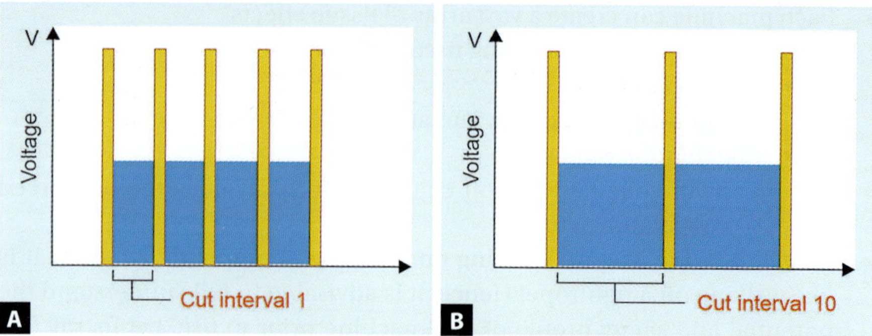

Figs. 19A and B: Cutting interval.

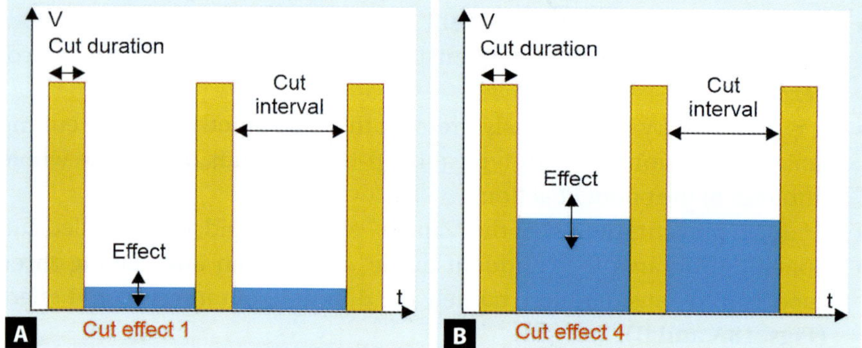

Figs. 20A and B: Cutting effect.

poor hemostasis. A cut interval of 10 means a slower beep sound with a slower cut, resulting in better hemostasis **(Figs. 19A and B)**.

- Effect (1–4) essentially determines the degree of hemostasis. The effect of four means better hemostasis. Effect one means poor hemostasis **(Figs. 20A and B)**

- So, by choosing these three variables wisely, we should be able to achieve precise predetermined tissue effects with less risk of bleeding or perforation.
- All diathermy machines can store programs with predetermined diathermy settings for various functions and hence are useful for repeated use.
  - *Examples of ERBE programs*:
    - *Endocut Q*: For snare polypectomy **(Fig. 21)**
    - *Endocut I*: For sphincterotomy **(Fig. 22)**

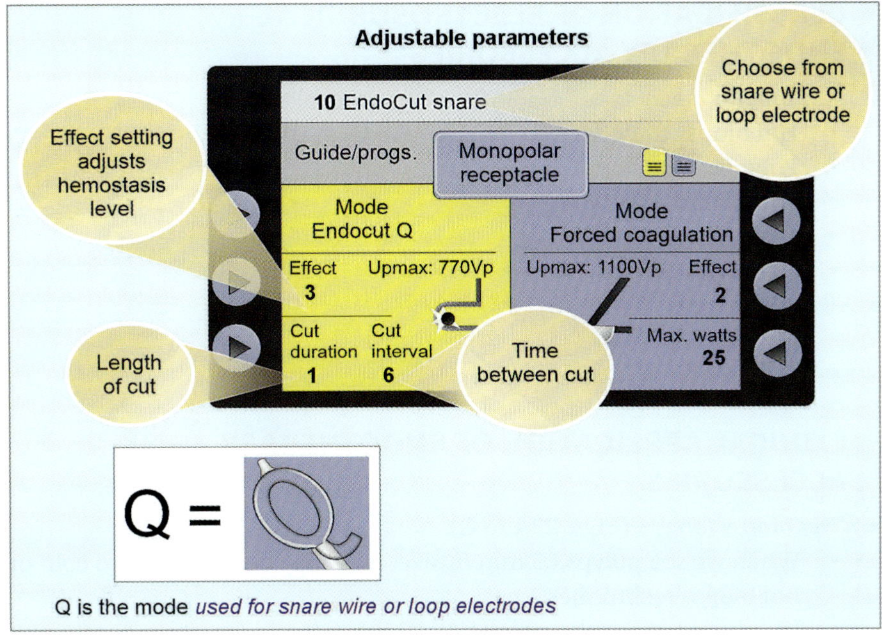

Fig. 21: Endocut Q.

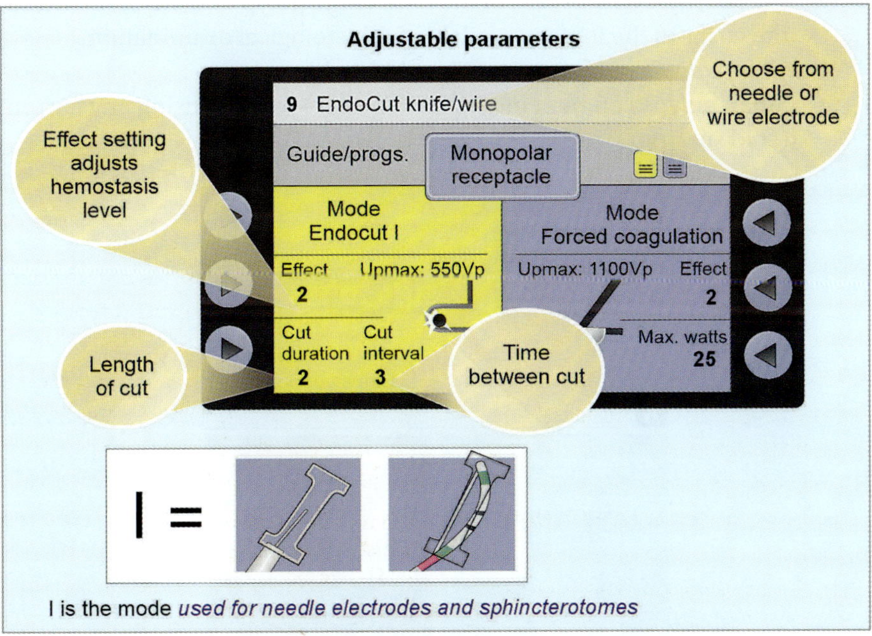

Fig. 22: Endocut I.

CLASSIFICATION OF ELECTROSURGICAL ENDOTHERAPY ACCESSORIES

- *Monopolar devices:*
  - Hot biopsy forceps
  - Polypectomy snare
  - Sphincterotomy wires
  - Coagulation forceps
  - Hybrid knife
- *Bipolar devices:*
  - Heater probe
  - Gold probe

CLINICAL APPLICATION OF ENDOTHERAPY ACCESSORIES

- *Hot biopsy forceps* **(Figs. 23A to C)***:*
  - When we see polyps <5 mm in size, they may be amenable to cold or hot biopsy techniques.
  - We should grasp the polyp with the hot biopsy forceps, gently pull it toward the lumen, and apply forced coagulation using 60 watts (effect 2).
  - This ensures hemostasis of the base of the polyp and the tissue within the cusps of the forceps available for histological examination.
- *Snare for colonic polypectomy* ***(Figs. 24A to F):***
  - Small polyps can be removed with a snare without using any current (cold snaring).

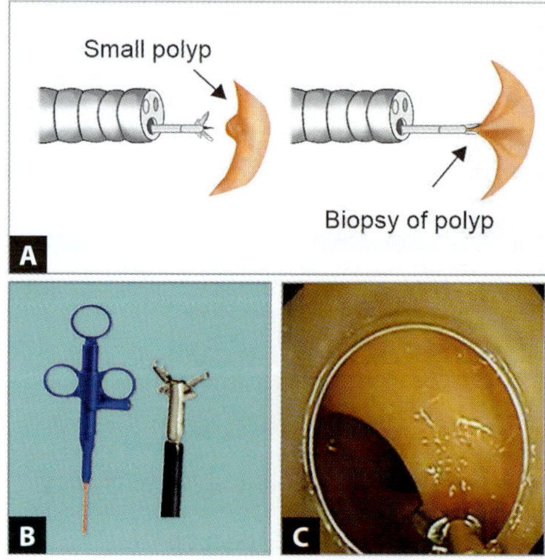

Figs. 23A to C: Hot biopsy forceps.

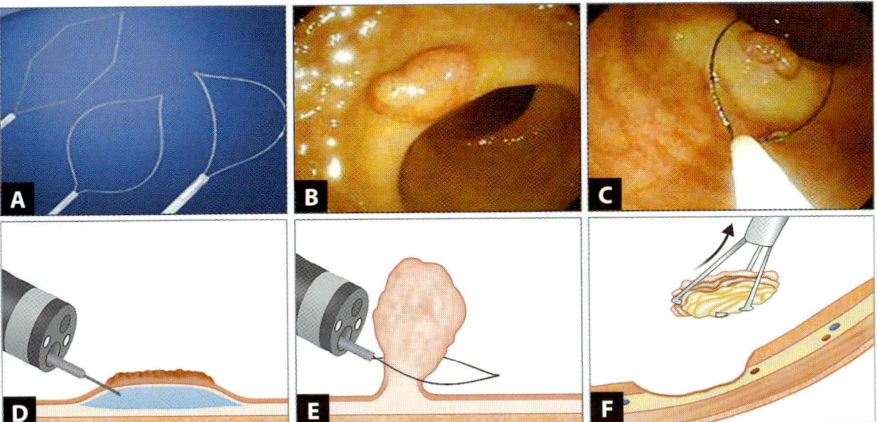

Figs. 24A to F: Snare for colonic polypectomy.

- Most of the pedunculated polyps can be easily removed by garlanding and chopping the stalk by using properly chosen, appropriately sized monopolar snares.
- Large polyps with thick stalks and sessile polyps need a submucosal saline cushion to prevent any risk of bleeding or perforation.
- Snare polypectomy can be done using endocut, pure cut, and coagulation current, or even alternate cut and coagulation mode current. The risk of immediate bleeding is high with pure cut or endocut, while the risk of delayed bleeding is higher with the use of a coagulation current!
- *ERBE program setting for polypectomy is endocut Q:*
    - *Effect*: 3
    - *Cut duration*: 1
    - *Cut interval*: 6
- The faster the cut speed, the higher the risk of bleeding.
- More the tissue within the snare or the closer the distance between the snare and the colonic wall, the higher the risk of thermal damage to the bowel wall.
- Thin snare wire with a short nose is more precise and safe to use.
- Use of CO_2 during polypectomy is advisable to prevent carbonization and any risk of explosion.
- When planning to remove a large pedunculated polyp, prevent any contact of the polyp head touching the opposite bowel wall and hence the risk of coupling current injury is minimized.
- Prior endoloop application at the base of the polyp is often done for large polyps with thick stalks, but beware that this causes current concentration with risk of perforation.

- Avoid contact with any nearby hemoclips during snare polypectomy to prevent direct coupling.
- I-snare is a special type of snare that has a hidden needle that can be brought out if required. Hence, it has the luxury of a dual function of creation of saline cushion and snare polypectomy, thus minimizing multiple unwarranted exchanges of devices.

▪ *Sphincterotome wires* **(*Figs. 25A to C*)**:
- Precut and bow wire sphincterotomes are widely used during ERCP.
- *ERBE program setting for papillotomy is endocut I*:
  - *Effect*: 2
  - *Cut duration*: 3
  - *Cut interval*: 3
- In addition to preventing zipper cuts, there is also less risk of pancreatitis and bleeding with this mode.
- Aim toward 10 o'clock for biliary Sphincterotomy and 2 o'clock for pancreatic sphincterotomy.
- Limit the length of the cut to the bulging part of the papilla to avoid the risk of perforation.

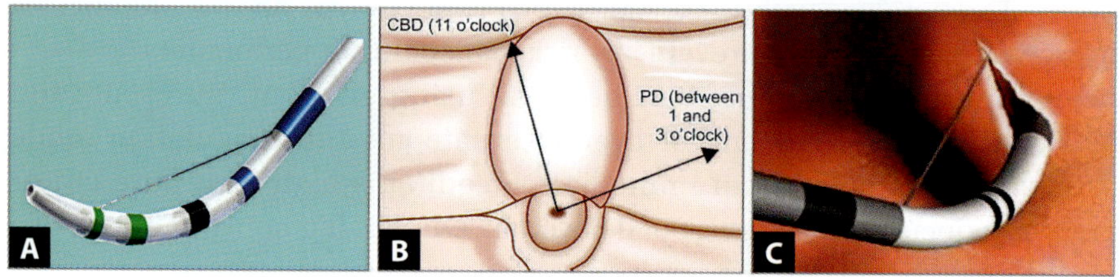

Figs. 25A to C: Sphincterotome wires. (CBD: common bile duct; PD: pancreatic duct)

▪ *Coagulation forceps* **(*Fig. 26*)**:
- Monopolar coagulation forceps are used for achieving effective hemostasis during any endotherapy, such as POEM and ESD.
- *ERBE setting*: Soft coagulation, 80 watts, effect 4.
- The irrigation pump helps us with the precise location of bleeding and its control.

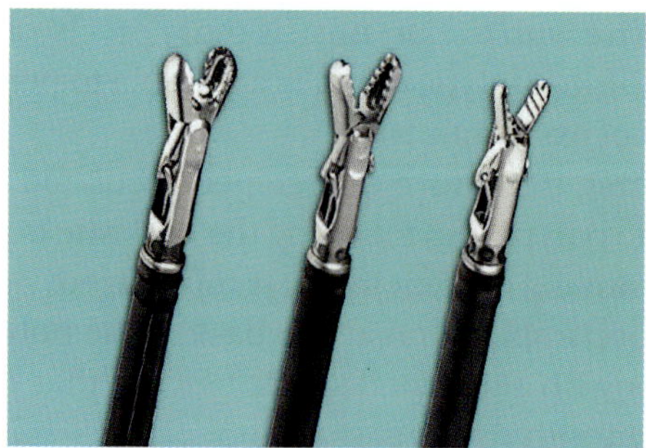

Fig. 26: Coagulation forceps.

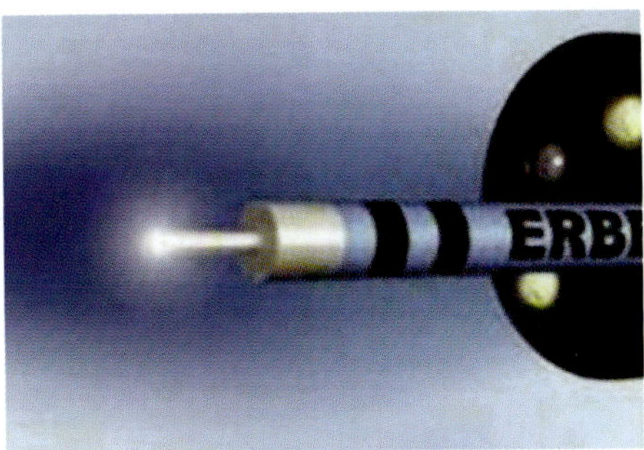

Fig. 27: Hybrid knife.

- *Hybrid knife* ***(Fig. 27)****:*
  - It is essentially an electrohydro thermo probe with provision for irrigation.
  - It is also armed with an antistick coating to aid seamless dissection.
  - ESD is done in the following five classical steps **(Figs. 28A to F)**:
    1. Marking
    2. Injection
    3. Incision
    4. Dissection
    5. Specimen acquisition
  - *ERBE setting for ESD*:
    - Endocut Q
      - *Effect*: 2
      - *Cut duration*: 4
      - *Cut interval*: 3
  - We should be vigilant to look for any breach in the muscularis propria (target sign) and consider pre-emptive application of hemoclips in such cases to prevent perforation.

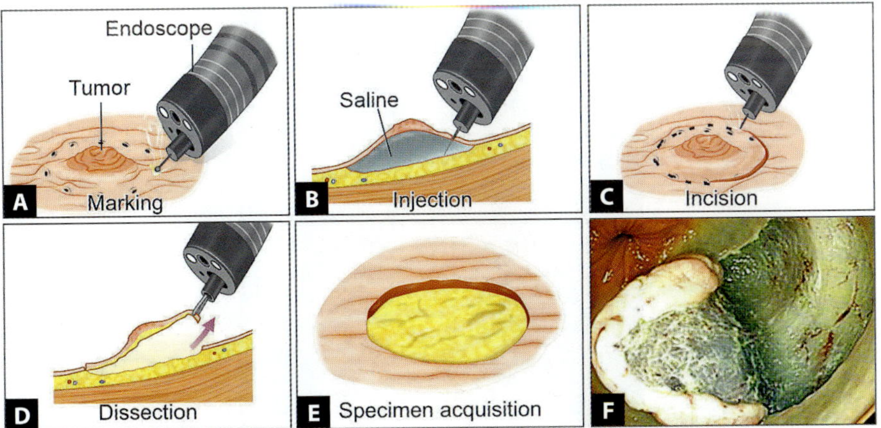

Figs. 28A to F: Endoscopic submucosal dissection steps.

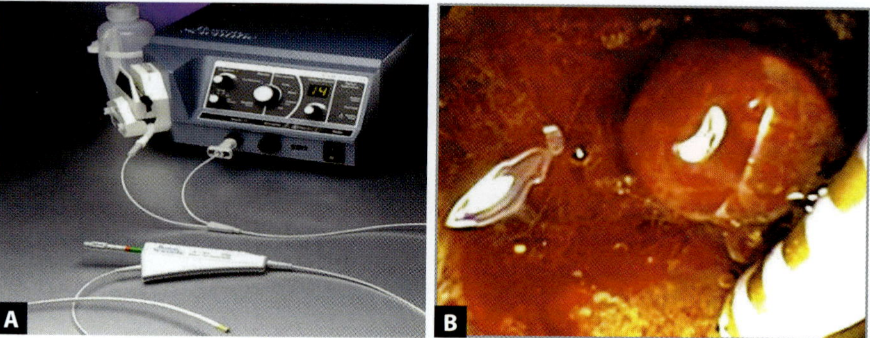

Figs. 29A and B: Bipolar gold probe.

- *Bipolar gold probe* ***(Figs. 29A and B):***
  - It is a bipolar probe with provision for irrigation through the nozzle at its tip.
  - It has a special gold coating on the surface (hence the name) to avoid sticking to the bowel surface.
  - It works on the principle of coaptive coagulation using a precise temperature control mechanism.
  - Useful for control of bleeding from lesions like arteriovenous (AV) malformations.

DIATHERMY IN A PATIENT WITH IMPLANTABLE CARDIAC ELECTRONIC DEVICE

In cases of any need for diathermy in a patient with a pacemaker or other implantable cardiac electronic device (ICED), we should take the following precautions to prevent any complications **(Fig. 30)**.

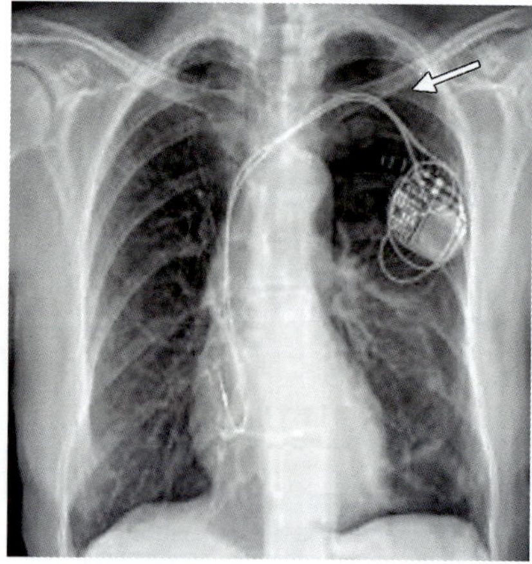

Fig. 30: Cardiac pacemaker.

- One should understand the type of ICED in the patient and consult with a cardiologist before endotherapy.
- Closely monitor the patient with ECG, saturation of peripheral oxygen (SpO_2), and noninvasive blood pressure (BP) measurements during the procedure.
- Prefer to use bipolar, if suitable
- *If a monopolar is needed, then refer to the following guidelines:*
  - Use the lowest power setting
  - Use short bursts of current
  - Ensure that the return pad and cables are far from the ICED device.
  - Keep the defibrillator and external pacing devices ready

USE OF ARGON PLASMA COAGULATION (FIG. 31)

- It is a monopolar electrosurgical device where in flow of inert argon gas drives the current. (Flow of electrons).
- Hence, it works in a noncontact mode without any drag **(Figs. 32A and B)**
- *Choose the appropriate type of probe*: End firing/side firing.
- Set the wattage and argon gas flow rate as required.

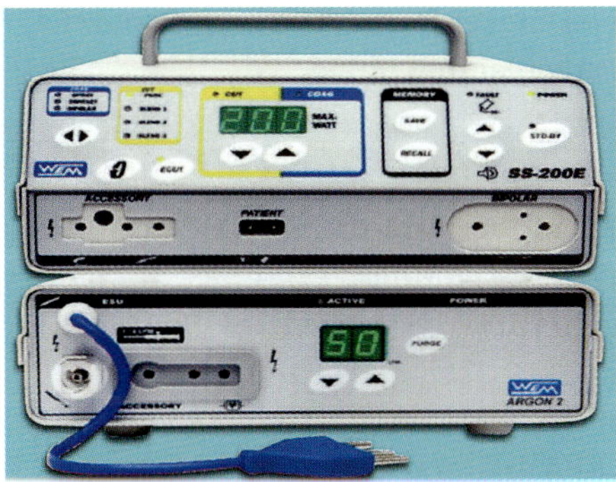

Fig. 31: Argon plasma coagulation.

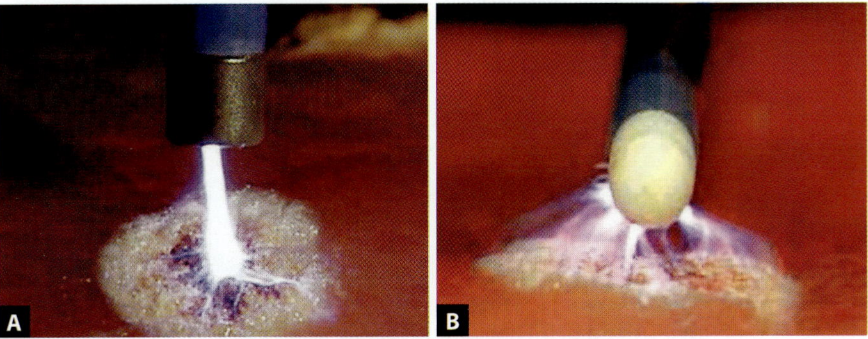

Figs. 32A and B: (A) End; and (B) Side firing probes.

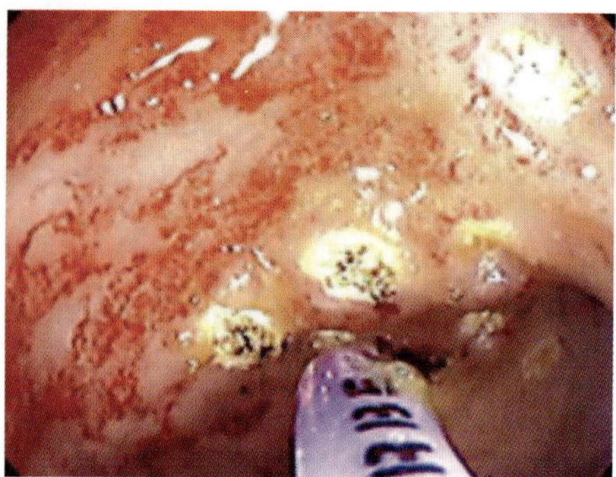

Fig. 33: APC for radiation proctitis.

- Keep the APC probe constantly projecting just 1 cm outside the scope tip.
- Activate and apply the APC to control the movement of the scope tip. This ensures the precise application of APC on the intended target. This is also known as the "Paintbrush" technique.
- APC is useful in the following conditions during colonoscopic endotherapy.
  - Radiation proctitis **(Fig. 33)**.
  - Angiodysplasia causes lower gastrointestinal (GI) bleeding.
  - To pulverize any residual polyp.

RADIOFREQUENCY ABLATION (FIGS. 34A AND B)

- It uses 450–500 kHz RF generator/bipolar electrodes.
- The following are some common examples of RFA devices, namely:
  - HALOFlex generator or similar for Barrett's esophagus/radiation proctitis.
  - Habib RFA biliary catheter for cholangiocarcinoma.
  - EUS-guided RFA ablation of a pancreatic lesion.

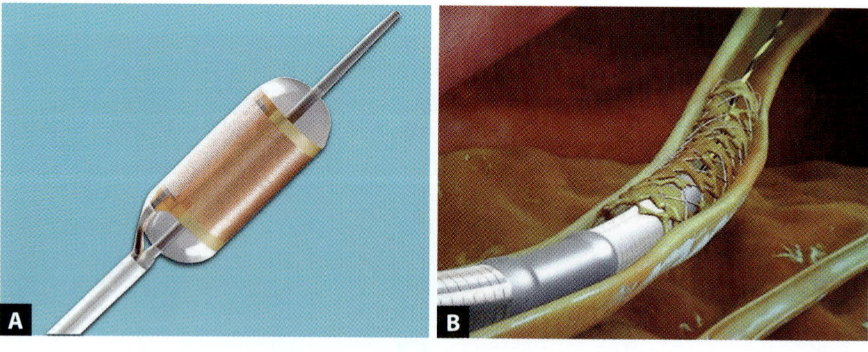

Figs. 34A and B: (A) Radiofrequency ablation (RFA) balloon catheter; and (B) Habib RFA biliary catheter.

USE OF LASER FOR ENDOTHERAPY (FIG. 35)

- Light amplification and stimulated emission of radiation
- It is a monochromatic coherent beam of photons useful for endotherapy in several clinical conditions.
- *Common indications for use:*
  - Ablation of esophageal and rectal tumors
  - Hemostasis for bleeding lesions
  - Photodynamic therapy
  - Laser lithotripsy
    - Blasting of CBD stone with a holmium laser **(Fig. 36)**
    - In SpyGlass cholangioscopy **(Figs. 37A and B)**
- *Demerits:*
  - Rather expensive gadget!
  - It is not versatile and has only a limited application

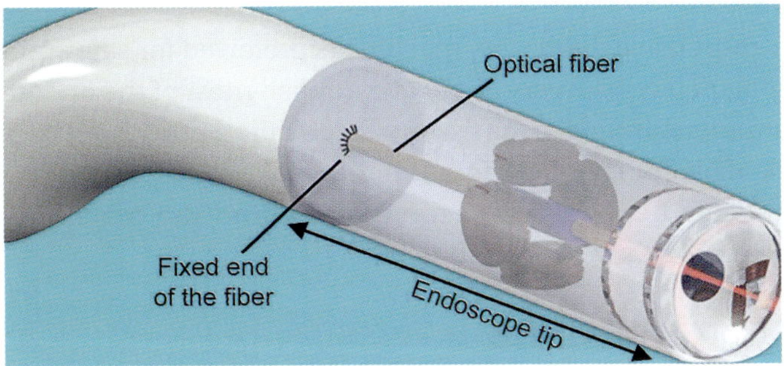

Fig. 35: Laser in endotherapy.

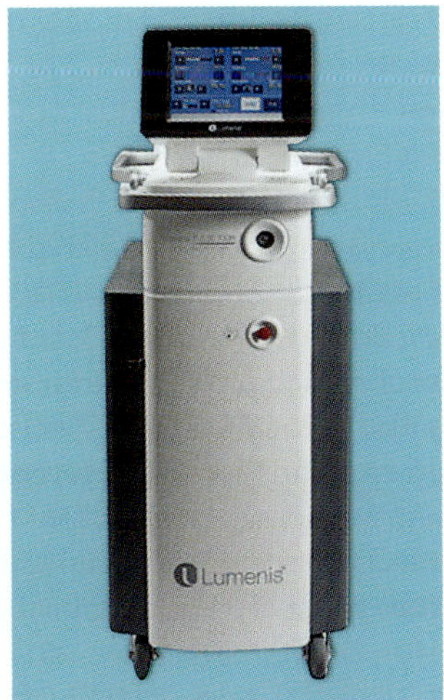

Fig. 36: Holmium laser.

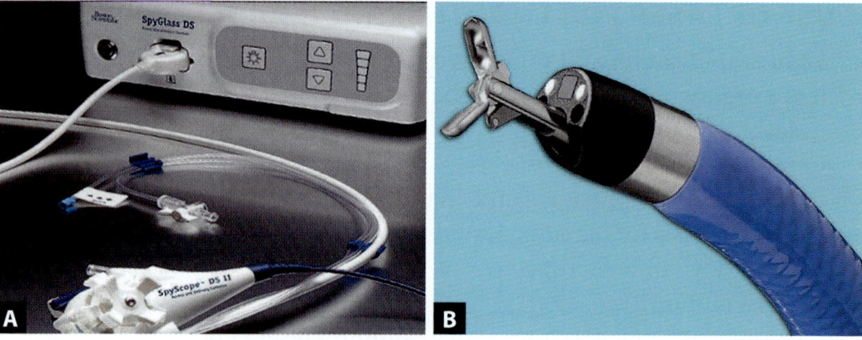

Figs. 37A and B: SpyGlass cholangioscopy.

- Needs special training to handle
- Poor visibility due to excessive smoke generation

KEY MESSAGES

- Tissue-responsive diathermy machine is preferred for safe endotherapy.
- Monopolar electrosurgery could accomplish most of the endotherapy.
- A clear understanding of the tissue effects of diathermy is key to preventing the risk of bleeding and perforation.
- Safety solely depends upon the man behind the machine, who has adequate knowledge and experience!

SUGGESTED READING

1. Barlow DE. Endoscopic applications of electrosurgery: a review of basic principles. Gastrointest Endosc. 1982;28:73-6.
2. Chino A, Karasawa T, Uragami N, Endo Y, Takahashi H, Fujita R. A comparison of depth of tissue injury caused by different modes of electrosurgical current in a pig colon model. Gastrointest Endosc. 2004;59:374-9.
3. Curtiss LE. High frequency currents in endoscopy: a review of principles and precautions. Gastrointest Endosc. 1973;20:9-12.
4. Deprez PH, Bergman JJ, Meisner S, Ponchon T, Repici A, Dinis-Ribeiro M, et al. Current practice with endoscopic submucosal dissection in Europe: position statement from a panel of experts. Endoscopy. 2010;42:853-8.
5. Ginsberg GG, Barkun AN, Bosco JJ, Burdick JS, Isenberg GA, Nakao NL, et al. The argon plasma coagulator: February 2002. Gastrointest Endosc. 2002;55:807-10.
6. Kimmey MB, Al-Kawas FH, Burnett DA, Carr-Locke DL, DiMarino AJ, Gannon RM, et al. Technology Assessment: Electrocautery use in patients with implanted cardiac devices. Gastrointest Endosc. 1994;40:794.
7. Morris M, Norton ID. Electrosurgery in Therapeutic Endoscopy. In: Ginsberg GG, Kochman ML, Norton ID, et al. (Eds). Clinical gastrointestinal endoscopy. 2nd edition. St. Louis (Mo): Saunders/Elsevier; 2011. pp. 69-77.
8. Morris ML, Tucker RD, Baron TH, Song LM. Electrosurgery in gastrointestinal endoscopy: principles to practice. Am J Gastroenterol. 2009;104:1563-74.

9. Nelson DB, Barkun AN, Block KP, Burdick JS, Ginsberg GG, Greenwald DA, et al. Technology status evaluation report. Endoscopic hemostatic devices. May 2001. Gastrointest Endosc. 2001;54:833-40.
10. Petersen BT, Hussain N, Marine JE, Trohman RG, Carpenter S, Chuttani R, et al. Endoscopy in patients with implanted electronic devices. Gastrointest Endosc. 2007;65:561-8.
11. Rey JF, Beilenhoff U, Neumann CS, Dumonceau JM. European Society of Gastrointestinal Endoscopy (ESGE) guideline: the use of electrosurgical units. Endoscopy. 2010;42:764-72.
12. Shaheen NJ, Overholt BF, Sampliner RE, Wolfsen HC, Wang KK, Fleischer DE, et al. Durability of radiofrequency ablation in Barrett's esophagus with dysplasia. Gastroenterology. 2011;141:460-8.
13. Tucker R. Principles of electrosurgery. In: Sivak MV (Eds). Gastroenterologic endoscopy. 2nd edition. Philadelphia (Pa): WB Saunders; 2000. pp. 125-35.

Expert's Comment

The energy sources are invaluable tools for surgeons. Electrosurgery remains the primary energy source used by the endoscopic surgeons. The surgeon must understand the basic principles of how they work, the physics behind them, the electrical waveforms in each mode, and their effects on the cells.

Various companies produce excellent electrosurgical units, but each has its own unique controls and functions. The surgeon must be familiar with the machine he will use and teach himself all the functions and controls. For example, the blend settings may be different between the Valley Lab and an ERBE machine. Similarly, one must learn how the argon plasma coagulator or the laser works.

Endoscopy is done in a closed and very delicate environment, and there is little room for error, which could lead to disastrous consequences. This chapter explains all these in excellent detail and should be studied thoroughly by an endoscopic surgeon.

Dr Amol Bapaye
Pune

CHAPTER 17

Guidelines for Cleaning and Disinfection of Flexible Endoscopes

Chapter Outline

- Sterilization Versus Disinfection
- Design of Cleaning and Disinfection Area in the Endoscopy Suite
- Steps of Endoscopy Reprocessing
    - Precleaning
    - Leak Test
    - Manual Cleaning
    - Disinfection Process
    - Rinsing and Drying
- Safe Transfer of Endoscope
- Storage of Endoscope and Accessories
- Automated Washer and Disinfector
- Guidelines for Ultrasonic Cleaning
- Staff Protection during Cleaning and Disinfection of Endoscopes
- Common Problems in Endoscopy Reprocessing
- Quality Control of Disinfection Process

Keywords: Spaulding classification, precleaning, chemical disinfection, glutaraldehyde, gas plasma sterilization

INTRODUCTION

There is always some risk of transmission of infection from patient to patient, patient to staffs, and rarely from staffs to patient. We ought to adhere to strict guidelines for cleaning and disinfection to protect our patients, staffs, and also all our expensive and delicate endoscopic equipment.

STERILIZATION VERSUS DISINFECTION

- Sterilization is the process of eliminating all microorganisms including all spores.
    - Autoclave, ethylene oxide, γ-rays, and gas plasma
- High-level disinfection is the process of eliminating all microorganisms except some spores.
    - Chemical disinfection using glutaraldehyde/peracetic acid

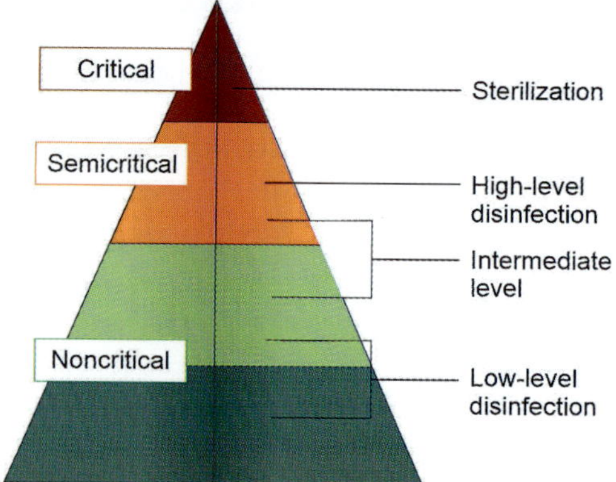

Critical devices	Enter normally sterile body cavity or tissue	*Example:* Biopsy forceps, snares, injecting needles, dilators, stents	Sterilization
Semicritical devices	Contact with mucous membranes	*Example:* Flexible endoscopes, mouth guard	Sterilization/ high-level disinfection
Noncritical devices	Contact with intact skin	*Example:* Stethoscopes, ECG leads	Intermediate or low-level disinfection

Fig. 1: Spaulding classification.

Spaulding has classified **(Fig. 1)** the medical devices into three major types based on their risk of infection. Endoscope is classified as "semicritical equipment" and hence needs high-level disinfection while most of the accessories are "critical" equipment and so they are either disposable or need sterilization process.

DESIGN OF CLEANING AND DISINFECTION AREA IN THE ENDOSCOPY SUITE

Designated areas for cleaning, disinfection, and storage:

- Spacious and ventilated
- Double sinks and multiple work tops
- Separate handwashing basin
- Automatic endoscope reprocessing unit (optional)
- Ultrasonic cleaner (optional)

STEPS OF ENDOSCOPY REPROCESSING

- Precleaning
- Leak test
- Manual cleaning
- Disinfection or automatic machine reprocessing
- Rinsing and drying
- Storage

Precleaning

- As soon as the endoscopy procedure is over, wipe down the insertion tube with a soft, disposable cloth/sponge **(Fig. 2)**.
- Before the endoscope is detached from the light source and/or video processor, suck detergent through the working channel (minimum 250 mL).
- Ensure that the working channel is not blocked. Flush the air/water channel with water from the water bottle.
- Check the outer surface of the endoscope for any damage
- Detach the endoscope from the light source and/ or video processor
- Transport the endoscope for leak test **(Fig. 3)**.

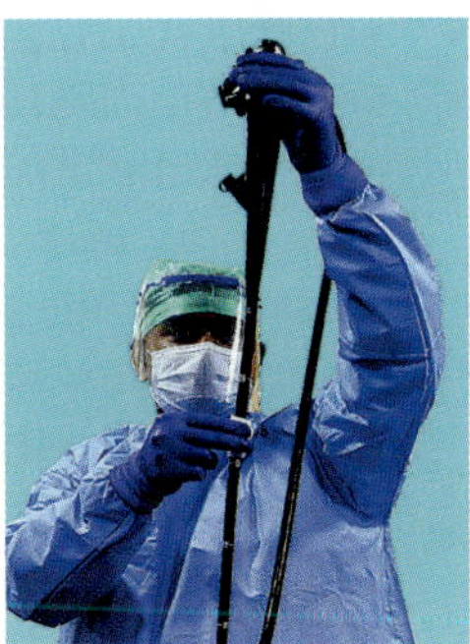

Fig. 2: Precleaning.

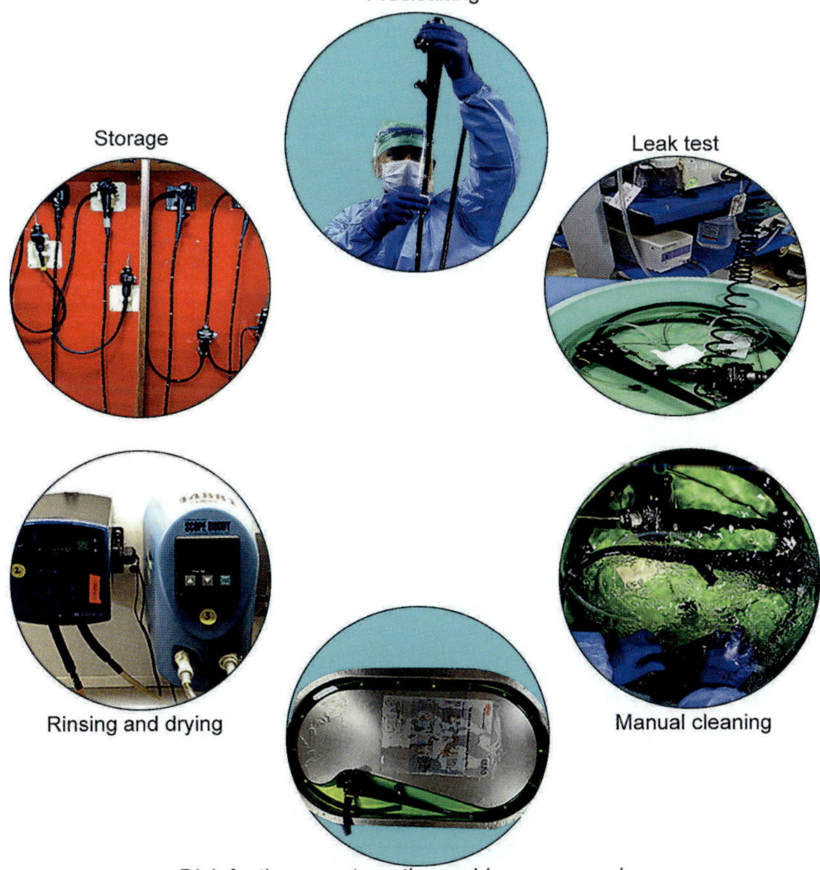

Fig. 3: Steps of endoscopy processing.

Leak Test (Fig. 4)

- Dismantle all detachable parts of the endoscope, e.g., suction valves and air/water valves, biopsy caps
- Attach a soaking cap if necessary
- Perform the leakage test according to manufacturer's instructions in order to check the inner and outer surfaces of the endoscope for any damage. Attach the leak testing device to pressurize the endoscope. Watch the pressure gauge to note that there is no drop in the pressure implying absence of any leak anywhere. But if there is any drop in pressure shown, then immerse the scope in a basin of water to look for site and size of the leak which is invariably in the bending section. Bubbling air denotes definite leak. Turn both big and small wheels to stretch the bending section rubber to look for any subtle damage. Ensure all the pressure is removed from the scope before removing the leak testing device.
- If the leakage test is positive, the reprocessing procedure must be interrupted immediately and repair of the endoscope must be initiated. Contact the service engineer.

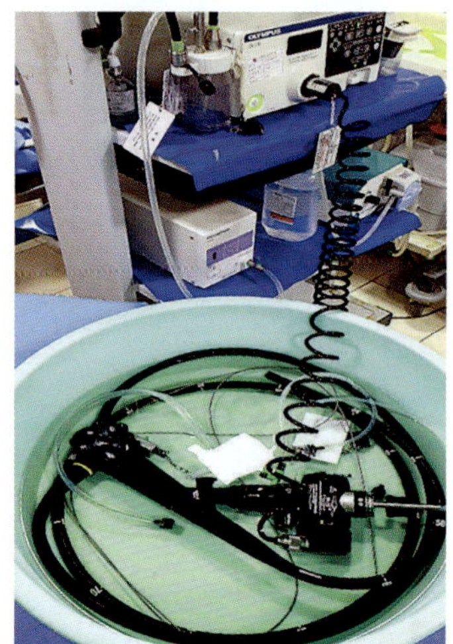

Fig. 4: Leak test.

Manual Cleaning (Figs. 5A to C)

- Scrupulous manual cleaning is the most effective way to bring down the bioburden.
- Never underestimate the importance of manual cleaning of the flexible endoscopy. Brushing and flushing are two most important aspects of reprocessing process. Even prolonged disinfection or automatic machine reprocessing will not compensate for inadequate cleaning.

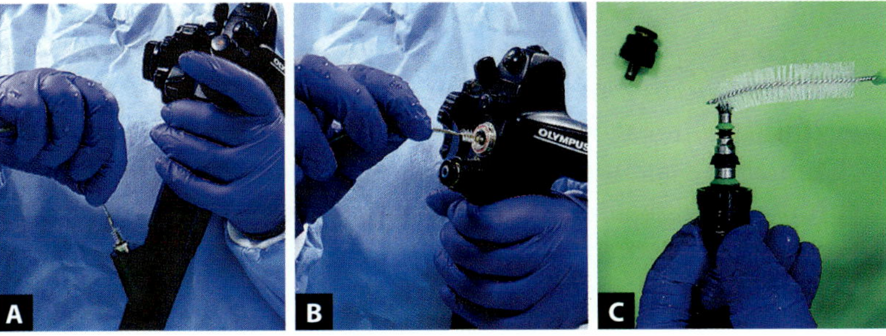

Figs. 5A to C: Manual cleaning.

- It should be done by an experienced certified person dutifully adhering to all the steps of cleaning process. He or she should be familiar with the structure of endoscope and already studied the manufacturer's advice.
- *Following are the steps of manual cleaning:*
  - Immerse the endoscope completely in water with detergent
  - Fill all channels with cleaning solution
  - Clean all external surfaces, valve ports, and channel openings using a soft, disposable cloth/sponge, and brushes
  - The distal end is brushed with a soft toothbrush and special attention is paid to the air/water outlet nozzle and the ridge/elevator.
  - Brush all accessible channels with a flexible, purpose designed brush

Disinfection Process

- *Types of disinfectants used:*
  - 2.4% glutaraldehyde
  - 3.4% glutaraldehyde
  - Ortho-phthalaldehyde
  - Peracetic acid
  - Hydrogen peroxide
- *Effectiveness of disinfectants:*
  - The common microorganisms of greatest concern to endoscopy, particularly hepatitis B virus (HBV) and human immunodeficiency virus (HIV), are among the most sensitive of all microbiological agents to chemical disinfection
  - Hepatitis C virus (HCV), being a lipid containing virus, is predicted to have a similar sensitivity to HBV.
  - Intermediate levels of resistance are shown by common vegetative bacteria like *Pseudomonas*.
  - Some increased resistance is present with mycobacteria and nonlipid-containing viruses, e.g., poliovirus and hepatitis A virus but still could easily eliminated following good manual washing and dwelling in the disinfectant solution for the recommended duration.

- There has been concern also regarding cross infection due to *Helicobacter pylori, Clostridioides difficile,* methicillin-resistant *Staphylococcus aureus* (MRSA), vancomycin-resistant *Enterococcus* (VRE), multidrug-resistant tuberculosis (MDR-TB) and prions like Creutzfeldt–Jakob disease (CJD). Proper cleaning and disinfection protocol clears all the above pathogens except prions which need special attention. Avoid endoscopy in proven cases of CJD or else use a backup scopes specifically designated for such cases.

Cidex 2% (Figs. 6A and B)

- *Dwelling time:* 20 minutes
- *Shelf life:* 2 weeks
- *Advantages:*
  - Once activated, it is stable for 14 days.
  - Excellent compatibility with materials does not damage the scope.
- *Disadvantages:*
  - Slow action against bacterial spores and mycobacteria
  - Sensitizing, irritant to skin, eyes, and respiratory tract/stains skin
  - Adverse effects for patients after insufficient rinsing of devices
  - Fixative, tends to create residue film on the scope
  - Environmental health and safety measures are expensive.

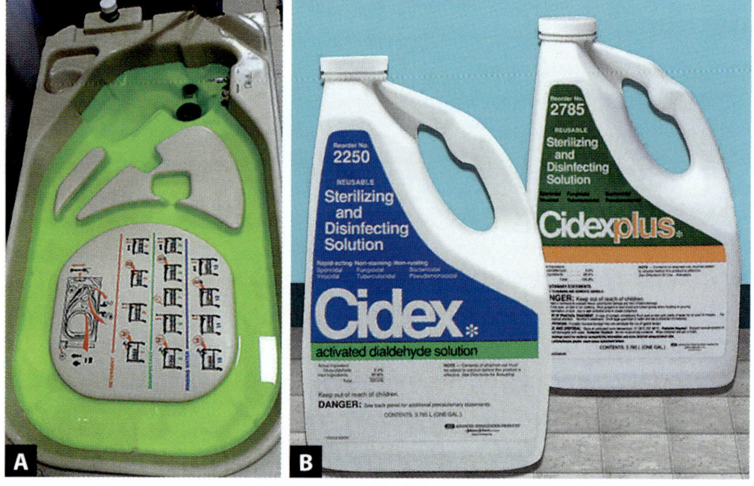

Figs. 6A and B: Cidex.

Peracetic Acid (Figs. 7A and B)

- *Dwelling time:* 10 minutes
- *Shelf life:* 24 hours

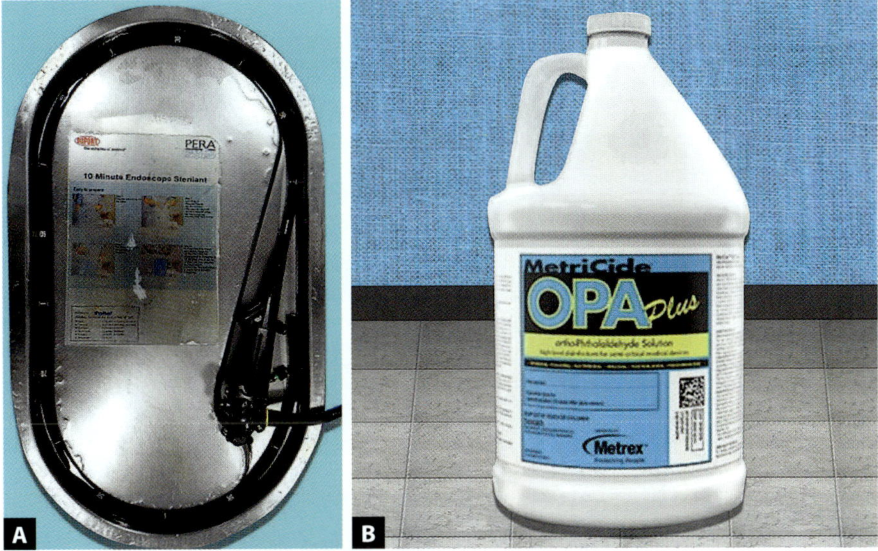

Figs. 7A and B: Peracetic acid.

- *Advantages of peracetic acid:*
  - Fast high-level disinfection and sporicidal activity
  - Preferably single-shot use
  - Environmentally friendly substance
  - No chemical crosslinking of protein residues
- *Disadvantages:*
  - Depending on pH value, irritant to skin, eyes, and respiratory tract
  - Strong odor of vinegar

Rinsing and Drying (Figs. 8A and B)

- Rinse the scope with sterile water. Use either RO water or autoclaved water.
- Dry the endoscope externally and flush each channel with air
- The drying process may be supported by flushing 70% isopropyl alcohol through the endoscope channels.
- Fit the disinfected and rinsed buttons and valves

SAFE TRANSFER OF ENDOSCOPE

Ensure that control head, umbilical cord, and the endoscope tip are all held in single or two hands to avoid any damage to these complexes and expensive equipment.

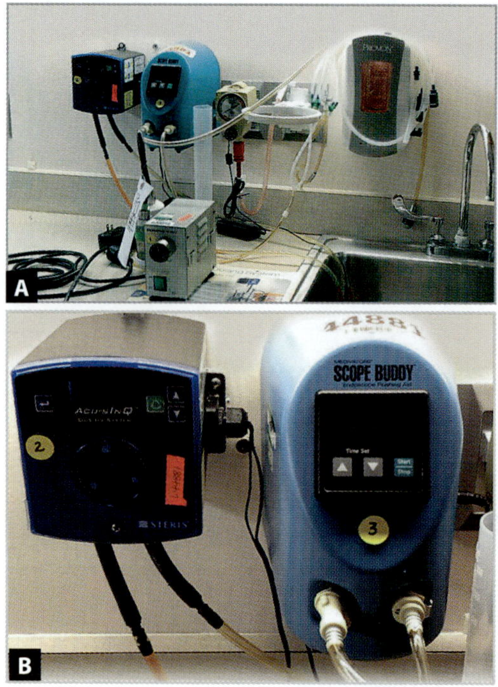

Figs. 8A and B: Rinsing and drying.

STORAGE OF ENDOSCOPE AND ACCESSORIES (FIGS. 9A TO C)

Store the endoscopes vertically hung in ventilated cupboard. Never store in the original suitcase. Keep them clean and dry. Consider reprocessing the scope again prior to use if >4 hours since disinfected.

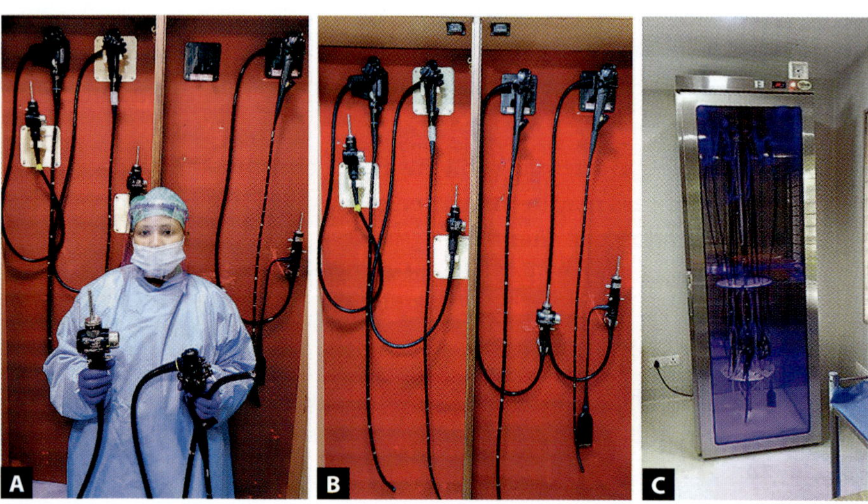

Figs. 9A to C: Storage of colonoscopy.

Accessories can be disposable or reusable. Consider ethical, medical, and economical issues prior to considering reprocessing of disposable items. Ensure protection against dust, moisture, temperature, and humidity extremes. Reprocessed items should be labeled to indicate the load number, the date of sterilization, and the expiration date (if applicable).

AUTOMATED WASHER AND DISINFECTOR (FIGS. 10A AND B)

- *Advantages:*
  - High level of standardization in reprocessing
  - Low risk of staff infection

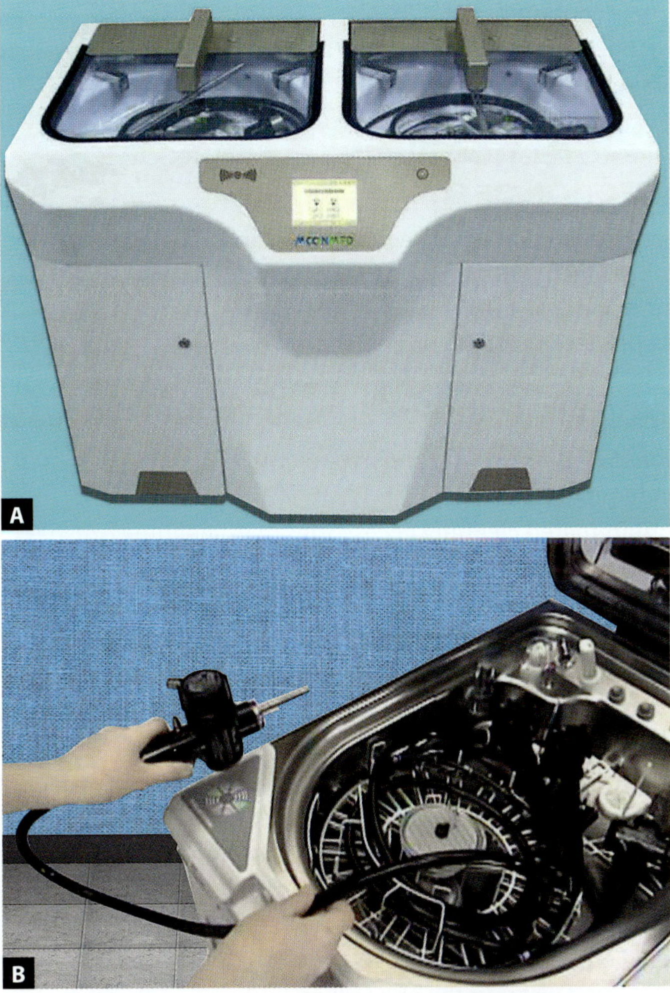

Figs. 10A and B: Automated washer and disinfector.

    - Complete documentation
    - Economic use of chemicals and other resources
    - More user-friendly and reliable
- *Disadvantages:*
    - High cost
    - Dedicated user skills and knowledge are still required.

GUIDELINES FOR ULTRASONIC CLEANING

- Use a medical grade ultrasonic cleaner with a frequency range over 30 kHz (38–47 kHz) and a maximum operating temperature of 45°C, following the manufacturer's instructions.
- Ensure that the detergent used is a nonfoaming solution.
- Renew the cleaning solution at least daily or more frequently if the solution is contaminated.
- Ensure that the tray is large enough and deep enough to allow for complete immersion of the devices.

STAFF PROTECTION DURING CLEANING AND DISINFECTION OF ENDOSCOPES

- Universal protection with gowns, gloves, and goggles
- Vaccine protection for hepatitis B and TB
- Frequent handwashing
- Safe disposal of soiled items and sharps

COMMON PROBLEMS IN ENDOSCOPY REPROCESSING

- *Inadequate reprocessing of endoscopes and accessories:*
    - Inadequate cleaning
    - Contaminated cleaning accessories (e.g., cleaning brushes)
    - Use of unsuitable or incompatible detergents and disinfectants
    - Inadequate concentrations, contact time of disinfecting agents
    - Contaminated rinsing water
    - Fixed organic material in endoscopes or washer-disinfectors
    - Inadequate reprocessing of water bottles (e.g., no sterilization)
    - Use of tap water in water bottles
- *Inadequate transport and storage of endoscopes:*
    - Insufficient drying before storage (e.g., *Pseudomonas*)
    - Inappropriate storage conditions (do not keep the scope inside a suitcase)
- Contaminated or defective washer-disinfector unit
- Damaged endoscopes
- Contaminated water in the endoscopy unit

QUALITY CONTROL OF DISINFECTION PROCESS (FIGS. 11A TO C)

- Keep records of cleaning and disinfection process
- Periodic bacteriological surveillance of endoscopes and the endoscopy washing and cleaning units. Transmission of *Mycobacterium tuberculosis* by bronchoscopes and *Pseudomonas* by ERCP scopes are distinct possibilities.
- Beware of water contamination leading to *Pseudomonas* and atypical mycobacteria infection
- Follow clearly written infection control policy
- Document any incidence of infection. Risk of infection depends on type and virulence of organism, host immunity, and type of endoscopy procedure performed. Risk of transmission of infection is higher during various therapeutic interventions such as POEM, ERCP, and sclerotherapy. Hence, administration of prophylactic antibiotics is recommended.

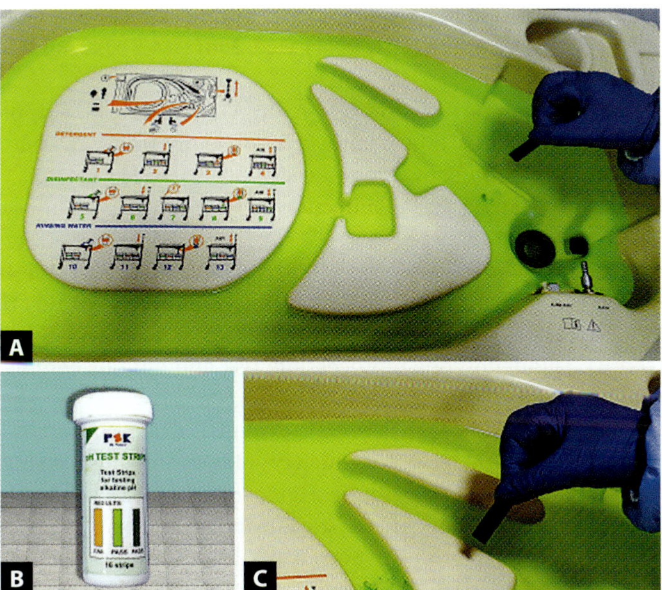

Figs. 11A to C: Quality control in disinfection process.

KEY MESSAGE

- Endoscope needs high-level disinfection prior to use.
- Accessories are ought to be disposable. If reusable, then proper sterilization has to be done.
- Adhere to local quality control policy for disinfection process.

SUGGESTED READING

1. ANSI webstore. (2021). ANSI/AAMI ST91:2015. Flexible and semi-rigid endoscope processing in health care facilities. [online]. Available from https://webstore.ansi.org/standards/AAMI/ansiaamist912015 [Last accessed April, 2025].
2. Becker B, Brill FHH, Todt D, Steinmann E, Lenz J, Paulmann D, et al. Virucidal efficacy of peracetic acid for instrument disinfection. Antimicrob Resist Infect Control. 2017;6:114.
3. Beilenhoff U, Neumann CS, Rey JF, Biering H, Blum R, Cimbro M, et al. ESGE-ESGENA Guideline: cleaning and disinfection in gastrointestinal endoscopy. Endoscopy. 2008;40(11):939-57.
4. Birnie GG, Quigley EM, Clements GB, Follet EA, Watkinson G. Endoscopic transmission of hepatitis B virus. Gut. 1983;24(2):171-4.
5. British Society of Gastroenterology. (2020). BSG Guidance on Decontamination of Equipment for Gastrointestinal Endoscopy: The Report of a Working Party of the BSG Endoscopy Committee. [online] Available from https://www.bsg.org.uk/BSG/media/BSG-Media/BSG-Decontamination-guidance-2020-update.pdf [Last accessed April, 2025].
6. Bronowicki JP, Venard V, Botté C, Monhoven N, Gastin I, Choné L, et al. Patient-to-patient transmission of hepatitis C virus during colonoscopy. N Engl J Med. 1997;337(4):237-40. Erratum in: N Engl J Med. 2001;344(5):392. Rhin B [corrected to Rihn B].
7. Cowan RE, Manning AP, Ayliffe GA, Axon AT, Causton JS, Cripps NF, et al. Aldehyde disinfectants and health in endoscopy units. British Society of Gastroenterology Endoscopy Committee. Gut. 1993;34(11):1641-5.
8. Guidelines on cleaning and disinfection in GI endoscopy. Endoscopy. 2000; 32:76-83.
9. Muscarella LF. Risk of transmission of carbapenem-resistant Enterobactericeae and related "superbugs" during gastrointestinal endoscopy. World J Gastrointest Endosc. 2014;6:457-74.
10. Petersen BT. Duodenoscope reprocessing: risk and options coming into view. Gastrointest Endosc. 2015;82:484-6.
11. Reprocessing Guideline Task Force; Petersen BT, Cohen J, Hambrick RD 3rd, Buttar N, Greenwald DA, et al. Multisociety guideline on reprocessing flexible GI endoscopes: 2016 update. Gastrointest Endosc. 2017;85(2):282-94.e1.
12. Rey JF, Kruse A, Neumann C; ESGE (European Society of Gastrointestinal Endoscopy); ESGENA (European Society of Gastrointestinal Endoscopy Nurses and Associates). ESGE/ESGENA technical note on cleaning and disinfection. Endoscopy. 2003;35(10):869-77.
13. Santos LX, Souza Dias MB, Borrasca VL, Cavassin LT, Deso di Lobo R, Bozza Schwenck RC, et al. Improving hand hygiene adherence in an endoscopy unit. Endoscopy. 2013;45(6):421-5.
14. Schmelzer M, Daniels G, Hough H. Safe storage time for reprocessed flexible endoscopes: a systematic review. JBI Database System Rev Implement Rep. 2015;13(9):187-243.

Expert's Comment

Reprocessing of flexible endoscopes is a cornerstone of infection prevention in gastrointestinal endoscopy. Owing to their intricate design, multiple channels, and repeated use across patients, flexible endoscopes represent a unique challenge for decontamination. Numerous reports have established the risk of transmission of pathogens such as hepatitis B, hepatitis C, *Pseudomonas aeruginosa*, and multidrug-resistant organisms when reprocessing protocols are inadequately followed.

A systematic approach comprising bedside precleaning, leak testing, meticulous manual cleaning, and high-level disinfection is essential. Among these, manual cleaning remains the most critical step, as inadequate removal of organic debris compromises subsequent disinfection, even when automated systems are employed. The use of glutaraldehyde, ortho-phthalaldehyde, or peracetic acid–based solutions achieves effective high-level disinfection, though each carries advantages and limitations. Automated washer-disinfectors enhance standardization and reduce occupational exposure, yet they are not a substitute for rigorous manual cleaning.

Post-disinfection measures, including proper rinsing with sterile or filtered water, alcohol flushing, forced air drying, and vertical storage in ventilated cabinets, are equally vital to prevent recontamination. Comprehensive staff training, appropriate use of protective equipment, vaccination, and adherence to institutional quality-control policies further reinforce safety.

Storage of disinfected endoscopes in well-ventilated cabinets in the hung-up state will avoid any moisture, formation of biofilms, and subsequent *Pseudomonas* superinfection.

I like to emphasize the importance of proper sterilization of endoscopic accessories, either using ETO or gas plasma, before reuse.

Ultimately, strict adherence to evidence-based reprocessing protocols ensures patient safety, protects healthcare personnel, and preserves the functional integrity of valuable endoscopic equipment.

The safety of the endoscopic procedure and longevity of endoscopes depend on proper cleaning and disinfection protocols.

I really appreciate the efforts taken by the author to highlight the importance of cleaning, disinfection and sterilization (CDS) in this *Manual of Endoscopy*.

Dr M Senthil
Hosur

CHAPTER

Training in the Art of Endoscopy

Chapter Outline

- Aim of the Endoscopy Training
- Achieving Competency in Endoscopy
- Cognitive Aspects of Endoscopy
- Technical Aspects of Endoscopy
- Modes of Training in Endoscopy
- Importance of Intensive Short Fellowship Courses in Flexible Endoscopy
- Indian Association of Gastrointestinal Endosurgeons Endoscopy Training Courses
    - Key Components of Indian Association of Gastrointestinal Endosurgeons Endoscopy Training Courses
- Types of Indian Association of Gastrointestinal Endosurgeons Endoscopy Training Courses
    - Endoscopy Fellowship of the Indian Association of Gastrointestinal Endosurgeons Course Curriculum (Basic Endoscopy Fellowship of IAGES)
    - FAGIE Colonoscopy Training Course
    - Fellowship in Advanced Gastrointestinal Endoscopy and Endoscopic Retrograde Cholangiopancreatography Training Course
    - Fellowship in Advanced Gastrointestinal Endoscopy UGI Therapeutic Endoscopy Course
- Quality Indicators of Good Endoscopy Practice
- Qualities of a Good Endoscopy Trainer

Keywords: Competence in endoscopy, cognitive skills, technical skills, virtual simulator

AIM OF THE ENDOSCOPY TRAINING

To teach the trainees to obtain the knowledge and technical skills so that he/she is:

- Able to take good history and relevant clinical examinations.
- Decide the need and urgency of any endoscopic examination.
- Able to do preprocedure patient checklist and Instrument checklist.

- Be able to obtain informed consent.
- Capable of using various drugs needed during endoscopy.
- Can perform the endoscopic procedure safely, swiftly, and completely.
- Able to correctly interpret the findings with standard terminology, correlate them with the clinical diagnosis, and initiate further relevant investigation.
- Recognize various possible complications and manage them competently.
- Able to understand various troubleshooting tricks during endoscopy and also know when to ask for a senior's help.
- Capable of proper documentation and reporting of the procedures and auditing the work in the department.
- Always willing to learn and strive to improve the quality of work.

ACHIEVING COMPETENCY IN ENDOSCOPY

Just by performing a threshold number of endoscopies (say 140 cases), one cannot claim to be an expert in endoscopy. Competency depends on both cognitive and technical skills, which can only be achieved by well-structured, flexible endoscopy fellowship courses.

COGNITIVE ASPECTS OF ENDOSCOPY

- Knowledge about when to do and when not to do endoscopy.
- Patient checklist and endoscopy workstation checklist before the procedure.
- Good knowledge about sedation/monitoring.
- Correct pathology interpretation and use of image enhancement and other innovative methods.
- Ability to do suitable therapeutic intervention.
- Competency in making and communicating appropriate clinical decisions.

TECHNICAL ASPECTS OF ENDOSCOPY

- Proper navigation techniques
- Loop recognition and loop reduction ability in colonoscopy
- Retroflexion
- Traversing a sphincter/ileoscopy during colonoscopy
- Management of suction and insufflation
- Appropriate use of abdominal wall pressure and position change
- Thorough mucosal evaluation
- Ability to properly target lesions for biopsy/removal

MODES OF TRAINING IN ENDOSCOPY

- By attending short-duration (3–5 days) or long-duration (6–12 months) endoscopy training courses.
- Refer to ASGE guidelines on various endoscopy and colonoscopic topics to study to improve the cognitive skillset.
- *Refer to various endoscopy atlases and videos*:
    - Dave's project for ASGE
        - Digital Atlas of Video Education
    - YouTube videos and several PPTs available on Google search
- Simulator-based training using both low-fidelity and high-fidelity simulators
- Apprentice-type training with live cases

IMPORTANCE OF INTENSIVE SHORT FELLOWSHIP COURSES IN FLEXIBLE ENDOSCOPY

Endoscopy skills are not optional but essential for every surgeon in this era of minimally invasive surgery. The diagnostic potential of high-definition (HD) endoscopy are quite obvious. In addition, surgeons would be able to perform the removal of polyps, control of bleeding, and closure of perforations on this flexible endoscopy platform without any need for surgery. Though surgeons are exposed to endoscopic procedures during their postgraduate training, often, it is not well structured and hence inefficient in skill transfer. The Joint Advisory Group in Gastrointestinal Endoscopy (JAG) highlighted the inadequacy of endoscopy training for Higher Surgical trainees in the UK (HST). Similarly, SAGES (Society of American Gastrointestinal Endo Surgeons) also realized the importance of endoscopy training for surgeons and initiated the Flexible Endoscopic Surgery program (FES). American Board of Surgery (ABS) now warrants every surgeon to complete the FES program before becoming board-certified.

Indian Association of Gastrointestinal Endosurgeons (IAGES) realized the need for similar short-structured endoscopic training and assessment courses for young surgeons in India. The curriculum working group, comprising of the IAGES endoscopy board adviser, conveners, and members, came out with a Pilot training module in 2016 and has now successfully implemented various short structured, flexible endoscopy fellowship courses as given below.

- *EFIAGES (Endoscopy fellowship of IAGES):*
    - 3-day basic endoscopy training and assessment course.
    - Aimed at both cognitive and technical skill training.
        - Key lecture modules.
        - Hands-on simulation module.
        - Live session with the option of performing endoscopy under supervision.

        - *Assessment module:*
            - 50 questions/1-hour MCQ.
            - Viva on technical and cognitive skill aspects.
    - *Aims to provide level 1 training:*
        - Mainly diagnostic upper gastrointestinal (GI) endoscopy/flexible sigmoidoscopy.
        - Basic therapeutic procedures.
        - Banding, injection of a bleeding ulcer, and FB removal.
- *FAGIE (Fellowship of Advanced Gastrointestinal Endoscopy):*
    - 3-day advanced endoscopy training and assessment course.
    - Aim to provide Level 2 training.
        - *FAGIE upper GI therapeutic endoscopy course:* Dilatation, self-expanding metallic (SEM) stenting, place a feeding tube (PEG) tube insertion.
        - *FAGIE colonoscopy training course:* Diagnostic colonoscopy, basics on polypectomy, image enhancement
        - *FAGIE endoscopic retrograde cholangiopancreatography (ERCP) course:* Biliary and pancreatic endotherapy for benign and malignant disorders and introduction to SpyGlass cholangioscopy and ABC of EUS-guided ERCP.

How many cases do you have to do to become a competent endoscopist?

- At least 100–130 gastroscopy procedure
- 25–30 flexible sigmoidoscopy
- 200 colonoscopy procedures
- 150–200 ERCP

The above threshold numbers for training are only an arbitrary and rough guide. We should realize that the procedure competency varies between individuals and also, competency in one procedure does not translate to competency in another procedure. Even after certification, the trainee should be willing to fine-tune and improve their skills by attending further training programs periodically.

Joint Advisory Group in Gastrointestinal Endoscopy (UK) approved the DOPS (Direct observed performance score) assessment based on the following abilities of trainees:

- Assessment, consent, and communication
- Safety and sedation
- Technical skills during endoscopy
- Knowledge about the Diagnostic and therapeutic ability of endotherapy

Similarly, SAGES has come out with GAGES (Global Assessment of Gastrointestinal Endoscopic Skills). Participation in the FES course by SAGES and a Score of >17/25 in GAGES, along with a minimum threshold number of 50 endoscopy cases, are a must for becoming an American board-certified surgeon. MCSAT (Mayo Colonoscopy Skill Assessment Tool) is also a well-known valid tool for the assessment of cognitive and technical skills of colonoscopy.

INDIAN ASSOCIATION OF GASTROINTESTINAL ENDOSURGEONS ENDOSCOPY TRAINING COURSES

Key Components of Indian Association of Gastrointestinal Endosurgeons Endoscopy Training Courses

- Lecture modules
- Simulation module
- Live demonstration module
- Assessment module

TYPES OF INDIAN ASSOCIATION OF GASTROINTESTINAL ENDOSURGEONS ENDOSCOPY TRAINING COURSES

- EFIAGES (basic endoscopy fellowship of IAGES)
- FAGIE Colonoscopy
- FAGIE ERCP
- FAGIE UGI therapeutic endoscopy

Endoscopy Fellowship of the Indian Association of Gastrointestinal Endosurgeons Course Curriculum (Basic Endoscopy Fellowship of IAGES)

Endoscopy Fellowship of the Indian Association of Gastrointestinal Endosurgeons Lecture Modules

- Endoscopy hardware/room setup
- *Endoscopy:* When to do and when not to do/informed consent.
- Endoscopy step-by-step
- Endoscopic atlas of upper GI pathology
- Role of endoscopy in upper GI bleeding
- Role of endoscopy in gastroesophageal reflux disease (GERD) and achalasia.
- Role of endoscopy in FB upper GI tract.
- Therapeutic upper GI endoscopy and role of endoscopy in upper GI malignancy.
- Prevention and management of complications of upper GI endoscopy.
- Colonoscopy hardware/indications/bowel preparation/room setup.
- Colonoscopy step-by-step and outline list of complications.
- Colonoscopic image atlas.
- Image-enhanced endoscopy and colonoscopy.
- Role of EUS in today's diagnosis and management.
- ABC of ERCP.

Live Demonstration Module

- Demonstration of diagnostic upper GI endoscopy and colonoscopy.
- Live transmission of therapeutic endoscopic procedures from centers of excellence in endoscopy.
- By a competent and passionate set of faculties teaching all the tricks in the art of endoscopy and allowing the trainee to do the procedure step-by-step.
  - *Step 1:* Allow them to watch all the steps closely and recognize and describe various lesions.
  - *Step 2:* Make them handle the endoscopy during withdrawal, then allow them to do various parts of the procedure.
  - *Step 3:* Allow them to do the whole procedure himself/herself under direct supervision.
- Teach the importance of patient safety and comfort.
- Teach how to monitor the patients and recognize any complications.
- Teach standard procedures initially and once he/she is competent, then proceed with more advanced procedures later.

Hands-on Simulation Module

- *Hands-on simulation exercises:* Static models/animal models/virtual simulators can be used.
- Use static plastic models for teaching hand-eye coordination and scope handling (e.g., Classen's upper GI plastic dummy) **(Fig. 1)**.
- Use animal models (pig or goat and teach therapeutic interventions (e.g., EASIE animal model) **(Fig. 2)**.
- *Live animal model:* Porcine model for peroral endoscopic myotomy (POEM) **(Fig. 3)**.
- Computer-aided training, e.g., GI mentor by Simbionix **(Fig. 4)**

FAGIE Colonoscopy Training Course

Lecture Modules for the FAGIE Colonoscopy Course

- About colonoscopes and accessories
- Setting up a colonoscopy suite
- Indication, contraindication, and consent
- Bowel preparation
- Colonoscopy step-by-step
- Atlas of colorectal pathology
- Tips and tricks during a difficult colonoscopy
- Cleaning and disinfection of colonoscopes
- ABC of therapeutic colonoscopy
- Recent advances in colonoscopy
- Complications of colonoscopy

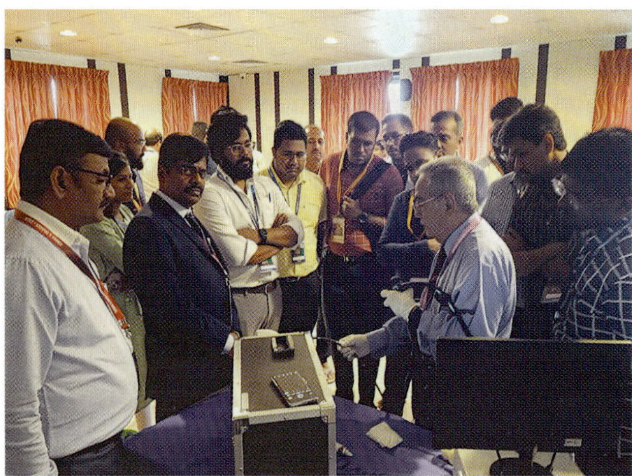

Fig. 1: Upper GI plastic model for endoscopy training.

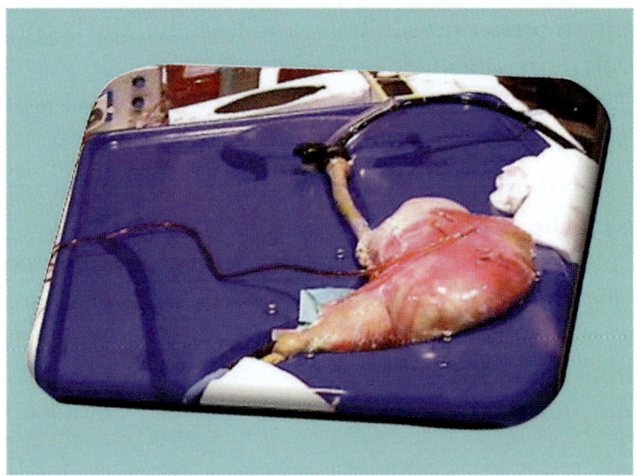

Fig. 2: EASIE animal model.

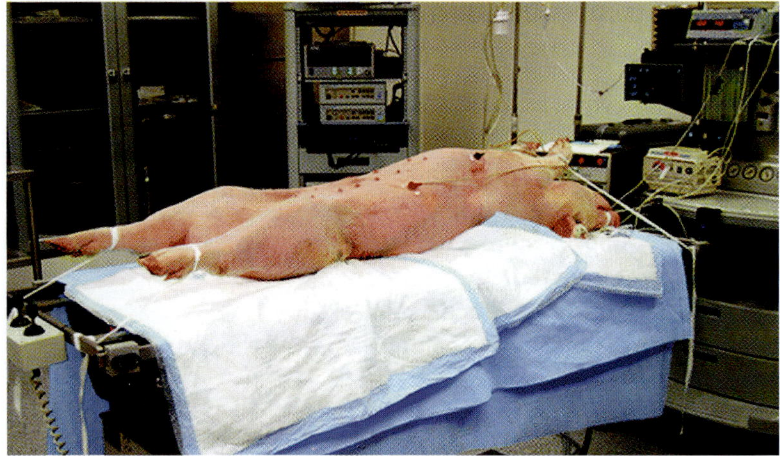

Fig. 3: Live animal model.

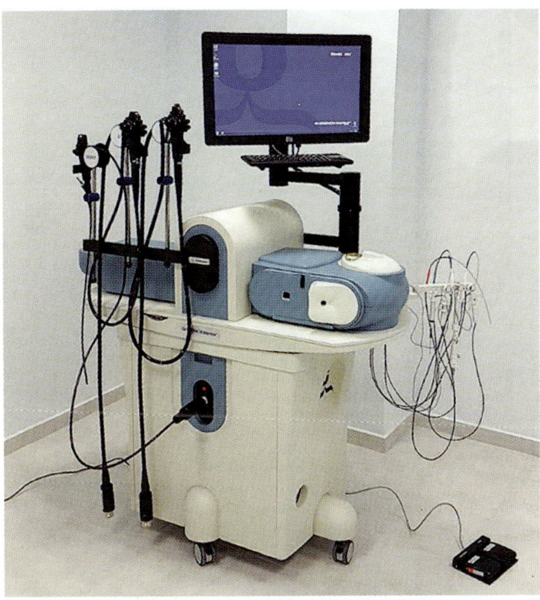

Fig. 4: Simbionix virtual endoscopy.

Hands-on Colonoscopy Simulation Module

- Perform and demonstrate various steps of colonoscopy using plastic models and computer simulators.
- Use static plastic models for teaching hand-eye coordination and scope handling.
    - St Mark's colonoscopy plastic tubing simulator **(Fig. 5)**.
    - Tubingen model using a wax-like substance, namely Artitex
    - Mikoto colonoscopy simulator **(Figs. 6A and B)**.

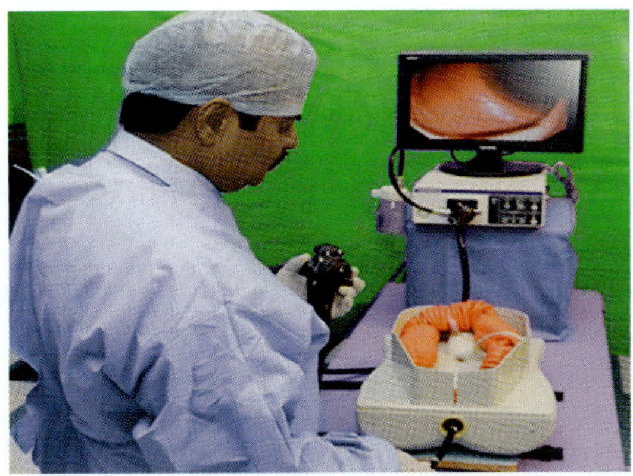

Fig. 5: St Mark's colonoscopy model.

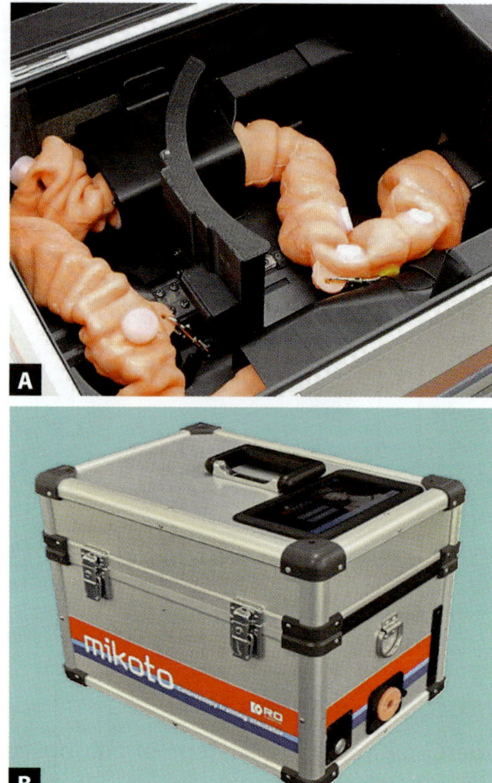

Figs. 6A and B: Mikoto colonoscopy simulator.

- *Use of animal models:*
  - *Ex vivo animal models:*
    - Useful to teach therapeutic interventions, such as polypectomy and ESD.
    - EASIE animal model in Erlangen Endo trainer developed by Hochberger et al. (Germany).
    - Colo EASIE ex vivo porcine model with external spiral support.
    - Bovine colon model by Sedlack et al.

Computer-aided Training (e.g., Gastrointestinal Mentor by Simbionix)

- *Benefits:*
  - 10 hours of training could shorten the learning curve of colonoscopy for real beginners.
  - Both cognitive and technical aspects can be taught.
  - With self-taught modules, training can be mostly unsupervised.
  - Provide us with a dependable, objective assessment of the competency of a trainee surgeon.

- *With near real-life experience in performing colonoscopies:*
    - Actual colonoscope with wheels and buttons
    - Simulation of insufflation and suction
    - Force feedback
    - Ability to see the tip location and loop formation
    - Could be a good assessment tool also.
- *Disadvantages:*
    - Very expensive
    - Not much to offer for more advanced training at present

Live Colonoscopy Demonstration Module

- By a set of competent and passionate faculty teaching all the tricks in the art of colonoscopy and allowing the trainee to do the procedure step-by-step.
    - *Step 1:* Allow them to watch all the steps closely and recognize and describe various lesions.
    - *Step 2:* Make them handle the scope during withdrawal then allow them to do various parts of the procedure.
    - *Step 3:* Allow them to do the whole procedure himself/herself under direct supervision.
- Teach the importance of patient safety and comfort.
- Teach how to monitor the patients and recognize any complications.
- Teach standard procedures initially and once he/she is competent, then proceed with more advanced procedures later.

Self-Learning Module

- Web-based learning, e.g., YouTube videos, various colonoscopy picture atlases and image galleries, and Webcasts.
- Standard textbooks, DVDs with various procedures, and endoscopy journals.

Assessment Module (Figs. 7A to C)

Both knowledge and technical skills are assessed by various components of this module:

- *Written assessment:* Employing MCQ and short essay papers.
- Oral presentation of various topics by the trainee.
- Viva by external faculty to assess the competency of the trainee and the quality of training.
- *Practical assessment:* With simulators and during a real clinical setting.
- Logbook submission with documentation of all the procedures seen or done under supervision.

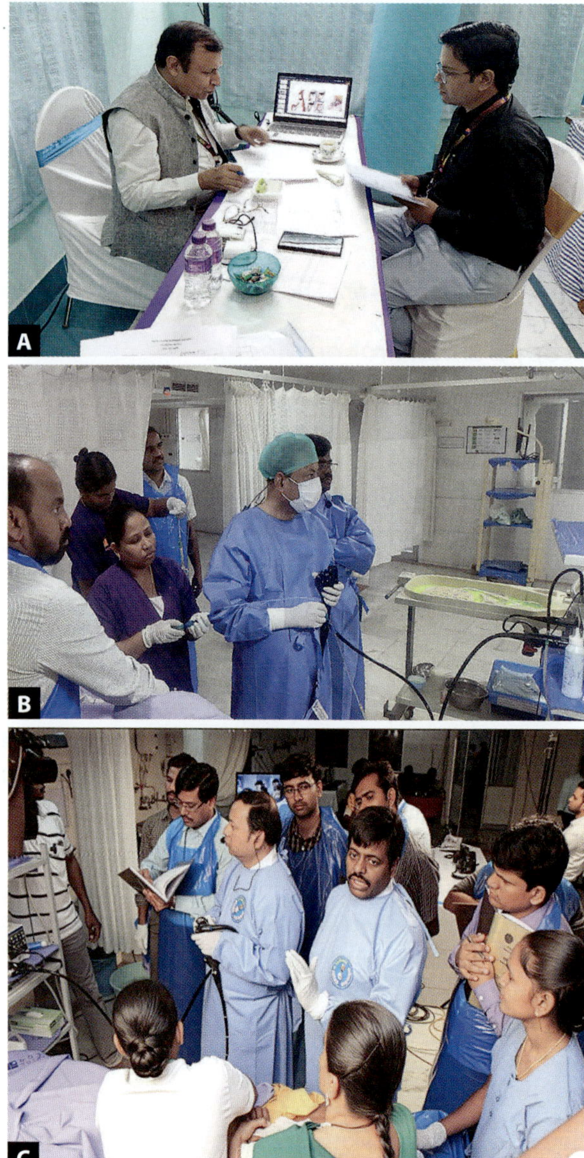

Figs. 7A to C: Assessment module.

Fellowship in Advanced Gastrointestinal Endoscopy and Endoscopic Retrograde Cholangiopancreatography Training Course

Endoscopic Retrograde Cholangiopancreatography Lecture Modules

- About Duodenoscope hardware and ERCP theatre setup.
- About Image intensifier and ERCP image interpretation.

- Indications, cautions, preparation, and consent for ERCP.
- *ERCP step-by-step to reach ampulla:* Tips and tricks in challenging situations.
- *Selective biliary cannulation:* Tips and tricks.
- Overview of biliary endotherapy accessories and techniques.
- *Precut sphincterotomy:* When and how to perform?
- Role of ERCP in malignant jaundice
- Role of ERCP in postlap chole complications
- Panel discussion on complications of ERCP
- Overview of pancreatic endotherapy
- *SpyGlass cholangioscopy:* When and how?
- Interesting case capsules with practice tips
- EUS with ERCP
- Intraoperative ERCP

Hands-on ERCP Simulation Module

- Easie animal model
- Simbionix virtual simulator
- Costamagna ERCP mechanical simulator **(Fig. 8)**

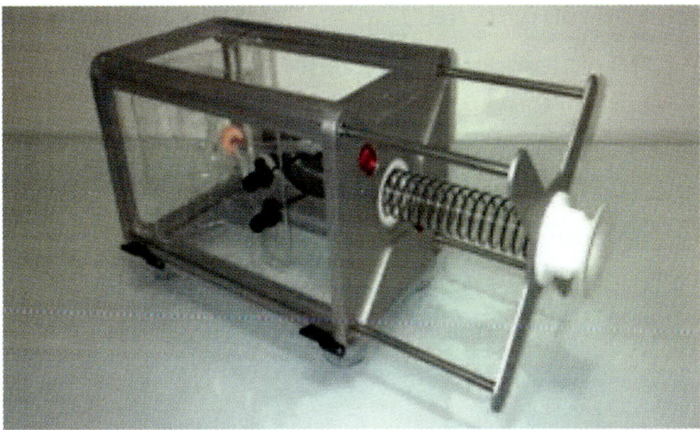

Fig. 8: Costa Magna endoscopic retrograde cholangiopancreatography (ERCP) simulator.

Endoscopic Retrograde Cholangiopancreatography Live Modules

- ERCP for biliary calculi
- ERCP and precut
- ERCP for residual stones
- ERCP and SpyGlass
- ERCP/EUS
- ERCP rendezvous
- Minor duct sphincterotomy

Fellowship in Advanced Gastrointestinal Endoscopy UGI Therapeutic Endoscopy Course

Lecture Modules

- About HD endoscopes, Image enhancement, and magnification endoscopes
- Top 10 tips for setting of advanced endoscopy unit
- Key aspects of energy sources, CO_2 insufflator, and irrigation device.
- Management of esophageal varices
- Endotherapy for gastric varices
- *Gastric EMR:* How do I do?
- Overview of POEM
- Endoscopic management of non-variceal Upper GI bleeding
- Overview of SEM stenting for esophageal carcinoma
- Endotherapy for GERD
- Role Endoscopy in Bariatric surgery
- Endoscopic rescue of anastomotic leaks and fistula and perforations
- Endoscopic management of Barrett's esophagus
- *Complications of therapeutic UGIE:* Panel discussion
- *Difficult FB upper GI tract:* Tips and tricks

Group Discussion: 30 Minutes Each

- Know your HD endoscope and accessories
- Meet the expert for Questions and Answers session

Hands-On Simulation Module

- EASIE animal model
- Simbionix virtual simulator
- Stomach plastic model mechanical simulator

Live Modules

- Chromoendoscopy
- Endotherapy for Barrett's esophagus
- Banding of esophageal varices
- Glue injection for gastric varices
- APC for gastropathy
- Snare polypectomy
- EMR for sessile gastric polyp
- Savary-Gilliard (SG) dilatation of corrosive stricture esophagus
- SEM stenting of carcinoma esophagus
- Antireflux mucosal ablation (ARMA) for GERD
- POEM for achalasia cardia

QUALITY INDICATORS OF GOOD ENDOSCOPY PRACTICE

Following proper structured training in colonoscopy, we should strive to maintain and also improve our skills by performing a minimum threshold number of at least 25 colonoscopy cases per year. Learning is a lifelong experience.

As we know, learning is a four-stage process, namely:

- Stage 1 of unconscious incompetence (Novice)
- Stage 2 of Conscious incompetence
- Stage 3 of Conscious competence
- Stage 4 of unconscious competence (Expert)

The training course helps us to move from stages 1 and 2–3, and lifelong committed learning would make us the real experts. Hard work always pays dividends.

QUALITIES OF A GOOD ENDOSCOPY TRAINER

- Designs a curriculum to train the candidate satisfactorily.
- Constantly monitors his/her progress in acquiring various technical skills.
- Willing to tailor the program as per the needs of the trainees and their skill level.
- Ready to change the program as per the feedback from the previous trainees.
- Willing to guide them with necessary reading materials and CDs.
- Always available and willing to listen and clarify any doubts from the trainee **(Figs. 9A and B)**.

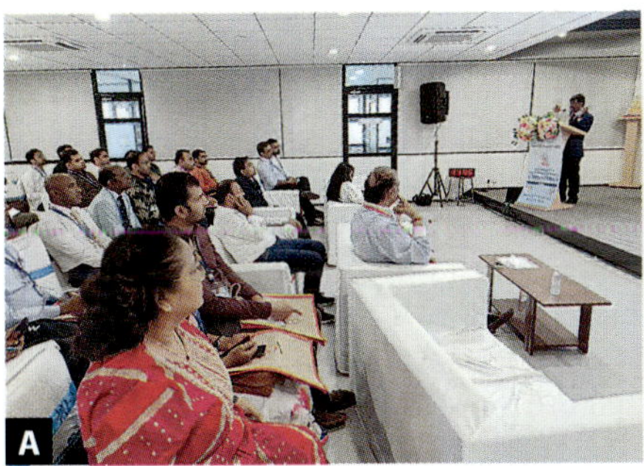

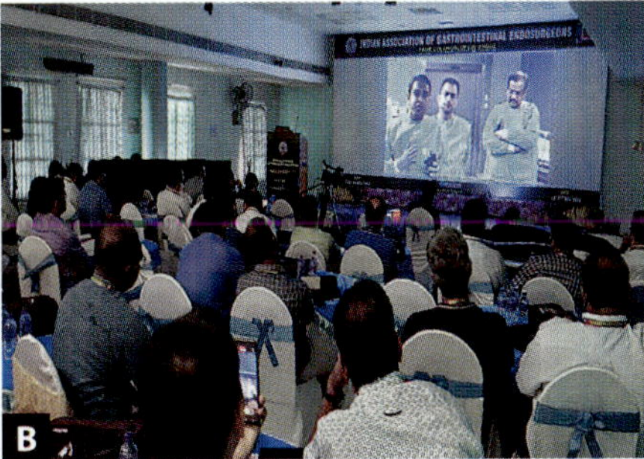

Figs. 9A and B: Endoscopy trainer.

CONCLUSION

- Structured endoscopy training program for surgeons is the need of the hour.
- The success and quality of any training program depends both on dedicated trainers and interested trainees.
- Accredited endoscopy training should be a key part of the general surgeon's training curriculum.

SUGGESTED READING

1. Ahlberg G, Hultcrantz R, Jaramillo E, Lindblom A, Arvidsson D. Virtual reality colonoscopy simulation: a compulsory practice for the future colonoscopist? Endoscopy. 2005;37(12):1198-204.
2. Armstrong D, Enns R, Ponich T, Romagnuolo J, Springer J, Barkun AN. Canadian credentialing guidelines for endoscopic privileges: an overview. Can J Gastroenterol. 2007;21(12):797-801.
3. Armstrong D, Hollingworth R, Gardiner T, Klassen M, Smith W, Hunt RH, et al. Practice Audit in Gastroenterology (PAGE) program: a novel approach to continuing professional development. Can J Gastroenterol. 2006;20(6):405-10.
4. Baillie J, Ravich WJ. On endoscopic training and procedural competence. Ann Intern Med. 1993;118(1):73-4.
5. Barton JR, Corbett S, van der Vleuten CP; English Bowel Cancer Screening Programme; UK Joint Advisory Group for Gastrointestinal Endoscopy. The validity and reliability of a Direct Observation of Procedural Skills assessment tool: assessing colonoscopic skills of senior endoscopists. Gastrointest Endosc. 2012;75(3):591-7.
6. Chung JI, Kim N, Um MS, Kang KP, Lee D, Na JC, et al. Learning curves for colonoscopy: a prospective evaluation of gastroenterology fellows at a single center. Gut Liver. 2010;4(1):31-5.
7. Cohen J, Cohen SA, Vora KC, Xue X, Burdick JS, Bank S, et al. Multicenter, randomized, controlled trial of virtual-reality simulator training in acquisition of competency in colonoscopy. Gastrointest Endosc. 2006;64(3):361-8.
8. Dunkin BJ. Flexible endoscopy simulators. Semin Laparosc Surg. 2003; 10(1):29-35.
9. Dunphy BC, Williamson SL. In pursuit of expertise. Toward an educational model for expertise development. Adv Health Sci Educ Theory Pract. 2004;9(2):107-27.
10. Ekkelenkamp VE, Koch AD, Man RA, Kuipers EJ. Training and competence assessment in GI endoscopy: a systematic review. Gut. 2016;65(4):607-15.
11. Grover SC, Garg A, Scaffidi MA, Yu JJ, Plener IS, Yong E, et al. Impact of a simulation training curriculum on technical and nontechnical skills in colonoscopy: a randomized trial. Gastrointest Endosc. 2015;82(6):1072-9.
12. Koch AD, Haringsma J, Schoon EJ, de Man RA, Kuipers EJ. Competence measurement during colonoscopy training: the use of self-assessment of performance measures. Am J Gastroenterol. 2012;107(7):971-5.
13. Rex DK, Petrini JL, Baron TH, Chak A, Cohen J, Deal SE, et al. Quality indicators for colonoscopy. Am J Gastroenterol. 2006;101(4):873-85.
14. Rex DK, Schoenfeld PS, Cohen J, Pike IM, Adler DG, Fennerty MB, et al. Quality indicators for colonoscopy. Am J Gastroenterol. 2015;110(1):72-90.
15. Rex DK. Quality in colonoscopy: cecal intubation first, then what? Am J Gastroenterol. 2006;101(4):732-4.
16. Sedlack RE, Kolars JC. Computer simulator training enhances the competency of gastroenterology fellows at colonoscopy: results of a pilot study. Am J Gastroenterol. 2004;99(1):33-7.
17. Vozenilek J, Huff JS, Reznek M, Gordon JA. See one, do one, teach one: advanced technology in medical education. Acad Emerg Med. 2004;11(11):1149-54.
18. Wilkins T, Jester D, Kenrick J, Dahl J. The current state of colonoscopy training in family medicine residency programs. Fam Med. 2004;36(6):407-11.

Expert's Comment

An endoscopic skillset is essential for all surgeons in this era of minimal access surgery. The diagnostic and therapeutic potentials of flexible endoscopy are plentiful.

Despite the need and necessity for an endoscopy skillset, many surgeons lack the competence in performing even diagnostic endoscopy nowadays. Although the endoscopy training curriculum exists for postgraduate surgical students, properly structured training by competent and interested trainers is not widely available in India. The Joint Advisory Committee in the UK has also mentioned that endoscopic training for higher surgical trainees is far from satisfactory. The American Board of Surgeons (ABS) has noticed similar inadequacies in their surgical trainees and hence advised them to take the Flexible Endoscopy Surgery Training Course (FES) conducted by the Society of American Gastrointestinal and Endoscopic Surgeons.

Now, surgeons have come to realize the importance of flexible endoscopy skills and look for any training opportunities. The apprenticeship model of yesteryears is not ideal and will not be practicable for busy practicing surgeons. Competence in the endoscopic skillset needs to be acquired through both technical and cognitive skillset training. Most of the surgeons possess a three-dimensional (3D) understanding of anatomy and good knowledge of various gastrointestinal (GI) pathologies. They also possess good hand and eye coordination. Hence, the diagnostic endoscopy skillset could be easily taught to the interested surgeons with properly structured endoscopy training courses conducted by competent and experienced senior surgeons. Competence in the endoscopy skillset can be measured reliably with direct observation of procedure skill (DOPS) or any similar assessment method.

Endoscopy training should ideally be a lifelong learning experience. The learners should know when to seek advice from experienced seniors to abate the risks from inadequate completion of the procedure.

It is heartening to note that IAGES has been conducting both basic and advanced flexible endoscopy courses for several years, benefiting hundreds of surgeons. The author has wonderfully summarized various such courses available and their curriculum.

Future surgeons are better placed if they possess both laparoscopic and endoscopic skillsets.

Dr Ganni Bhaskara Rao
Rajahmundry

CHAPTER 19

Drugs used in Endoscopy Unit

Chapter Outline

Keywords: Conscious sedation, propofol infusion, procedural monitoring

INTRODUCTION

Endoscopy plays a significant role in the diagnosis and treatment of gastrointestinal diseases. Sedation has been used in clinical practice to make the procedure more comfortable and improve patient satisfaction by helping patients feel relaxed. Although sedation is widely used for these benefits, it continues to pose some potential risks, requiring medical teams to monitor patients closely during the procedure.

All the endoscopists and staff in the endoscopy suite should be well-versed in all the knowledge about commonly used drugs in the endoscopic unit.

We shall enumerate the list and details of all the commonly used drugs in the endoscopy unit. Informed written consent for administering sedatives is essential.

LOCAL ANESTHETIC SPRAY (XYLOCAINE 10% SPRAY) OR LIQUID (FIG. 1)

Indication

Pharyngeal anesthesia can be used in any upper gastrointestinal (GI) endoscopic procedure.

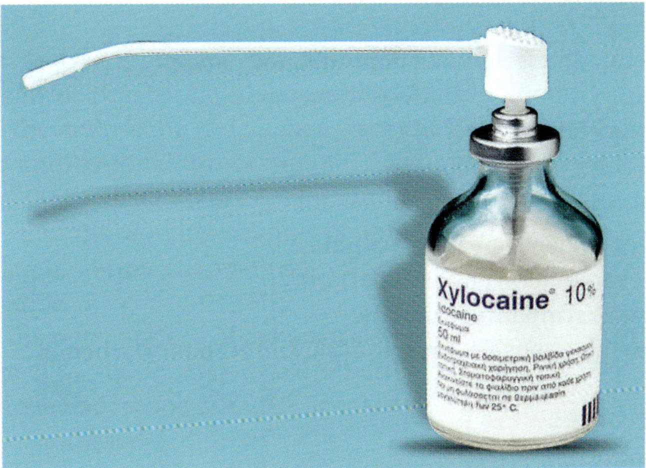

Fig. 1: Xylocaine spray.

Contraindications

- Emergency endoscopy (increased risk of aspiration)
- Known hypersensitivity

Advantage

Better patient tolerance of the examination.

Disadvantages

- Increased risk of aspiration
- Allergic reaction
- Bad taste
- Cough
- Swallowing difficulties after the examination

Method

Two squirts of lidocaine sprayed into the pharynx or 5–10 mL of liquid solution.

Precautions

Nothing by mouth from 30 minutes to 1 hour after the examination.

SEDATION DURING ENDOSCOPY

Indications

- Requested by the patient
- Very anxious patient

Contraindications

- Emergency endoscopy in a nonintubated patient
- Respiratory failure
- Circulatory failure

Advantages

- Improves subjective patient tolerance
- Makes examination easier to perform
- Suppresses sympathetic outflow
- Reduces hypertension, arrhythmias, and coronary ischemia

Disadvantages

- Respiratory depression
- Less cooperative patient
- Paradoxical reaction
- Risk of aspiration

Endoscopy Performed without any Sedation

- Selected patients may be able to undergo endoscopic procedures without sedation.
- Small-diameter endoscopes (<6 mm) can improve the tolerability of upper endoscopy when sedation is not used. In general, topical anesthesia is used during unsedated endoscopy.
- A successful colonoscopy may be performed in selected patients who receive no sedation or sedation only if needed. Older patients, men, patients who are not anxious, or patients without a history of abdominal pain may have better tolerance of colonoscopy with little or no sedation.

Endoscopy Performed Under Sedation

- The level of sedation required to perform a successful procedure may range from minimal sedation to general anesthesia.
- Patient age, health status, concurrent medications, preprocedural anxiety, and pain tolerance influence the level of sedation required to achieve the desired result.
- The procedural variables include the degree of invasiveness, the level of procedure-related discomfort, the need for the patient to lie relatively motionless [e.g., endoscopic ultrasound-guided fine-needle aspiration (EUS-FNA)], and the duration of the examination. Typically, diagnostic and uncomplicated therapeutic upper endoscopy and colonoscopy are successfully performed with moderate sedation. Deeper levels of sedation may be considered for longer and more complex procedures, including,

but not limited to, endoscopic retrograde cholangiopancreatography (ERCP) and EUS. Additionally, deep sedation or general anesthesia should be considered for patients who have been difficult to manage with moderate sedation and are anticipated to be poorly responsive to sedatives. This includes patients who have had long-term use of narcotics, benzodiazepines, alcohol, or neuropsychiatric medications.

Drugs used Commonly for Sedation

- Midazolam
- Diazepam

Precautions

- Close patient surveillance with pulse oximetry
- Intravenous line
- Nasal O_2 available
- *Have antagonists available:* IV flumazenil for midazolam overdose

Levels of Sedation

1. *Minimal sedation (anxiolysis):* The patient responds normally to verbal commands. Cognitive function may be impaired, but ventilatory and cardiovascular functions are unaffected.
2. *Moderate sedation (conscious sedation):* The patient responds purposefully to verbal commands with or without light tactile stimulation. Spontaneous ventilation is adequate, and cardiovascular function is maintained.
3. *Deep sedation:* The patient is not easily aroused but responds purposefully to painful stimulation. Patients may not be able to maintain a patent airway, and spontaneous ventilation may be inadequate. Cardiovascular function usually is maintained
4. *Anesthesia:* Consists of general anesthesia and spinal or major regional anesthesia. It does not include local anesthesia. Patients are not arousable, even by painful stimulation. The patient often requires assistance in maintaining a patent airway and positive pressure ventilation. Cardiovascular function may be impaired.

During endoscopy, the patient has to be in a level of conscious sedation. It means:

- The patient can make a purposeful response to verbal or tactile stimulation
- Both the ventilatory and cardiovascular functions are maintained.

Midazolam (Fig. 2)

- Short-acting benzodiazepine
- *Merits:* Sedation, anxiolytic, and amnesia for the procedure

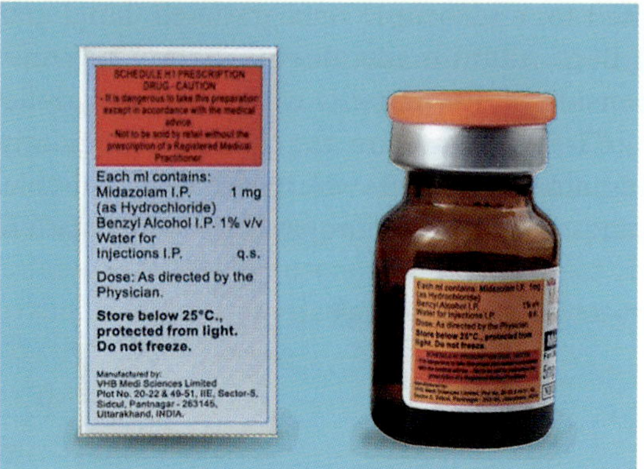

Fig. 2: Midazolam.

- *Onset:* In 2–3 minutes
- *Duration of action:* For about 30 minutes
- *Dose:*
    - *Adult:* 1–5 mg/slow IV
    - *Child:* 0.05–0.1 mg/kg
- *Side effects:*
    - Hypotension
    - Apnea
    - Paradoxical reaction
    - Local pain and induration (IM)
- *Advice:* Monitor the patient closely until recovery
- *Antidote:* Flumazenil 0.1–0.2 mg **(Fig. 3)**

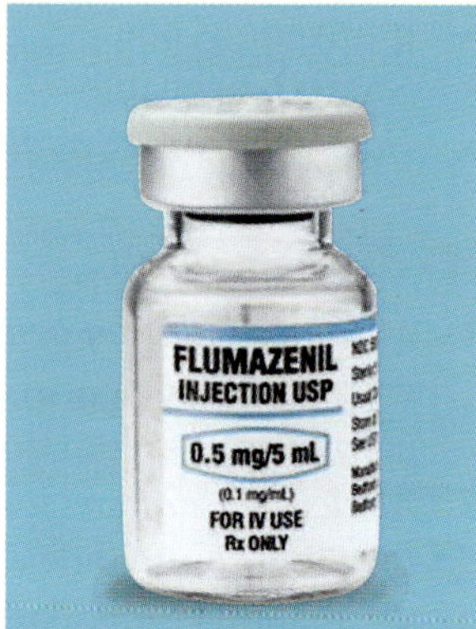

Fig. 3: Flumazenil.

Diazepam

- Short-acting benzodiazepine
- *Merits:* Sedation and anxiolytic
- *Onset:* 2–3 minutes
- *Duration of action:* Usually 30 minutes but half-life could be up to 30 hours.
- *Dose:*
    - *Adult:* 5–10 mg/slow IV
    - *Child:* 0.05–0.1 mg/kg
- *Side effects:*
    - Hypotension
    - Apnea
    - Paradoxical reaction
    - Local pain and induration
- *Advice:* Monitor the patient who had diazepam until recovery.
- *Antidote:* None available

When do We Need an Anesthetist during Endoscopy?

- Prolonged or therapeutic endoscopic procedure requiring deep sedation
- Anticipated intolerance to standard sedatives
- Increased risk for complication because of severe comorbidity [American Society of Anesthesiologists (ASA) class III and above]
- Increased risk for airway obstruction
- Endoscopy in children and unstable sick patients

Use of Propofol Infusion for Endoscopic Procedures (Fig. 4)

- Propofol (2,6-diisopropylphenol) is classified as an ultra-short-acting hypnotic agent that provides sedative, amnestic, and hypnotic effects with no analgesic properties. Typically, the time from injection to the onset of sedation is 30–60 seconds. Its duration of effect is 4–8 minutes.
- Pain on injection is frequent. The cardiovascular effects of propofol include decreases in cardiac output, systemic vascular resistance, and arterial pressure. Negative cardiac inotropy and respiratory depression can be seen with the use of propofol. These effects reverse rapidly with dose reduction or interruption of drug infusion and rarely require temporary ventilatory support. There is no reversal agent for propofol.
- Personnel specifically trained in the administration of propofol with expertise in emergency airway management must be present during the use of this agent, and the patient's physiologic parameters must be continuously monitored.
- Additional anesthetic agents that have been used for endoscopic procedures include ketamine, dexmedetomidine, and inhalational agents.
- Propofol infusion has become routine for advanced endoscopic procedures such as ERCP and EUS. It is advisable to have an anesthetist during such complex procedures.

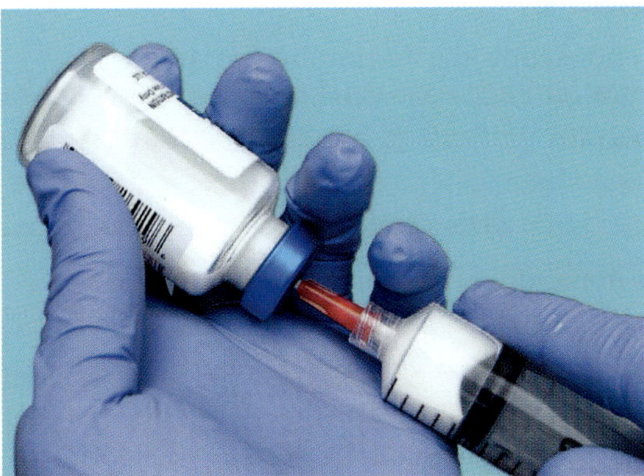

Fig. 4: Propofol infusion.

Beware of Some Common Causes for Difficult Airways

- Patients with previous problems with anesthesia or sedation
- Patients with a history of stridor, snoring, or sleep apnea
- Patients with dysmorphic facial features, such as Pierre–Robin syndrome or trisomy 21
- Patients with oral abnormalities, such as a small opening (<3 cm in an adult), edentulous, protruding incisors, loose or capped teeth, high-arched palate, macroglossia, tonsillar hypertrophy, or a nonvisible uvula
- Patients with neck abnormalities, such as obesity involving the neck and facial structures, short neck, limited neck extension, decreased hyoid-mental distance (<3 cm in an adult), neck mass, cervical spine disease or trauma, tracheal deviation, or advanced rheumatoid arthritis.
- Patients with jaw abnormalities such as micrognathia, trismus, or significant malocclusion.

ANALGESIC DRUGS

Common Drugs used

- *Pethidine:* 50–100 mg IV
- *Tramadol:* 50 mg/IV
- *Fentanyl:* 50–100 µg/IV
- *Ketamine:* 1–2 mg/kg (under anesthetist supervision) **(Fig. 5)**

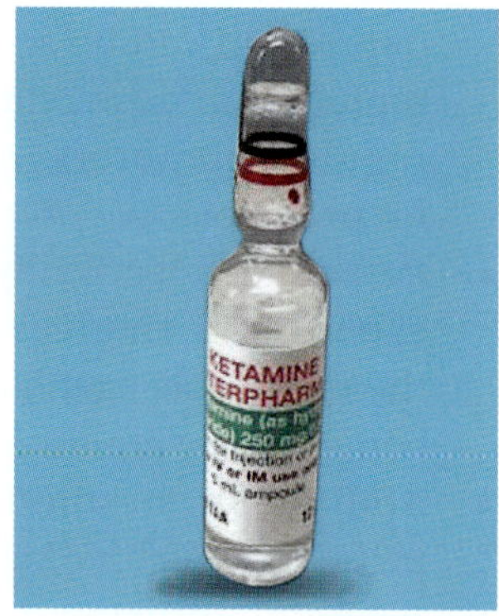

Fig. 5: Ketamine.

Indications

Indicated only for painful procedures, e.g., bougie or balloon dilatation, percutaneous endoscopic gastrostomy (PEG) placement.

Contraindications

- Emergency endoscopy in a nonintubated patient
- Respiratory failure
- Circulatory failure

Advantage

Better tolerance of painful procedures.

Disadvantages

- Respiratory depression
- Circulatory depression
- Bradycardia

ANTISPASMODIC DRUGS

Drug Commonly used

Butylscopolamine, 5–20 mg IV **(Fig. 6)**.

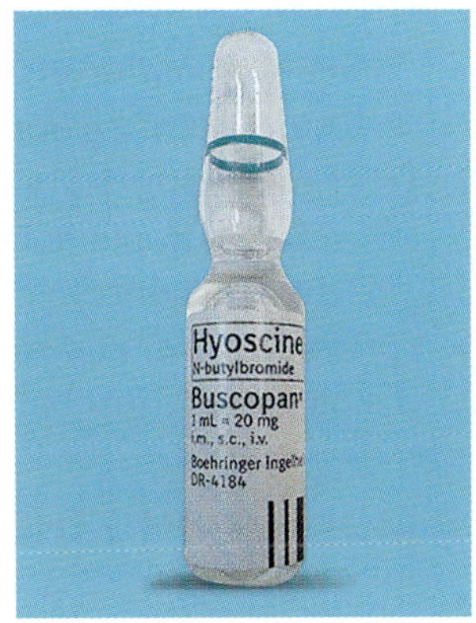

Fig. 6: Butylscopolamine.

Indications

- Pyloric spasm
- During duodenal biopsy
- For visualization of duodenal diverticula/ampulla of Vater

Contraindications

- Glaucoma
- Prostatic hypertrophy
- Arrhythmias

Advantage

Eliminates possible interference from peristalsis.

Disadvantage

Its side effects like dry mouth, tachycardia, etc.

TRANSMISSION OF INFECTION DURING ENDOSCOPY

Nature of the Procedure

- *During diagnostic endoscopy:* Less likely
- *During therapeutic endoscopy:* More common, e.g., tissue or fluid sampling, polypectomy, injection sclerotherapy, bougie or balloon dilatation, stenting, and prosthesis insertion.

Modes of Transmission of Infectious Organisms

- From the previously examined patient
- Endogenous transmission (bacteremia)
- From the contaminated endoscope

Patients with a Higher-risk for Transmission of Infection

- Cardiac valve defects
- Artificial heart valve
- Indwelling venous catheter and port
- Hematological disease
- Patient on immune-suppressing drugs
- Human immunodeficiency virus (HIV) infection
- Advanced liver or kidney disease

Drugs for Antibiotic Prophylaxis, Recommended for High-risk Patients

- *Diagnostic endoscopy:*
  - Ampicillin, 2 g orally 60 minutes before the procedure
  - Ampicillin, 1.5 g orally 6 hours after the procedure (for patients allergic to penicillin, give clindamycin, 600 mg orally 1 hour before the procedure)
- *Interventional endoscopy:* Also, add 80 mg of gentamycin IV or 2 g of cefotaxime IV just before starting the procedure

MONITORING THE PATIENT DURING ENDOSCOPY

- *Clinical monitoring:*
  - Vigilance by the endoscopists and all the staff
  - Trained to recognize the symptoms of cardiorespiratory distress
- *Electronic monitors:*
  - Pulse oximeter **(Fig. 7)**
  - ECG
  - Capnograph
  - BP

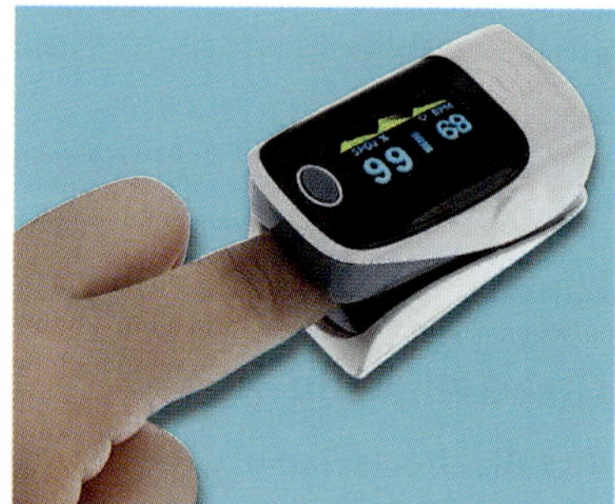

Fig. 7: Pulse oximeter.

ROLE OF RECOVERY ROOM NURSE (FIG. 8)

- Close monitoring of patients
- Monitor and record the patient's conscious status and vitals
- Consider administering flumazenil if drowsiness is due to an overdose of midazolam.
- Administer naloxone in case of morphine overdose
- Advice regarding when to eat and drink

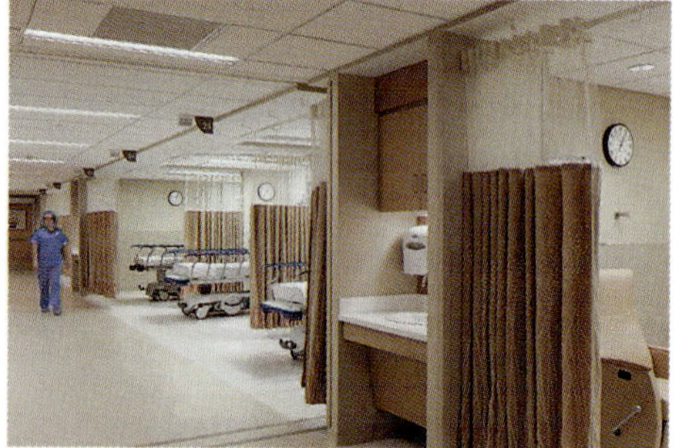

Fig. 8: Recovery room.

- Patients are usually allowed to take liquids after 30 minutes and solids after 1 hour.
- Following banding of varices, patients are advised to be on a liquid diet for 24–48 hours before going for a soft and sloppy diet.
- Following dilatation or stenting, patients may be kept nil oral for a few more hours before the liquid or liquidized diet.
- It is preferable to give clear written instructions to the patient and relatives.

DECIDE ON THE TIMING OF DISCHARGE OF THE PATIENT

- Usually after 1–2 hours, when the patient is alert, comfortable, and no undue pain or bleeding.
- Able to go home if they have come with a competent companion or relative.
- He/she has received the written discharge summary.

ARRANGING FOR A WRITTEN DISCHARGE SUMMARY

- Give a copy of the report with all endoscopic findings
- Advice on further treatment and biopsy report
- Contact details if the patient develops any trouble such as persisting throat or chest pain, dysphagia, hematemesis, melena, and fever after reaching home

SUMMARY OF RECOMMENDATIONS FOR ENDOSCOPY SUITE

- Resuscitation equipment and sedation reversing/antagonist drugs must be available in the endoscopy room and recovery area.
- Drugs and equipment necessary for the maintenance of airway, breathing, and circulation should be present in the endoscopy room and recovery area and be checked regularly.
- A qualified nurse trained in endoscopic techniques and resuscitation techniques should monitor the patient's condition during procedures.
- *Principles of usage of drugs during endoscopy:*
    - The dosage of benzodiazepines and opiates should be kept to a minimum to achieve sedation and should be within the manufacturer's guidelines.
    - Opioids should, whenever possible, be given before benzodiazepines, and their effect observed before proceeding.
    - Most endoscopic practices recommend that 5 mg of midazolam should usually be the maximum dose given and that elderly patients are given 1–2 mg initially with a sensible pause to observe the effect. All sedated patients must have a flexible (not "butterfly") intravenous cannula in situ throughout the procedure and recovery period.
- Nasal oxygen should be given to all sedated patients and selected unsedated patients throughout the procedure and recovery period.
- Pulse oximetry monitoring should be used in all sedated patients, and ECG and blood pressure monitoring should be readily available for high-risk patients.
- Clinical monitoring must be continued in the recovery area.
- Endoscopy is sometimes an emergency procedure, so high-risk patients should be resuscitated as much as possible before attempting the procedure.

- Records of management outcomes and adverse events should be taken as part of the patient plan and kept and used for audit of departmental practice.
- The endoscopist/surgeon is not just a technician and is responsible for the health and safety of the patient throughout the procedure.

SUGGESTED READING

1. Aisenberg J, Cohen LB, Piorkowski JD. Propofol use under the direction of trained gastroenterologists: an analysis of the medicolegal implications. Am J Gastroenterol. 2007;101:707-13.
2. American Society of Anesthesiologists Task Force on Sedation and Analgesia by Non-Anesthesiologists. Practice guidelines for sedation and analgesia by non-anesthesiologists. Anesthesiology. 2002;96(4):1004-17.
3. Evans LT, Saberi S, Kim HM, Elta GH, Schoenfeld P. Pharyngeal anesthesia during sedated EGDs: is "the spray" beneficial? A meta-analysis and systematic review. Gastrointest Endosc. 2006;63(6):761-6.
4. Faigel DO, Baron TH, Goldstein JL, Hirota WK, Jacobson BC, Johanson JF, et al. Guidelines for the use of deep sedation and anesthesia for GI endoscopy. Gastrointest Endosc. 2002;56(5):613-7.
5. Godwin SA, Caro DA, Wolf SJ, Jagoda AS, Charles R, Marett BE, et al. Clinical policy: procedural sedation and analgesia in the emergency department. Ann Emerg Med. 2005;45(2):177-96.
6. Horiuchi A, Nakayama Y. Unsedated ultrathin EGD by using a 5.2-mm-diameter videoscope: evaluation of acceptability and diagnostic accuracy. Gastrointest Endosc. 2006;64:868-73.
7. Leung FW, Mann SK, Salera R, Toomsen L, Cabrera H, Prather D, et al. Options for screening colonoscopy without sedation: sequel to a pilot study in U.S. veterans. Gastrointest Endosc. 2008;67(4):712-7.
8. Nelson DB, Block KP, Bosco JJ, Burdick JS, Curtis WD, Faigel DO, et al. Technology status evaluation report: ultrathin endoscopes esophagogastroduodenoscopy: March 2000. Gastrointest Endosc. 2000;51(6):786-9.
9. Rex DK, Imperiale TF, Portish V. Patients willing to try colonoscopy without sedation: associated clinical factors and results of a randomized controlled trial. Gastrointest Endosc. 1999;49:554-9.
10. Training Committee. American Society for Gastrointestinal Endoscopy. Training guideline for use of propofol in gastrointestinal endoscopy. Gastrointest Endosc. 2004;60(2):167-72.
11. Waring JP, Baron TH, Hirota WK, Goldstein JL, Jacobson BC, Leighton JA, et al. Guidelines for conscious sedation and monitoring during gastrointestinal endoscopy. Gastrointest Endosc. 2003;58(3):317-22.
12. Wille RT, Barnett JL, Chey WD, Scheiman JM, Elta GH. Routine droperidol pre-medication improves sedation for ERCP. Gastrointest Endosc. 2000;52(3):362-6.
13. Zakko SF, Seifert HA, Gross JB. A comparison of midazolam and diazepam for conscious sedation during colonoscopy in a prospective double-blind study. Gastrointest Endosc. 1999;49:684-9.

Expert's Comment

The chapter "Drugs used in Endoscopic Units" provides a comprehensive overview of the medications commonly utilized in endoscopy suites. The author has effectively highlighted the importance of sedation, analgesia, and topical anesthesia in ensuring patient comfort and safety during endoscopic procedures.

The discussion on the pharmacology of these agents, including their mechanisms of action, dosing, and potential side effects, is particularly valuable. Additionally, the emphasis on patient monitoring and the need for trained personnel to administer these medications is crucial. Overall, this chapter serves as a valuable resource for healthcare professionals involved in endoscopic procedures, providing essential knowledge on the safe and effective use of drugs in this setting.

The term "Conscious Sedation" has been beautifully explained by the author. It is key for the beginner to imbibe the knowledge and importance of conscious sedation before any endoscopic procedures.

Dr Sakthivel Chandrasekar
Erode

CHAPTER 20

Adverse Events during Flexible Endoscopy

Chapter Outline

- Causes for the Unplanned Events
  - Guidelines for Preventing or Minimizing Complications
  - General Guidelines for Managing any Unplanned Events
  - Adverse Events during Upper Gastrointestinal Endoscopy
  - Adverse Events during Colonoscopy
  - Adverse Events during Endoscopic Retrograde Cholangiopancreatography

Keywords: Unplanned events, perforation, bleeding after endoscopy, postpolypectomy syndrome, and missed diagnosis

INTRODUCTION

Endoscopy has become an essential diagnostic and therapeutic tool for every surgeon. Endoscopy can never be completely safe. However, potential benefits should far exceed the perceived risks of any procedure. Unexpected events can happen even in the hands of an experienced endoscopist. To prevent medicolegal consequences, we should describe any adverse events developing during endoscopy as "unplanned events" rather than as "complications".

While cardiopulmonary events related to sedation are probably the most common unplanned events, medicolegal claims arise more often from perforation and failure to diagnose or missing pathology. Hence, it is better to mention these risks in the informed consent process.

CAUSES FOR THE UNPLANNED EVENTS

- *High-risk endoscopy team:* Poor technical or cognitive skillset of the endoscopy team
- *High-risk patient:* Note the American Society of Anesthesiologists (ASA) grading of each patient for risk assessment
- *High-risk procedure:* Interventions like dilatation, endoscopic submucosal dissection (ESD), peroral endoscopic myotomy (POEM), etc.

Guidelines for Preventing or Minimizing Complications

- Experienced endoscopist
- Educated and agile staff
- Follow strict protocols in every procedure
- Stop aspirin/clopidogrel 5 days before any endoscopic therapy
- Stop warfarin 3 days prior and keep the patient on low molecular weight heparin (LMWH) (consult the cardiologist)
- Appropriate electronic monitoring of all patients (pulse oximetry, ECG, $ETCO_2$)
- Administer antibiotic prophylaxis when indicated
- Training of staff in advanced cardiac life support
- Resuscitation trolley and emergency drugs are always available
- Risk assessment and risk reduction of your patient [diabetes mellitus/hypertension/ischemic heart disease (DM/HT/IHD)]
- Continuous quality improvement in endoscopy service

General Guidelines for Managing any Unplanned Events

- Vigilance
- Early recognition of any complication
- *Prompt action:* Delay is dangerous both medically and legally
- Proper communication with patients and relatives
  - Be frank and truthful
  - Care with compassion
  - Be present and answerable
  - Document everything in clear and chronological order
- Perform appropriate investigation
- Involve senior colleagues and surgeons in expert care
- Audit the outcome of all unplanned events

Adverse events during endoscopy can be discussed in the following subheadings:

- Adverse events during upper gastrointestinal (GI) endoscopy
- Adverse events during colonoscopy
- Adverse events during endoscopic retrograde cholangiopancreatography (ERCP)

Adverse Events during Upper Gastrointestinal Endoscopy

Summary of Unplanned Events during Upper Gastrointestinal Endoscopy

- *Overall incidence of unplanned events:* 0.1%
- *Mortality rate:* 0.01%
- *Cardiac complications:* Ischemia and arrhythmias

- *Pulmonary complications:*
  - Hypoxia and aspiration
  - Bleeding
  - Perforation
  - Infection
- *Complications from medications used during the procedure:*
  - *Pharyngeal anesthesia:* Allergy and aspiration
  - *Sedation:* Respiratory depression and hypotension
- *Specific complications of therapeutic endoscopy:*
  - *Due to polypectomy:* Bleeding
  - *After dilatation:* Perforation
- *Failure to diagnose*:
  - Failure to follow-up suspicious gastric ulcer with repeat endoscopy
  - Failure to recognize a tumor or polyp during endoscopy

Risk Factors for Bleeding during Upper Gastrointestinal Endoscopy

- *Instrument tip damaging the bowel wall:*
  - From pre-existing varices or ulcer
  - Due to retching (Mallory–Weiss tear)
  - Coagulopathy
- *Following various therapeutic interventions:*
  - Snare polypectomy
  - ERCP and sphincterotomy
  - Banding or sclerotherapy for varices

Risk Factors for Perforation during Upper Gastrointestinal Endoscopy

- *During diagnostic endoscopy:*
  - Zenker's diverticulum
  - Postcricoid web
  - False passage through carcinoma esophagus
  - Corrosive injury
- *During therapeutic endoscopy:*
  - Endoscopic dilatation of esophageal stricture
  - Pneumatic dilatation for achalasia
  - Polypectomy and ESD

Management of Endoscopic Perforation of the Esophagus and Stomach

- Persisting chest pain, abdominal distention, dyspnea, and subcutaneous emphysema with crepitus and tachycardia. Fever and hypotension are usually due to late presentation

- Cervical esophageal perforation can be managed conservatively if there is no mediastinal contamination. Keep the patient with nil oral intake, Intravenous fluids, and antibiotics. Consider parenteral nutrition in a malnourished individual.
- Imaging modalities such as abdominal plain film radiography or CT scan are commonly performed in the case of clinically suspected or diagnosed perforation, to verify the presence of gas or fluid collections. Cross-sectional imaging has an improved sensitivity and specificity over conventional radiography in detecting small amounts of free gas, liquids, and small pneumothorax. Moreover, a CT scan can assess whether a previously performed endoscopic closure was successful. For suspected upper GI perforations, the ingestion of water-soluble contrast medium before a CT scan adds accuracy because it may display the site of extravasation or it may confirm the effective closure of the defect.
- Endoscopic closure should be considered depending on the type of iatrogenic perforation, its size, and the endoscopist's expertise available. Immediate, endoscopic closure results in the prevention of peritonitis or mediastinitis and reduces the need for surgical intervention. Through-the-Scope (TTS) clips can be used for perforations <10 mm, and Over the Scope (OTS) clips are recommended for perforations >10 mm. Covered Stents can be used for larger defects (>20 mm).
- Switch to carbon dioxide (CO_2) endoscopic insufflation, diversion of digestive luminal content, and decompression of tension pneumoperitoneum or pneumothorax should also be performed
- Endoscopic dilations and mucosal resection/submucosal dissection are the common reasons for gastric iatrogenic perforation. If perforation is large or if there is sepsis syndrome, surgical intervention and omental patch are warranted.

Adverse Events during Colonoscopy

Types of Unplanned Events during Colonoscopy

- *Cardiopulmonary events:*
  - Arrhythmia and myocardial infarction (MI)
  - Hypoxia and aspiration
- Drug-related events
  - Respiratory depression
  - Allergy
- Fluid and electrolyte imbalance
- Risk of infection
- Bleeding
- Perforation
- Postpolypectomy syndrome

- Gas explosion
- *Failure to diagnose:*
  - Failure to reach the cecum
  - *Failure to recall the patient:* For repeat colonoscopy for surveillance, e.g., after polypectomy

Issues Related to Bowel Preparations

- *Polyethylene glycol:*
  - No fluid or electrolyte imbalance
  - Large volume and difficult to tolerate
  - Abdominal bloating and nausea
- *Sodium phosphate preparation:*
  - Less volume/better tolerated
  - But risk of fluid overload and acute phosphate nephropathy
  - Risk in renal failure, elderly, and cardiac patients

Colonoscopic Perforation

- *How common is it?*
  - During diagnostic colonoscopy (0.1–0.01%)
  - More common with therapeutic colonoscopy (up to 5%)
  - But perforations are larger in diagnostic colonoscopy and smaller with therapeutic colonoscopy.
- *When does it happen?*
  - *During diagnostic colonoscopy* **(Fig. 1)**:
    - Due to inadequate experience
    - Use of excessive and blind force
    - Excessive air insufflation (barotrauma)
    - Inappropriate use of biopsy forceps (like a dart)

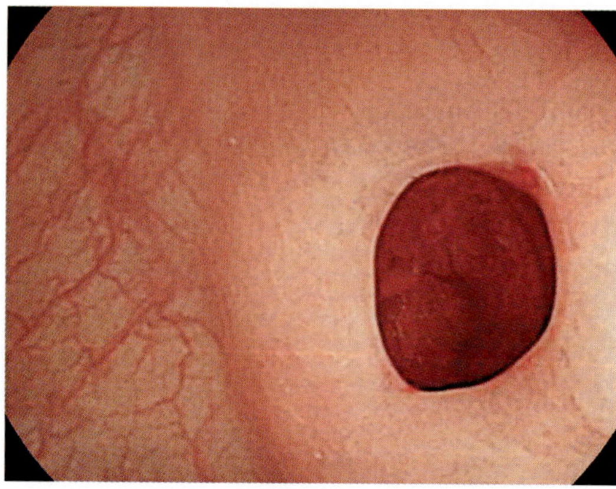

Fig. 1: Diagnostic perforation.

        - *High-risk cases:*
            - Pathologically fixed bowel loops
            - Inflamed and ulcerated colon
            - Ischemic or necrotic lesions
            - Severe diverticulosis
    - *During therapeutic colonoscopy* **(Fig. 2)**:
        - Polypectomy, e.g., flat polyps
        - *ESD:*
            - Look for a "target sign" after the procedure. It indicates a breach in muscularis propria
            - Immediate recognition and closure with hemoclips are the treatment of choice
        - Dilatation of stricture
        - Argon plasma coagulation

Mechanism of perforation during colonoscopy **(Fig. 3)**:

- *Who is the culprit?*
    - Tip of the scope
    - Shaft of the scope
    - Diathermy
    - Biopsy forceps
    - Snare
    - Dilatation balloon
- *Site of perforation* **(Fig. 4)**: Rectosigmoid region is the common site of perforation
- *Symptoms:*
    - Persisting pain abdomen
    - Painful distension of the abdomen
- *Signs:*
    - Fever

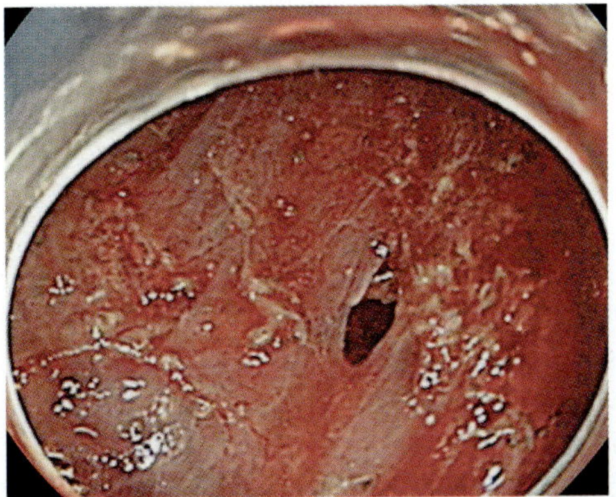

Fig. 2: Therapeutic perforation.

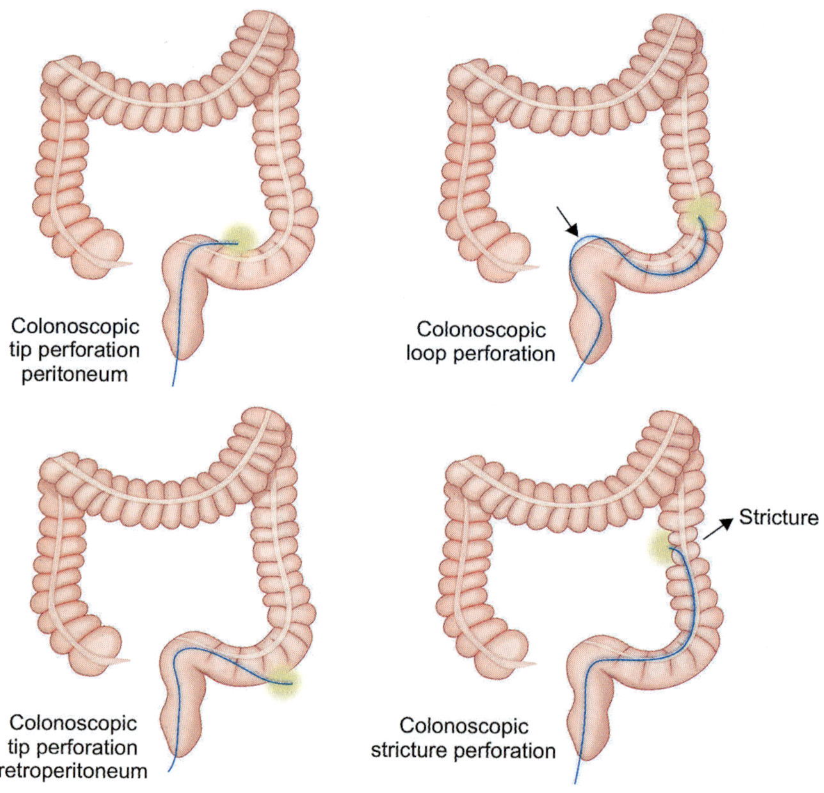

Fig. 3: Mechanism of perforation.

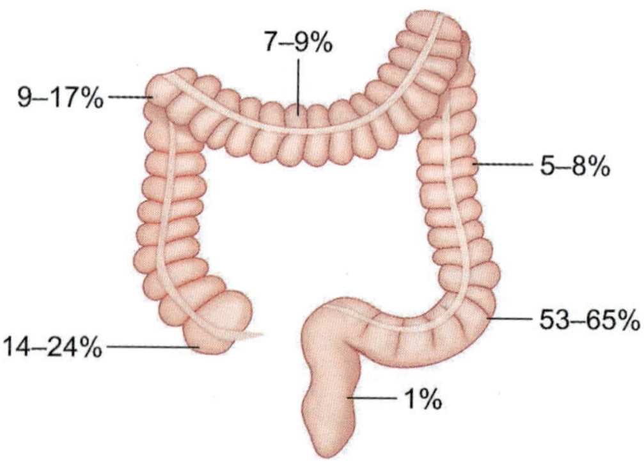

Fig. 4: Sites of perforation.

    - Tachycardia
    - Tender and rigid abdomen
- *Investigations:*
    - Leukocytosis
    - *X-ray abdomen:* Free gas under the diaphragm (65–87% cases)
    - CT abdomen with water-soluble contrast

- *Treatment:*
  - *Factors to be considered to plan treatment:*
    - Mechanism, site, and size of perforation
    - Nature of bowel preparation
    - Time between procedure and diagnosis of perforation
    - Clinical status and comorbid conditions
  - *Conservative treatment:*
    - Only in a stable patient with minimal abdominal signs following small perforation in an otherwise well-prepared colon.
    - Active observation, IV fluids, bowel rest, and broad-spectrum antibiotics
    - Low threshold for surgery in case of any deterioration in patient's condition
  - *Endoscopic intervention **(Figs. 5A and B)**:* Hemoclip and over-the-scope clip (OTSC) have been successfully tried.
  - *Surgical intervention:* Usual course of action
    - Early intervention is essential for better outcome.
    - *Laparoscopic or open surgery **(Fig. 6)**:*
      - Primary sutured repair in early cases of perforation
      - Resection and anastomosis in cases of perforation with associated pathology like diverticular stricture or tumor
      - Diverting colostomy and lavage in delayed cases or gross soiling of the peritoneal cavity

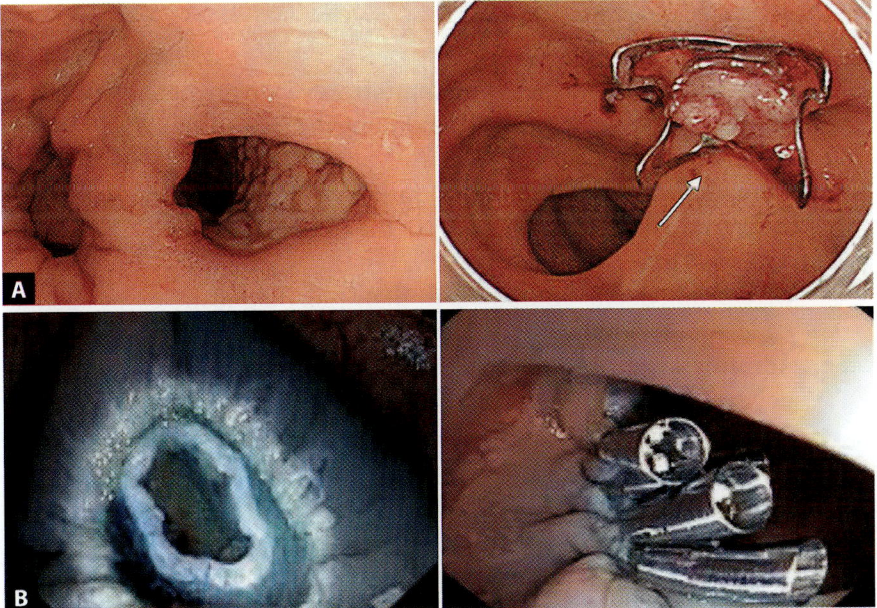

Figs. 5A and B: (A) Over the scope clip (OTSC) application; and (B) Hemoclip application.

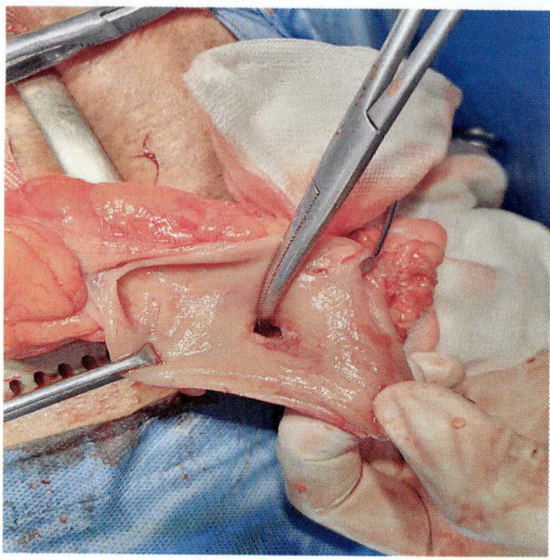

Fig. 6: Diagnostic colonoscopic perforation.

- Delayed diagnosis and therapy could lead to unacceptable morbidity (20–50%) and mortality (0–26%).
- Prompt diagnosis and individualized management are the key factors for better outcome.

- *Measures to prevent colonoscopic perforation:*
  - Be slow and gentle during colonoscopy
  - Do not blindly push with force
  - Be sensitive to the patient's discomfort. Severe pain means we have to halt and decide about even abandoning the procedure.
  - Avoid oversedation
  - Consider virtual colonoscopy rather than persevering with your attempts in total colonoscopy with the risk of perforation
- *Prevention of infection:*
  - Give prophylactic antibiotics in high-risk diagnostic cases such as endocarditis prophylaxis, e.g., patients with heart valve replacement
  - Administer antibiotics in all cases involving intervention, e.g., polypectomy
  - Proper cleaning and disinfection of colonoscopes

Bleeding (Fig. 7)

- *Causes:*
  - Instrument tip damaging bowel wall
  - Coagulopathy

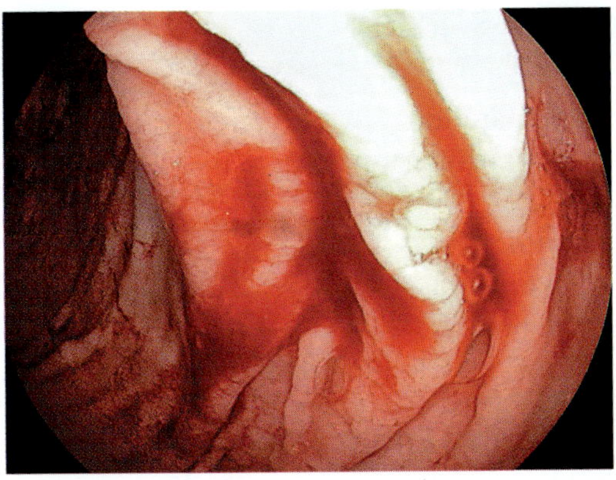

Fig. 7: Bleeding during colonoscopy.

- *Therapeutic intervention:*
  - Polypectomy
  - ESD
- *Timing:*
  - Immediate
  - Delayed after 10–12 days
- *Treatment:*
  - Inject with dilute adrenaline 1/10,000
  - Hemoclip
  - Endo loop

Postpolypectomy Syndrome

- Present with localized pain, fever with abdominal tenderness, and some guarding
- Suggestive of full-thickness thermal damage to bowel wall following polypectomy
- No free gas under the diaphragm in X-ray abdomen
- Manage conservatively with antibiotics and analgesics

Gas Explosion

- *Risk factors:*
  - Poor bowel preparation
  - Bowel prepared using mannitol/lactulose
  - Use of energy sources/advanced process control (APC)
- *Cause:* Combustible level of hydrogen or methane
- *Prevention:*
  - Use of CO_2
  - Good bowel preparation

Missed Diagnosis

- *Causes:*
  - Poor bowel preparation
  - Failure to reach cecum
  - *Blind areas:*
    - Distal rectum
    - Splenic flexure
    - Ileocecal region
- *Management:* Consider CT colonography or repeat colonoscopy

Adverse Events during Endoscopic Retrograde Cholangiopancreatography

Pancreatitis

- Transient post-ERCP hyperamylasemia can be of no clinical consequence.
- *But serious pancreatitis could occur in the following situations:*
  - Difficult cannulation
  - Precut papillotomy
  - Repeated pancreatic duct cannulation and overfilling of the pancreatic duct with contrast (parenchymogram)
  - Sphincter of Oddi dysfunction
  - Cases of pancreatic duct therapeutic interventions

Management:

- Aggressive fluid therapy and analgesics
- Pre-emptive administration of indomethacin (100 mg) or diclofenac (75 mg) suppositories
- Pancreatic stenting **(Fig. 8)**

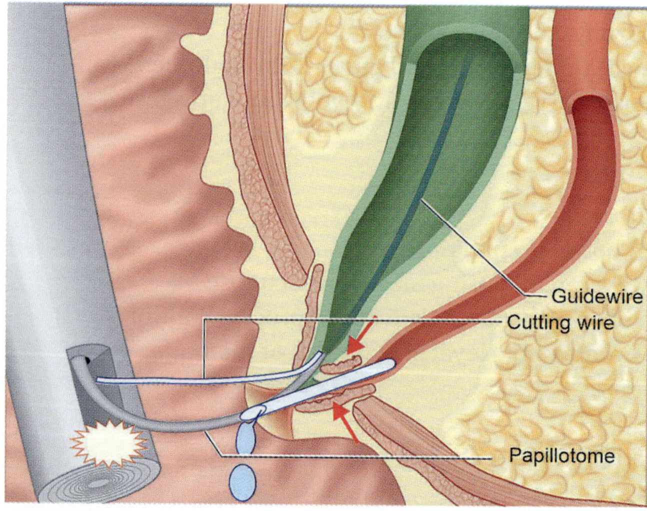

Fig. 8: Prophylactic pancreatic duct stenting (arrows) to minimize severity of pancreatitis.

Cholangitis

- Due to an obstructed and undrained biliary system caused by stones or stricture, over injection of contrast, or using improperly disinfected scope and accessories
- Gram-negative bacilli such as *Escherichia coli, Klebsiella, Enterobacter, Proteus,* and *Pseudomonas*

Prevention:

- Always aspirate the biliary system before any contrast injection
- Ensure wire-guided access to the proximal obstructed ducts before any injection of contrast
- Avoid forceful or overfilling of proximal obstructed system
- Prophylactic dose of antibiotic, e.g., IV cefotaxime

Bleeding

- In deviated or large sphincterotomy, especially in patients with coagulopathy
- Manage it by using an occlusion balloon for tamponade effect, injection of dilute adrenaline, diathermy, or even a hemoclip

Retroperitoneal Duodenal Perforation

- Due to deviated or excessive cuts at the papilla
- Retroperitoneal air better recognized by CT abdomen
- Mostly settle with conservative therapy

CONCLUSION

Misadventures mean unplanned events despite a good standard of care, while negligence is when an adverse event happens because of a poor standard of care. Adequate training, proper patient care, and expertise in treatment should ensure fewer chances for such medicolegal issues.

To err is human, but to fail to learn from such an event is indefensible.

SUGGESTED READING

1. ASGE Standards of Practice Committee; Fisher DA, Maple JT, Ben-Menachem T, Cash BD, Decker GA, et al. Complications of colonoscopy. Gastrointest Endosc. 2011;74(4):745-52. Erratum in: Gastrointest Endosc. 2016;84(5):883.
2. Cotton PB, Garrow DA, Gallagher J, Romagnuolo J. Risk factors for complications after ERCP: a multivariate analysis of 11,497 procedures over 12 years. Gastrointest Endosc. 2009;70(1):80-8.
3. Dafnis G, Ekbom A, Pahlman L, Blomqvist P. Complications of diagnostic and therapeutic colonoscopy within a defined population in Sweden. Gastrointest Endosc. 2001;54(3):302-9.
4. Dindo D, Demartines N, Clavien PA. Classification of surgical complications: a new proposal with evaluation in a cohort of 6336 patients and results of a survey. Ann Surg. 2004;240(2):205-13.

5. Dumonceau JM, Kapral C, Aabakken L, Papanikolaou IS, Tringali A, Vanbiervliet G, et al. ERCP-related adverse events: European Society of Gastrointestinal Endoscopy (ESGE) Guideline. Endoscopy. 2020;52(2):127-49.
6. Elmunzer BJ, Scheiman JM, Lehman GA, Chak A, Mosler P, Higgins PD, et al. A randomized trial of rectal indomethacin to prevent post-ERCP pancreatitis. N Engl J Med. 2012;366(15):1414-22.
7. Froehlich F, Gonvers JJ, Fried M. Conscious sedation, clinically relevant complications and monitoring of endoscopy: results of a nationwide survey in Switzerland. Endoscopy. 1994;26(2):231-4.
8. Ko CW, Dominitz JA. Complications of colonoscopy: magnitude and management. Gastrointest Endosc Clin N Am. 2010;20(4):659-71.
9. Ladas SD, Karamanolis G, Ben-Soussan E. Colonic gas explosion during therapeutic colonoscopy with electrocautery. World J Gastroenterol. 2007; 13(40):5295-8.
10. Reumkens A, Rondagh EJ, Bakker CM, Winkens B, Masclee AA, Sanduleanu S. Post-Colonoscopy Complications: A Systematic Review, Time Trends, and Meta-Analysis of Population-Based Studies. Am J Gastroenterol. 2016;111(8):1092-101.
11. Schulze S, Móller Pedersen V, Hóier-Madsen K. Iatrogenic perforation of the esophagus. Causes and management. Acta Chir Scand. 1982;148:679-82.
12. Sieg A, Hachmoeller-Eisenbach U, Eisenbach T. Prospective evaluation of complications in outpatient GI endoscopy: a survey among German gastroenterologists. Gastrointest Endosc. 2001;53(6):620-7.
13. Silvis SE, Nebel O, Rogers G, Sagawa C, Mandelstam P. Endoscopic complications. Results of the 1974 American Society for Gastrointestinal Endoscopy Survey. JAMA. 1976;235(9):928-30.
14. Wolfsen HC, Hemminger LL, Achem SR, Loeb DS, Stark ME, Bouras EP, et al. Complications of endoscopy of the upper gastrointestinal tract: a single-center experience. Mayo Clin Proc. 2004;79:1264-7.

Expert's Comment

Flexible endoscopy has emerged as an indispensable modality in contemporary gastroenterology and surgery, offering both diagnostic and therapeutic advantages. Yet, no procedure is entirely without risk, and adverse outcomes—better termed *unplanned events*—may occur even in expert hands. Such events may be related to patient comorbidities, high-risk procedures, or limitations in team preparedness.

The most common unplanned events include cardiopulmonary complications from sedation, bleeding, perforation, infection, and missed diagnosis. In upper gastrointestinal endoscopy, complications may involve aspiration, Mallory–Weiss tears, or perforation during dilatation and endoscopic submucosal dissection. Colonoscopy carries risks of diagnostic or therapeutic perforation, bleeding, postpolypectomy syndrome, and rarely gas explosion. Endoscopic retrograde cholangiopancreatography (ERCP), while invaluable, is associated with post-ERCP pancreatitis, cholangitis, bleeding, and retroperitoneal duodenal perforation.

The chapter underscores preventive strategies as the cornerstone of safe practice: Thorough risk assessment, rational anticoagulation management, adherence to antibiotic prophylaxis when indicated, vigilant monitoring, and readiness for resuscitation. Equally important are early recognition, decisive management, transparent communication with patients and families, and meticulous documentation to minimize both clinical harm and medicolegal risk.

Ultimately, the difference between misadventure and negligence lies in the quality of care delivered. With proper training, vigilance, teamwork, and continuous quality improvement, the frequency and impact of adverse events can be greatly reduced. The ultimate aim of the expert endoscopist should always be prevention rather than cure.

Professor Subhash Khanna
Guwahati

Index

Page numbers followed by *b* refer to box, *f* refer to figure, and *t* refer to table.

C

D

H

I

J

K

O

P

R

T

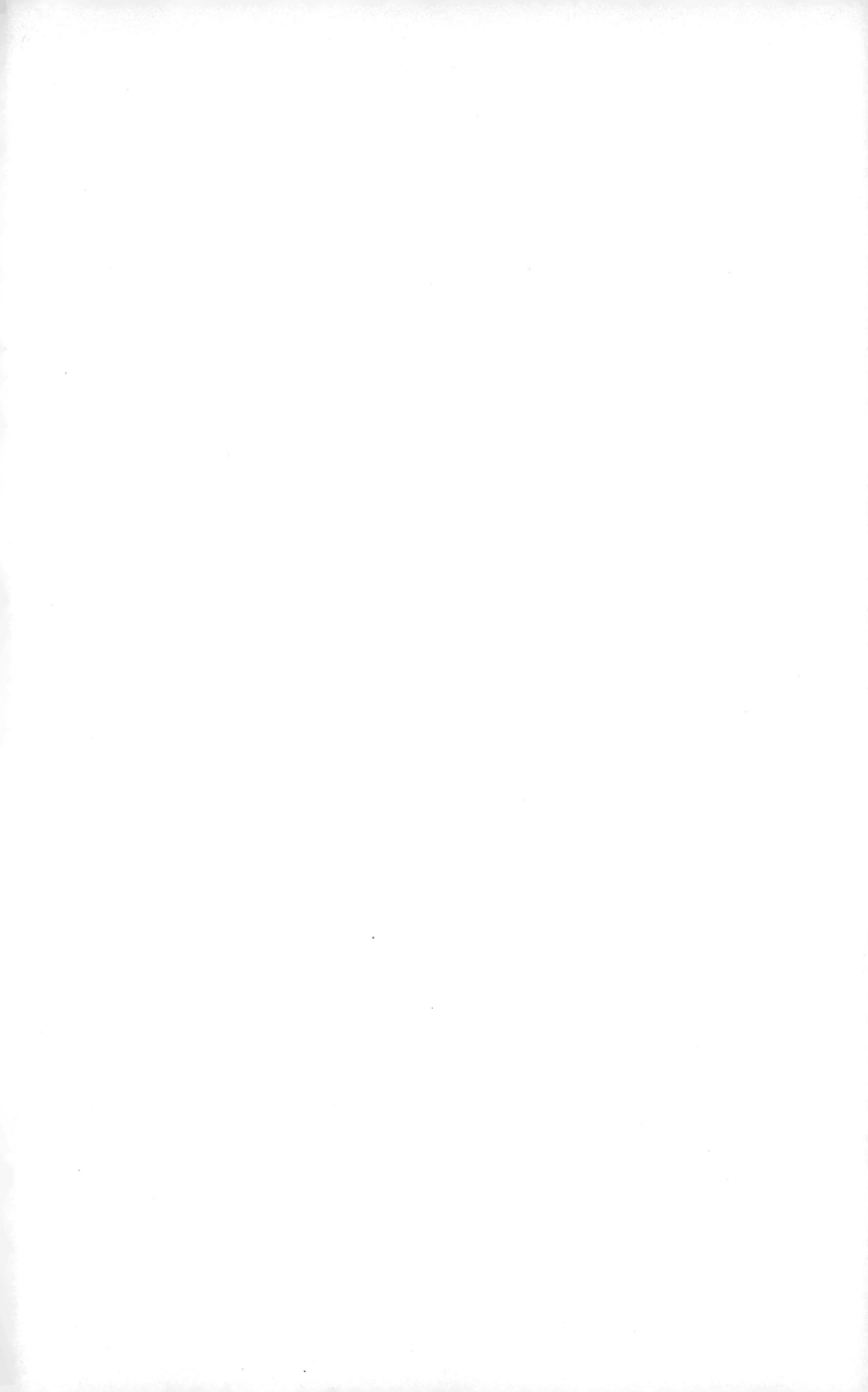